OXFORD MEDICAL PUBLICATIONS

Oxford Handbook of
Clinical Skills in
Adult Nursing

Published and forthcoming Oxford Handbooks

Oxford Handbook of
Clinical Skills in Adult Nursing

Jacqueline Randle

Associate Professor, School of Nursing,
Clinical Skills Lead for Masters of Nursing Science, School
of Nursing, Midwifery & Physiotherapy, University of
Nottingham, UK

Frank Coffey

Consultant in Emergency Medicine, Nottingham University
Hospitals NHS Trust, Associate Professor and Consultant
in Advanced Clinical Skills to the School of Nursing,
Midwifery & Physiotherapy, University of Nottingham, UK

Martyn Bradbury

Clinical Skills Network Lead, School of Nursing and
Community Studies, Faculty of Health and Social Work,
University of Plymouth, UK

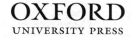

OXFORD
UNIVERSITY PRESS

OXFORD
UNIVERSITY PRESS

Great Clarendon Street, Oxford OX2 6DP

Oxford University Press is a department of the University of Oxford.
It furthers the University's objective of excellence in research, scholarship,
and education by publishing worldwide in

Oxford New York

Auckland Cape Town Dar es Salaam Hong Kong Karachi
Kuala Lumpur Madrid Melbourne Mexico City Nairobi
New Delhi Shanghai Taipei Toronto

With offices in

Argentina Austria Brazil Chile Czech Republic France Greece
Guatemala Hungary Italy Japan Poland Portugal Singapore
South Korea Switzerland Thailand Turkey Ukraine Vietnam

Oxford is a registered trade mark of Oxford University Press
in the UK and in certain other countries

Published in the United States
by Oxford University Press Inc., New York

British Library Cataloguing in Publication Data
Data available

Library of Congress Cataloging in Publication Data
Oxford handbook of Clinical Skills in Adult Nursing / Jacqueline Randle ... [et al.].

Typeset by Cepha Imaging Private Ltd., Bangalore, India
Printed in China
on acid-free paper by
Asia Pacific Offset Limited

ISBN 978–0–19–921104–3

10 9 8 7 6 5 4 3 2 1

Preface

The range of clinical skills performed by nurses is expanding rapidly and the boundaries that previously existed between healthcare workers are blurring. Procedures once the preserve of doctors, such as detailed patient assessment and complex practical procedures, are now being performed by nurses. Although this book is aimed primarily at nurses, many of the procedures are also undertaken by other healthcare workers. The range and complexity of clinical skills can be as daunting for experienced practitioners as they are for students and newly qualified practitioners. We hope that the body-systems framework, alongside detailed evidence based, step-by-step descriptions for each clinical procedure will enable this book to be a practical workplace aid as well as a valuable teaching and learning tool. We have endeavoured to incorporate many of the newer skills performed by healthcare workers while ensuring that the core skills, traditionally undertaken by nurses, are also included. The professional issues that underpin the performance of all clinical skills are outlined at the outset. The `practice tips' and `pitfalls' sections are a distinctive feature of the book. The `practice tips' offer helpful advice from the authors' experiences to facilitate perfromance of the skill. The `pitfalls' sections alert the reader to potential difficulties and complications that may be encountered.

Regardless of who is undertaking a clinial skill, it is paramount that the patient receives the highest standard of care. It is important to remember that clinical skills form part of the total care package and that concepts underpinning high quality care, such as effective communication, clinical governance and patient involvement should always be considered along with the performance of the actual skill itself. Local guidelines may differ for some of the procedures described in this book and we would urge you to follow local policies and be aware of, and understand the reasons for any differences. Finally, we hope that you learn as much from this book as we have from editing it and the ultimate beneficiaries will be the patients we care for.

JR
FC
MB

Contents

Contributors

Janet Barker
Associate Professor, Director of Undergraduate Diploma/BSc (Hons) in Nursing, School of Nursing, Midwifery & Physiotherapy, University of Nottingham, UK

Martyn Bradbury
Clinical Skills Network Lead, School of Nursing and Community Studies, Faculty of Health and Social Work, University of Plymouth, UK

Fiona Branch
Nurse Consultant, Critical Care Clinical Lead Specialist Support, Nottingham University Hospitals NHS Trust, UK

Brenda Clarke
Associate Lecturer, Open University, UK

Mitch Clarke
Infection Prevention and Control Nurse Specialist, Nottingham University Hospitals NHS Trust, UK

Frank Coffey
Consultant in Emergency Medicine, Emergency Department, Nottingham University Hospitals NHS Trust, Associate Professor and Consultant in Advanced Clinical Skills, School of Nursing, Midwifery & Physiotherapy, University of Nottingham, UK

Paul Crawford
Professor, School of Nursing, Midwifery & Physiotherapy, University of Nottingham, UK

Pat Frakes
Emergency Nurse Practitioner, Emergency Department, Nottingham University Hospitals NHS Trust, UK

Kate Johnson
Formerly Senior Lecturer in Cardiac Nursing, City University, London, UK

Keith Knox
Charge Nurse, Eye Casualty Department, Head and Neck Directorate, Nottingham University Hospitals NHS Trust, UK

Iain Neely
Clinical Nurse Trainer, Emergency Department, Nottingham University Hospitals NHS Trust, UK

Rachel Peto
Lecturer, School of Nursing, Midwifery & Physiotherapy, University of Nottingham, UK

Yvonne Powell-Richards
Registered Nurse, Nottingham University Hospitals NHS Trust, UK

Jacqueline Randle
Associate Professor, Clinical Skills Lead for Masters of Nursing Science, School of Nursing, Midwifery & Physiotherapy, University of Nottingham, UK

Louise Stayt
Senior Lecturer in Professional
Practice Skills, School of Health
& Social Care, Oxford Brookes
University, Oxford, UK

Ann Thurgood
Registered General Nurse,
University Hospital, Nottingham,
UK

Bob Tudor
Clinical Nurse Trainer and
Senior Staff Nurse, Emergency
Department, Nottingham
University Hospitals NHS Trust,
UK

Natalie Vaughan
Senior Nurse, Infection Prevention
and Control, Nottingham
University Hospitals NHS Trust,
Nottingham, UK

Jennifer Walker
Clinical Educator, Trauma and
Orthopaedics Department,
Nottingham University Hospitals
NHS Trust, UK

Alison Whitfield
Emergency Nurse Practitioner,
Clinical Educator in Emergency
Medicine, Trauma and
Orthapaedics Emergency
Department, Nottingham
University Hospitals NHS Trust, UK

Paula Wooldridge
Clinical Educator for
Neurosciences, Plymouth Hospitals
Trust, Derriford Hospital, UK

Abbreviations

ABCD	Airway, breathing, circulation, and disability
ABCDE	Airway, breathing, circulation, disability, exposure
ABG	Arterial blood gas
ABPI	Ankle–brachial pressure index
ACBT	Active cycle of breathing techniques
ACOP	Approved codes of practice
ADL	Activities of daily living
ADR	Adverse drug reaction
AED	Automated external defibrillator
AHR	Acute haemolytic reaction
ALS	Advanced life support
AMPLE	Allergies, medications, past medical history, last meal, events/environment related to the injury
ANTT	Aseptic non-touch technique
ASB	Anatomical snuff box
ATLS	Acute trauma life support
AVPU	Alert, responding to voice, pain, or unresponsive
BiPAP	Bilevel (or biphasic) positive airway pressure
BIPP	Bismuth iodoform paraffin paste
BLS	Basic life support
BMAT	Bone marrow apirate and trephine
BVM	Bag–valve–mask
CF	Count fingers
CNS	Central nervous system
CO	Cardiac output
COPD	Chronic obstructive pulmonary disease
CPAP	Continuous positive airway pressure
CPP	Cerebral perfusion pressure
CPR	Cardiopulmonary resuscitation
CRBI	Catheter-related bloodstream infection
CSF	Cerebrospinal fluid
CSU	Catheter specimen of urine
CVC	Central venous catheter
CVP	Central venous pressure
CVS	Cardiovascular system
CXR	Chest X-ray
DHx	Drug history

DIPJ	Distal interphalangeal joint
DoH	Department of Health
DPI	Dry powder inhaler
DVT	Deep venous thrombosis
ECG	Electrocardiogram
EEG	Electroencephalograph
ENT	Ear, nose, and throat
ET	Endotracheal
ETCO$_2$	End-tidal carbon dioxide monitoring
ETT	Endotracheal tube
EVD	External ventricular drain
EVM	Eye opening, verbal response, motor response
FHx	Family history
FLACC	Face, Legs, Activity, Cry, Consolability (Scale)
FVC	Forced vital capacity
GCS	Glasgow Coma Scale
GIT	Gastrointestinal
GUT	Genito-urinary tract
HCW	Health care worker
HIV	Human immunodeficiency virus
HM	Hand movements
HME	Heat–moisture exchanger
HSE	Health and Safety Executive
HxPC	History of the presenting complaint
I/M	Intramuscular
ICP	Intracranial pressure
ISC	Intermittent self-catheterization
ISMN	Isosorbide mononitrate
IV	Intravenous
IVI	Intravenous infusion
JVP	Jugular venous pressure
L&B	Lund and Browder (chart)
LMA	Laryngeal mask airway
LP	Lumbar puncture
mA	Milliamperes
MAP	Mean arterial pressure
MC&S	Microscopy, culture, and sensitivity
MCPJ	Metacarpophalangeal joint
MDI	Meter dose inhaler
MRSA	Meticillin-resistant *Staphylococcus aureus*

MS	Multiple sclerosis
MSU	Midstream urine
NG	Nasogastric
NHS	National Health Service
NIBP	Non-invasive blood pressure
NICE	National Institute for Health and Clinical Excellence
NMC	Nursing and Midwifery Council
NPA	Nasopharyngeal aspiration
NPL	No perception of light
NPSA	National Patient Safety Agency
NSAIDS	Non-steroidal anti-inflammatory drugs
NSFs	National Service Frameworks
ODP	Operating department practitioner
OPA	Oropharangeal airway
OSA	Obstructive sleep apnoea
PA	Pulmonary artery
PACU	Postanaesthetic care unit
PAWP	Pulmonary artery wedge pressure
PC	Presenting complaint
PCA	Patient-controlled analgesia
PE	Phenytoin equivalent
PEA	Pulseless electrical activity
PEEP	Positive end expiratory pressure
PEFR	Peak expiratory flow rate
PEG	Percutaneous endoscopic gastrostomy
PFT	Pulmonary function test
PHx	Past medical history
PIC	Posterior iliac crest
PIPJ	Proximal interphalangeal joint
PL	Perception of light
PMT	Premenstrual tension
PN	Parenteral nutrition
PND	Paroxysmal nocturnal dyspnoea
PPP	Personal professional profile
PREP	Post registration education and practice
prn	As required
RHF	Right-sided heart failure
RIDDOR	Reporting of Injuries, Diseases and Dangerous Occurrences Regulations
RN	Registered nurse
RTC	Road traffic collision

SOAP	Subjective, Objective, Assessment, Plan
S/C	Subcutaneous
S/l	Sublingual
SA	Sino-atrial
SABRE	Serious Adverse Blood Reactions and Events
SAH	Subarachnoid haemorrhage
SE	Status epilepticus
SHx	Personal and social history
SI	System Internationale
SLE	Systemic lupus erythematosis
SR	Systems review
SVC	Superior vena cava
TB	Tuberculosis
TBSA	Total body surface area
TD	Total drainage (from catheter)
TECP	Transcutaneous external cardiac pacing
TENS	Transcutaneous electrical nerve stimulation
TM	Tympanic membrane
TRAC™	Therapeutic regulated accurate care
TRALI	Transfusion-related acute lung injury
U&E	Urea and electrolytes
UTI	Urinary tract infection
V	Volts
V/Qe	Ventilation–perfusion
VAC	Vacuum-assisted closure
VAP	Ventilator-associated pneumonia
VF	Ventricular fibrillation
VT	Ventricular tachycardia

Principles

Janet Barker
Associate Professor, Director of Undergraduate Diploma/BSc
(Hons) in Nursing, School of Nursing, Midwifery & Physiotherapy,
University of Nottingham, UK

Jacqueline Randle
Associate Professor, Clinical Skills Lead for Masters of Nursing
Science, School of Nursing, Midwifery & Physiotherapy,
University of Nottingham, UK

Nursing and Midwifery Council (NMC) standards of proficiency

Background

Standards of proficiency (previously known as 'competencies') are over-arching principles that are considered central to safe and effective nursing practice. These standards were established in 2004 by the NMC and must be achieved by all those on the register of qualified nurses, midwives, and specialist community public health nurses. The standards set by the NMC apply to pre-registration nursing students.

Registered nurses, midwives, and specialist community public health nurses are expected to maintain their proficiency in relation to the standards, and they are expected to ensure their knowledge and skills are up to date and to the standard required for safe and effective practice. When renewing their registration, they are required to declare that they have met the post registration education and practice (PREP) requirements of the NMC. These requirements relate to two standards:

- PREP practice standard—registered nurses (RNs) must have worked, using their professional qualification, for a minimum of 450 hours in the previous 3-year period or undertaken a recognized return-to-practice course.
- PREP continuing professional development standard—they must have maintained a personal professional profile (PPP) recording of at least 35 hours of continuing professional development in the 3 years preceding re-registration.

RNs must comply with any request from the NMC to audit the PPP.

The standards of proficiency

Professional and ethical practice

- Manage oneself, one's practice, and others in accordance with the NMC Code of Professional Conduct (2008), recognizing one's own abilities and limitations.
- Practice in accordance with a legal and ethical framework, which ensures the primacy of patient interest and well-being and respects confidentiality.
- Practice in a fair and antidiscriminatory way, acknowledging the differences in beliefs and cultural practices of individuals and groups.

Care delivery

- Engage in, develop, and disengage from therapeutic relationships through the use of appropriate communication and interpersonal skills.
- Create and document a comprehensive, systematic, and accurate assessment of the physical, psychological, social, and spiritual needs of patients and communities.
- Formulate and document a plan of care, if possible in partnership with patients and their carers, family, and friends, within a framework of informed consent.
- Care should be delivered on the basis of the best available evidence— apply knowledge based on best available evidence and an appropriate repertoire of skills indicative of safe and effective practice.

- Evaluate and document the outcomes of interventions.
- Demonstrate sound clinical judgement across a range of differing professional and care-delivery settings.

Care management

- Contribute to public protection by creating and maintaining a safe environment of care through the use of quality assurance and risk-management strategies.
- Demonstrate knowledge of effective interprofessional working practices, which respect and use the contributions of others.
- Delegate duties to others, as appropriate, ensuring that they are supervised and monitored.
- Demonstrate key skills.

Personal and professional development

- Demonstrate a commitment to the need for continuing professional development and personal supervision activities, to enhance the knowledge, skills, values, and attitudes needed for safe and effective practice.
- Enhance the professional development and safe practice of others through peer support, leadership, supervision, and teaching.

Further reading

NMC Code of Professional Conduct (2008): http://www.nmc-org.uk.

Lifelong learning

Background

Evidence-based practice is an approach to the delivery of care aimed at ensuring all activities are based on rigorous evidence. The NMC Code of Conduct 2008 states that all care must be based on the best evidence available and reflect best practice. Pre-registration education provides a foundation for professional practice. However, practice is dynamic and there is a need to ensure registered nurses, midwives and specialist community public health nurses maintain and develop their proficiencies to meet the changing demands of health care through life long learning. This is more than simply keeping up to date, requiring a commitment to continuing professional development throughout your career as a HCW. NMC (2002) state that the principles of lifelong learning are central to professional practice and require all nurse to demonstrate these through various means.

Preceptorship

All newly qualified nurses are expected undertake a period of preceptorship (approximately 4 months) where a named, qualified nurse is identified to act as their supervisor, providing support and guidance during the transition from student to registered nurse.

Continuing professional development

PREP requirements require you to keep a portfolio of learning to demonstrate the continuing development of your knowledge and skills.

Clinical Supervision

Clinical supervision involves a skilled supervisor assisting a practitioner to reflect on practice facilitating problem-solving, on going learning and practice development. The NMC (2002) identify clinical supervision should be

- practice focussed supporting the improvement of care standards
- locally developed to meet local needs
- accessible to all nurse
- a formal, confidential process

NMC Supporting Nurses and Midwives through lifelong learning (2002)
http://www.nmc-org.uk

Responsibility and accountability

Background

'Responsibility' means to be obliged, being answerable for ones own actions a behaviour duty (NMC 2004)[1]. All healthcare workers (HCWs) have individual and collective responsibilities to protect the patient and are legally accountable for their actions or inactions.

'Accountability' refers to the concept that individuals are responsible for their actions and may be asked to justify them (NMC 2008).[2]

If you are a pre-registration student, you will not be held professionally accountable by the Nursing and Midwifery Council (NMC), but you can be called to account by your university or the law for the consequences of your actions. The registered HCW you are working with is professionally accountable for your actions or inactions and this is why you must work under the supervision of a registered HCW.

Procedure: underlying principles

- All HCWs should protect and care for the vulnerable individual and act as an advocate for them, as appropriate.
- HCWs are liable to be called to account for their actions or omissions.
- HCWs should work within their own scope of professional skill and proficiency.
- Reasonable actions should be taken to avoid acts or omissions that can be foreseen.
- Care should be delivered according to evidence-based practice and reasonable standards.
- If concerns are raised, HCWs will be questioned about their practice.
- The patient and family, as appropriate, should be involved in decision-making, treatment, and care.
- Work should not be delegated to others unless you are confident about the ability of others to carry out the work proficiently.
- Interprofessional communication and working should be co-ordinated and encouraged.

---

1   NMC Code of Professional Conduct advice on delegation for registered nurses or midwives. (2004): http://www.nmc-org.uk.

2   NMC Code of Professional Conduct advise on accountability for registered nurses or midwives (2008): http://www.nmc-org.uk.

Consent

Background

- Before any form of care is undertaken, a patient must consent to treatment. 'Consent' refers to a patient's agreement for a healthcare worker (HCW) to provide treatment. Consent can be given in the following ways:
- In writing
- Verbally
- Non-verbally

It is common practice for written consent to be obtained before surgery, complex treatments or procedures, and administration of a general anaesthetic or sedation if there are significant consequences for the patient's employment, social, or personal life or it is part of a research programme.

For consent to be valid, the following criteria must be met:
- Given by a competent person.
- Given voluntarily.
- Informed.

Procedure: underlying principles

- The best interests of the patient should be paramount, ensuring that consent is obtained before any care is provided.
- If for any reason a patient is unable to give consent (e.g. as the result of an accident or because they are unconscious), care can be provided if it is felt to be in the best interests of the patient or deemed to be life-saving (accounting for pre-existing instructions).
- All adults are deemed competent, unless identified as incompetent by an appropriately qualified HCW.
- Competent pregnant women may refuse treatment, even if the action causes harm to the unborn fetus.
- Children aged 16–17 years are able to give consent. Younger children in some circumstances can give consent if they fully understand the procedure, its consequences, and its risks.
- According to the Mental Capacity Act (2005), if an individual is shown to lack mental capacity, health professionals have a statutory duty to act in the best interests of the patient.
- Information should be provided in a clear and open way, recognizing that all patients have a right to receive information about their care, treatment, and condition and to be involved in decisions about their care.
- Patients need sufficient information to decide whether to give consent.
- Patients have the right to accept or decline treatment and care and their decisions should be respected.
- Patients can change their mind or withdraw their consent at any time.
- All actions relating to obtaining consent or refusal of consent should be documented.

Confidentiality

Background

Information concerning any patient is considered confidential and health-care workers (HCWs) have a duty to protect all patient information. In sharing personal information, the patient is demonstrating a high degree of trust, and any breach of this trust can seriously harm the HCW–patient relationship and have implications for the HCW's professional standing.

Procedure: underlying principles

- If information has to be shared with other HCWs, it is important that the patient is made aware of this.
- Information should not be shared with the patient's family or friends without first gaining consent of the patient. If for any reason a patient is incapable of giving such consent, this should be discussed with other HCWs.
- If consent to share information is refused or cannot be obtained for other reasons, information can be given in exceptional circumstances and only if it is in the public interest—to protect the patient or others from significant harm or required by law or order of a court.
- Before disclosing confidential information, it is advisable that you discuss the situation with senior HCWs, the Nursing and Midwifery Council (NMC), and/or your professional body.
- If a decision is taken to share confidential information, you will be held accountable for any disclosures and must be able to justify the actions taken.
- If you want to refer to a real-life situation in a written assignment, all information that could identify a patient should be removed.

Practice tip

- Beware in particular of breaching the confidentiality of celebrities and also other health care workers known within the practice setting.

Further reading

NMC Code of Professional Conduct (2008): http://www.nmc-org.uk.

Documentation

Background

Documentation is used to communicate the care provided and record any significant events. Documentation can function as evidence, to investigate a complaint or for criminal and other court proceedings, but it also has the following uses:
- Promotes high standards of care.
- Encourages continuity of care.
- Ensures good interprofessional communication.
- Provides detailed and accurate accounts of care delivery and management.
- Facilitates the detection of problems and monitoring of changes in the patient's condition.

Procedure: underlying principles

- You will be held accountable for what you write and record.
- Patients have a legal right to read their records. Information can only be withheld if it could seriously harm a patient or breaches the confidentiality of others.
- All documentation relating to patients must be kept securely and mechanisms must be in place to safeguard confidentiality.
- Professional judgement must be used when identifying the relevant information to record and frequency of entries.
- Records should be accurate, clearly written in black indelible ink (in terms that are easily understandable), dated (including the time) and signed, contain only relevant information, and exclude jargon, abbreviations, or offensive subjective statements. Documentation written by students should be countersigned by the qualified nurse supervising the student.
- Records should provide clear and full accounts of assessments and plans of care, appropriate information relating to the condition of the patient and the nature of interventions provided, evidence of safe and accountable practice, accounts of the arrangements for continuity of care, and evidence of patient involvement, as appropriate. In a court of law, care is not considered to have been given unless it has been documented.
- The names, designations and ideally bleep/pager numbers of health care workers involved in management decisions should be recorded in the patient records.
- Documentation should be regularly audited to ensure the required standards are achieved and areas for improvement are identified.

Legal frameworks and policies

Background

Healthcare workers (HCWs) are answerable for their actions and must be aware of their limits and powers in relation to the delivery of care. HCWs are required to ensure their practice is lawful, by being aware of legislation and local protocols that relate to care delivery.

Law

There are two sources of law:
- *Acts of Parliament and statutory instruments*—these are statutory requirements, such as the Care Standards Act (2000), Health Act (2006), Mental Incapacity Act (2005), and Disability Act (1998).
- *Common law*—this relates to individual judgments or interpretations in relation to statute law and the precedence these set in relation to statute law.

Policy

Policy provides guidance in relation to the activities undertaken in a particular setting. In the health care setting, two types of policies are in evidence: national and local.

The Government, through the Department of Health (DoH), provides the legislation and national policy relating to how the National Health Service (NHS) is structured, financed, and managed. The DoH also sets standards against which care provision will be measured. This, in turn, is interpreted in light of local needs and services, resulting in local policy, which provides guidance on how NHS trusts should implement health legislation and policy, operationalize standards of care, and develop practice protocols and policies. Policies change over time and may vary from organization to organization. Therefore it is important that your knowledge remains current and that you familiarize yourself with the policies relating to the organization within which you practise.

Standard-setting

Clinical governance

Clinical governance is advocated to ensure that quality health care is provided in an effective way. It aims to promote formal reporting and accountability systems, clinical audit, and clinical effectiveness. These are termed 'quality assurance and improvement approaches' and promote standard setting and evidence-based practice.

National Institute for Health and Clinical Excellence (NICE)

NICE is an independent organization commissioned by the Government to produce national standards in relation to specific areas of care. Using expert panels, NICE develops guidelines for best clinical practice and benchmarks for best practice.

National Service Frameworks (NSFs)

NSFs provide national standards for specific areas of care and identify goals to be achieved within set timeframes. NSFs are currently available for the following areas:

- Coronary heart disease.
- Cancer.
- Paediatric intensive care.
- Mental health.
- Older people.
- Diabetes.
- Long-term conditions.
- Renal services.
- Children.
- Chronic obstructive airway disease.

Health and safety

Background

The environment in which healthcare workers (HCWs) practise must, by law, be safe for both staff and patients. Each HCW has a responsibility for ensuring the safety of the environment in which they practise, minimizing the risk to others, and should be aware of health and safely legislation. The requirements for health and safety issues are usually found in three types of documents: regulations, guidance, and approved codes of practice (ACOPs).

Regulations

The Health and Safety at Work Act (1974) provides the basis for British law in this area, specifying the duties of employers and employees in maintaining a safe working environment. Further regulations have been added that outline the responsibilities placed on employers in relation to the management of health and safety issues. The main requirement outlined in these regulations is systematic risk assessments of work activities for the following reasons:

- To identify hazards.
- To identify who is at risk.
- To evaluate risk.
- To identify methods of managing risk.
- To record assessment.

Guidance

The Health and Safety Executive (HSE) provides guidance in relation to specific health and safety problems and general processes across a range of areas. The main purpose of the guidance is as follows:

- To help people interpret and understand the regulations.
- To help people adhere to the legal requirements.
- To provide technical advice.
- To provide a way of ensuring that legal requirements are met, although following the guidance is not compulsory.

ACOPs

These provide practical examples and advice on how the regulations can be met.

Untoward incidents

Background

All health care environments must have a system for reporting and investigating untoward incidents. According to the Reporting of Injuries, Diseases and Dangerous Occurrences Regulations (1985; RIDDORs), the Environmental Health department of the local authority must be notified in the following situations:

- Fatal injuries to employees or other people in an accident connected with the area.
- Major injuries to employees or other people.
- Any of the dangerous occurrences listed in the regulations.
- Any other injury to an employee that results in an absence from work for more than 3 days.
- Any cases of ill health resulting from exposure to toxic chemicals, occupational asthma, or any illness caused by a pathogen.

Procedure: underlying principles

- Reporting and recording untoward incidents is vital—it is considered as providing information that enables trends and management interventions to be identified.
- The procedure identified for recording such incidents must be followed and usually involves:
  - Reporting accidents or untoward incidents to the senior manager.
  - Completing an incident form.
  - Notifying the Health and Safety Officer
- An untoward incident form must include the following details:
  - Date of the report.
  - Date, time, and place of the incident.
  - Personal details of those involved.
  - Brief description of the event or incident and actions taken.

Communication skills

Paul Crawford
Professor, School of Nursing, Midwifery & Physiotherapy,
University of Nottingham, UK

Initiating communication

Background

Given the demands on healthcare workers (HCWs) and the limited time to carry out interventions, it is crucial that effective communication is initiated, maintained, and promoted in encounters or interactions. Additionally, communication should be non-jargonistic and tailored to the context, individual and situation.

How HCWs begin a clinical encounter will influence patient engagement. Inappropriate or 'cold' communication could alienate people.

Procedure: underpinning principles

- Greet the person using positive verbal and non-verbal communication.
- Assess and adapt communication in response to:
  - Language needs or sensory impairment.
  - Emotional and cognitive factors or barriers.
  - Cultural preferences.
- Use engaging (non-staring) eye contact.
- Maintain an open posture, facing the person and leaning slightly forwards.
- Ensure a level of proximity that responds to cues or signals from the person.
- Consider using legitimate touch that is sensitive to cues.
- Adopt a relaxed manner.

Practice tips

- If using touch, ensure you are sensitive to the situation and to the individual and keep to 'safe zones', such as hands, arms, or shoulders.
- Demonstrate consistency in your verbal and non-verbal communication.

Maintaining and promoting communication

Background

Effective communication involves dialogue and sensitivity to how language choices can maintain respectful interaction. There are multiple factors that can inhibit interaction with others. Healthcare workers (HCWs) will need to consider environmental factors and adopt a range of interpersonal techniques to help people enter into dialogue, thereby maximizing the exchange of information.

Procedure: underlying principles

- Remain open to communicating with others and avoid presenting yourself 'as too busy to talk'.
- During conversation, acknowledge and share the presence of others by using eye contact, smiling, nods, or other appropriate gestures.
- In conversation ensure balanced turn-taking and avoid interrupting the other person or making abrupt or curt statements.
- Tend towards non-jargonistic language and limit the use of specialist terms or acronyms.
- Avoid labels and phrases that could be considered stigmatizing, such as describing people as an illness, e.g. 'The cancer in the side room', using offensive colloquialisms such as 'grumpy old man', 'retard', 'nutter' or describing someone as 'allergic', 'diabetic' or 'schizophrenic' rather than as a person with an allergy, schizophrenia or diabetes.
- Use small talk and appropriate humour to develop a rapport.
- Demonstrate active listening, warmth (being approachable), honesty, and a genuine regard (respect).
- Use verbal and nonverbal prompts to show interest and encourage disclosure.
- Use silence selectively to facilitate further reflection and expression.
- Use open ('how' or 'what') questions to enable exploration of ideas and a rich exchange of information.
- Use closed questions to obtain simple responses ('yes' or 'no').
- Be hyper-polite (even apologetic), cautious or circumspect when asking sensitive questions, using the word 'just' to soften or downgrade the intrusion and opening up the possibility that a difficult question is about to be asked. For example: 'I'm sorry, I just need to ask a rather personal question if I may?'; 'Could I just ask…'; or 'This might seem a strange question but we just always have to sort of find out…'.
- Be cautious if asking 'why?' questions because these could seem judgemental.
- Avoid asking too many questions because this could seem rude or intrusive and can result in anxiety.
- Negotiate with and involve the person in decision-making.
- Offer clear, accurate advice, information, and opinion.
- Provide constructive feedback.
- Consider the feedback given by the person.

- End or close a conversation in a satisfying, respectful manner by clarifying what has been discussed and decided upon in terms of any goals that have been set, when further meetings will take place and 'signing off' in a pleasant friendly manner, for example: 'OK, that's great, so I will see you then. OK? Bye bye.'
- Keep brief, factual, and accurate care records, according to the standards set out in the Nursing and Midwifery Council (NMC) Professional Code of Conduct (2004).
- Consider the environment and adapt to ensure privacy, comfort, optimal room temperature and humidity, adequate lighting and reduction of ambient noise.
- During consultations that include the use of a computer, consider your position relative to the screen and the person, thereby maintaining a rapport.
- Answer telephone queries by identifying yourself, being polite, striving to reduce hostility, and resolving queries or concerns.
- Ensure confidentiality, according to the NMC Code of Professional Conduct (2004).

Practice tips

- Remember that even the briefest positive interaction or conversation with patients or colleagues can have profound impacts and help to 'warm-up' potentially alienating or 'cold' clinical environments.

Pitfalls

- Using derogatory terms to describe patients. No matter what your personal feelings are you should retain respect for the dignity of all patients.
- Labelling patients as diseases e.g. the diabetic, asthmatic, schizophrenic. This is done all too frequently.

Further reading

NMC Code of Professional Conduct (2004)http://www.nmc-org.uk.

Managing interpersonal communication

Background

Interpersonal conflict can occur for a number of reasons, such as a person feeling offended, misunderstood, frustrated or blocked in some way in achieving their goals. Conflict may be displayed in verbal or non-verbal behaviour and lead to aggression or violence if unresolved. Since health care environments can be stressful, healthcare workers (HCWs) need to possess the necessary skills to de-escalate and manage conflict situations and be able to apply local complaints procedures.

Procedure: underlying principles

- HCWs should be trained to deal with complaints.
- Avoid flashpoints by being aware of a person's appearance and mood.
- Match anger with concern and commitment to solve problems.
- Avoid 'cornering' a person in any sense.
- Regularly break eye contact.
- Avoid appearing too calm or uninterested.
- Move to a quiet space, if possible, but within view of others.
- Avoid standing over a person or being lower than them.
- Sensitively mirror the person's posture.
- Listen carefully without interrupting.
- Clarify using gentle, tentative paraphrasing and questioning.
- Avoid appearing defensive or patronizing.
- Depersonalize issues.
- Do not make deals that you cannot keep.
- Make clear arrangements if the person needs to speak to someone else.
- Provide information about the procedure for making complaints.

Breaking bad news

Background

Bad news is any information that a person may find upsetting or disruptive. Healthcare workers (HCWs) frequently have to break bad news to patients, their loved ones, and their carers. Bad news is often associated with a terminal illness, such as cancer, but is, in part, a perception by the person and not always linked to life and death issues.

Procedure: underlying principles

- Prepare all relevant information beforehand.
- Ensure privacy and avoid interruption.
- Encourage the attendance of a key relative, carer, or advocate.
- Seek out the person's current perspective of the situation or issue.
- Summarize actions, interventions, and progress to date.
- Use sensitive language and empathetic responses.
- Prepare the person to indicate that there is some bad news coming.
- Provide clear, steadily paced information in stages, taking cues from the patient as to whether or not to continue.
- Clarify understanding after each piece of information given.
- At each stage, be prepared for the person who simply doesn't want to know more and respect this decision.
- Empathize and be accepting of unique responses.
- Assess the person's reaction to information.
- Provide honest, but sensitively delivered responses to questions.
- Support through appropriate touch and proximity (if appropriate).
- Allow the person to express anger, silence, passivity, withdrawal, and loss of concentration (shutdown).
- Facilitate further exploration of issues, helping the person adapt to the news, make decisions and come to their own conclusions.
- Address concerns and emphasize your role or the role of others in support or further interventions.
- Consider and facilitate additional space and time for the person and relative or carer to absorb the bad news at their own pace and without direction.
- Provide written information where appropriate and offer to return and restate the information, not least to relatives and friends if the person wishes.
- Be able to provide answers to questions and a 'way forward' if necessary.
- Don't be afraid of saying 'I don't know' and returning with the answer at a later time.

Communicating via interpreters

Background

Often, communication between healthcare workers (HCWs) and patients takes place via interpreters. These may be professional interpreters of spoken language, non-professional or informal interpreters (e.g. family members, other members of staff) and sign-language interpreters.

Procedure: underlying principles

- Promote language and deaf awareness among HCWs.
- Assess a patient's level of English language proficiency.
- Establish which kind of interpreter is best suited to assist with communication in any given context.
- Whenever possible, and initially, use qualified, empathic, professional interpreters familiar with health care settings and procedures to ensure confidentiality.
- If a professional interpreter is not available use other healthcare workers familiar with the patient's first language or a shared language or ask the most appropriate adult family member to assist.
- Respect a patient's request to use family rather than professional interpreters.
- Avoid using children of parents as interpreters.
- In sign-language interpretation ensure that detailed information is provided to or received from the deaf patient, avoiding over-simplification.
- Where possible use the same interpreter on each occasion for any given patient to ensure consistency and to promote an ongoing, trusting relationship.

Pitfall

- Developing a rapport and interacting predominantly with the interpreter to the detriment of the clinician-patient relationship.

Chapter 3

Assessment of the patient

Frank Coffey
Consultant in Emergency Medicine, Emergency Department,
Nottingham University Hospitals NHS Trust, Associate Professor
and Consultant in Advanced Clinical Skills, School of Nursing,
Midwifery & Physiotherapy, University of Nottingham, UK

Iain Neely
Clinical Nurse Trainer, Emergency Department, Nottingham
University Hospitals NHS Trust, UK

Initial observation/impression of a patient

Background

A great deal of information can be gained on first encountering a patient. Health care workers (HCWs) should use their senses to become skilled observers of the patient and their environment.

Equipment

- Your eyes, ears, hands, and nose.

Procedure

Look

- The patient's demeanour:
  - Physical—is their appearance consistent with their age? Look at the body habitus—are they obese or underweight? Are they comfortable, in pain, or distressed? Is there respiratory compromise e.g. use of accessory muscles, recession of the intercostals muscles, tachypnoea, or purse-lip breathing? Is the patient limping or using mobility aids? Any tremor or involuntary movements? Any obvious deformities—e.g. kyphosis or hemiplegia? Do they have a hearing aid, prosthetic eye or limb prosthesis, tracheostomy, fistula for renal dialysis? Look at their skin for pallor, plethora, cyanosis, or jaundice. Does the patient have any rashes, scars, tar ('nicotine') staining, needle marks or tattoos? Note any alopecia or hirusitism.
  - Psychological—does the patient seem happy or anxious, depressed, or aggressive? Does the patient have a tic? Are they displaying exaggerated grimaces of pain?
  - Dress—is the patient dressed appropriately or dishevelled and unkempt? Observe the style of dress, including jewellery—e.g. ethnic or religious dress or a sports shirt (the team supported can provide topic of conversation).
- The environment:
  - Look for clues to the patient's health and personality—e.g. mobility aids, splints, medications, inhalers, sputum jars, oxygen, nebulizers, monitoring, drains and dialysis. Without being intrusive, note photographs, cards, reading materials (books, magazines, and newspapers), mobile phones, ipods®, computer games, and religious or spiritual objects.
- The patient's interaction with relatives and friends.

Listen
- Language spoken/fluency in English
- Regional accent, use of slang or swear words.
- Quality of voice—confident or nervous? Angry?
- Abnormalities of speech—e.g. stuttering, monotonous, or dysphasia.
- Vocal tics.
- Cough, wheeze, or stridor.
- Clicking of a mechanical valve?
- Music, radio, or TV that the patient is listening to.
- The noise of equipment—e.g. ventilator or suction drain.

Smell
- Evidence of poor or good hygiene.
- Alcohol on the breath.
- Infection—e.g. the foul smell of an anaerobic infection.
- Fruity odour on the breath—diabetic ketoacidosis.
- Foul-smelling (dark) stools—melaena.

Practice tip

- Shaking or holding the patient's hand (if appropriate) can provide important information. Note eye contact, firmness of the grip, or the presence of tremor. Note whether the skin feels sweaty (might indicate anxiety or a pathological process).

Pitfalls

- Not being aware of cultural behaviour for different ethnic groups. A handshake might be appropriate in some encounters but would be inappropriate if offered by a ♂ health care worker to a veiled Muslim ♀. Eye contact is considered rude in some cultures.
- Making snap judgements on the basis of a patient's appearance or social class.

The medical history

Background

The taking of a history is a crucial interaction between the health care worker (HCW) and the patient. The information obtained will yield a differential diagnosis and is essential for focusing subsequent examination, investigations, and treatment. History-taking is often the first interaction between the HCW and the patient and its quality will affect the subsequent relationship. The depth and focus of the history will vary, depending on the setting and the role and seniority of the clinician. Communication skills are addressed in more detail in Chapter 2 (📖 on p. 15).

Procedure

- Explain the procedure and gain consent.
- Ask the patient their age and occupation.
- Take a history following a system that covers all, or the appropriate, elements of a comprehensive health history.
  - Presenting complaint (PC) (📖 on p. 27).
  - History of the PC (HxPC) (📖 on p. 28).
  - Past medical history (PHx). (📖 on p. 30).
  - Medications/allergies (📖 on p. 32).
  - Personal and social history (SHx) (📖 on p. 36).
  - Systems review (SR) (📖 on p. 38).

Practice tips

- Allow the patient time to tell their story but be focused, if necessary, to obtain key information.
- Use silence appropriately. If a patient does not respond immediately to a question, allow them time to think.
- Recognize non-verbal cues. Note whether the body language does not match what the patient is saying.
- Explain to the patient that you don't mean to be rude if you interrupt them but that you must elicit certain information.
- A number of systems for more focused or abbreviated assessment have been described, often using acronyms, e.g. SOAP (Subjective, Objective, Assessment, Plan of treatment). Explore those relevant to your area of practice.
- Obtain collateral histories from relatives, friends, carers, or bystanders for patients who cannot give a full history because of mental incapacity or other reasons (e.g. loss of consciousness).

Pitfalls

- Not being systematic in taking the history, leading to omission of crucial elements.
- Converging (i.e. narrowing) the focus at an early stage and making the history fit a predetermined diagnosis.
- Ignoring vital clues in the history.
- Not requesting an interpreter, if appropriate.
- Failing to appreciate the importance of social and psychological factors.
- Not asking the patient about their perception of their health problem and their expectations of you and the health service.
- Not obtaining consent from patients who are mentally competent before discussing their health with other people.

Presenting complaint (PC)

Background
The PC is the one or more symptoms or concerns that have brought the patient to seek or need medical care. The PC is the gateway to the rest of the history and sets the scene for the reader or listener if the health history is written or presented.

Procedure

Eliciting the PC from the patient
- Build an initial rapport with the patient.
- Ask the patient what has brought them to the health care setting—general prompting questions, e.g. 'when were you last well?' or 'how can I help?' might encourage shy or nervous patients.
- Allow the patient to tell you the PC in their own words, without interruption. Listen attentively.
- Clarify the length of time that each problem has been present. If intermittent, ascertain the first occasion that it occurred.

Presenting the PC to another health care worker (HCW)
- Give the PC in the patient's own words and its duration—e.g. 'breathlessness for 10 days'.
- If the patient has multiple complaints, rank them in order of importance and give a duration for each one. Leave a pause before moving on to give the 'history of the PC'—📖 on p. 28).

Practice tips

Eliciting the PC from the patient
- The complaint that the patient seeks advice about might not be their main concern, e.g. a man embarrassed about impotence might come on the pretext of back pain. The true PC should be elucidated by an empathetic and skilled interviewer.

Presenting or recording the PC
- Although the PC is usually the first part of the history to be presented, it is often helpful to first give a relevant background, e.g. 'this 42-year-old lady with a history of severe asthma since childhood presents with a 2-hour history of breathlessness and wheeze'.
- It is preferable to say the number of hours or days that the patient has had the symptom(s) e.g. rather than saying since 'last Saturday' say the number of days the symptom(s) has been present. This makes it clearer for the listener.

Pitfalls

Presenting or recording the PC
- Not using the patient's own words, where appropriate.
- Not giving the duration of the symptom(s).
- Going into detail about the PC before pausing (i.e. including elements of the history of the presenting complaint [HxPC] in the PC).

History of the presenting complaint

Background

The history of the presenting complaint (HxPC) is an exploration and analysis of the patient's current problem(s), which helps to formulate a differential diagnosis and focus examination, investigations, and treatment. It is the health care worker's (HCW) responsibility to organize the information given by the patient into a coherent and comprehensive narrative.

Procedure

Taking the HxPC from the patient

- Clarify the nature of the presenting complaint (PC).
- Elucidate the baseline—when was the patient last well or what is their usual level of disability?
- Find out how and when the presenting symptom(s) started.
- Initially, allow the patient to tell their story and avoid leading questions. Then, ask more focused questions to ascertain essential information.
- Characterize the presenting symptom(s) systematically using the following headings, which can be applied to the majority of symptoms:
  - Onset.
  - Location.
  - Character.
  - Duration.
  - Frequency.
  - Periodicity.
  - Severity.
  - Aggravating or relieving factors.
- If the PC is pain, in addition to the above ask about radiation of the pain and score its severity at the time of onset and at the time of history taking.
- Ask about associated symptoms and their relationship to the PC— e.g. sweating associated with chest pain.
- Clarify what the patient means if they use medical terms without explanation, e.g. if a patient says they have 'gastritis' do they mean pain, reflux, or some other symptom?
- Ask about treatments to date.
- Ask about cardinal symptoms of the involved system.
- Ask about risk factors that are relevant to potential diagnoses e.g. recent immobility, operations or a history of thromboembolism in a patient with pleuritic chest pain where pulmonary embolism would be a differential.
- Ask questions relevant to the PC that would normally be covered in other sections of the history—e.g. whether there is a family history of heart disease in a patient presenting with chest pain or about relevant medications (e.g. non-steroidal anti-inflammatory drugs (NSAIDs) or warfarin in a patient with haematemesis).
- Ask the patient what they think the problem is and what their fears and expectations are.

Presenting the HxPC to another HCW
- Present the HxPC in a systematic fashion, giving a clear, concise, and chronological account.
- Give positive and negative findings in a way that suggests or rules out differential diagnoses. The listener should understand the thought processes behind your narrative.
- Present *relevant* factors from other sections of the history within the HxPC.

Pitfalls
- Not being systematic and thorough when taking and presenting the history, particularly if there are multiple symptoms. ▶ Ask or present all the facts relevant to one symptom before moving on to the next one—e.g. in a patient with chest pain and breathlessness, ask all the relevant questions about the chest pain before moving on to explore the onset, duration and other characteristics of the breathlessness.
- Asking leading questions—e.g. 'is it a crushing-type pain?' rather than 'tell me what the pain feels like'.
- Asking double questions—e.g. 'describe the pain and how long you have had it'. The patient will tend to only answer the second half of the question.
- Not clarifying the exact location of symptoms such as pain and paraesthesiae.

Past medical history

Background

The past medical history (PHx), in addition to 'the drug history and allergies' (📖 on p. 32), provides the background to the patient's current health or disease. It builds a picture of the health status and experience of the patient and might provide important diagnostic clues. A complete PHx, including childhood illnesses and a psychiatric and sexual history, is necessary if a comprehensive health history is being taken. An experienced clinician will focus on information that will affect the diagnosis or treatment.

Procedure

Taking the PHx from the patient

- Ask the patient whether they have had any medical problems, hospitalizations, accidents, or operations in the past. Record them in chronological order. If the patient has been hospitalized or had operations, find out the name of the hospital and their consultant.
- After giving the patient the opportunity to tell you their health history, ask focused questions to ensure that you have the full picture.

Ask about

- Childhood illnesses—e.g. mumps, whooping cough, chickenpox, rubella, and rheumatic fever.
- Previous illnesses or chronic (ongoing) medical problems— e.g. diabetes, asthma, tuberculosis (TB), high blood pressure, and heart disease.
- Cholesterol level (if known).
- Operations—dates and types.
- Accidents and injuries—dates, nature of injuries, and treatments.
- Psychiatric illnesses, hospitalizations, and treatments.

If relevant also ask about

- Sexual history—sexuality, number of partners, and sexually transmitted diseases.
- Obstetric and gynaecologic history—births, abortions, miscarriages, menstrual history, and contraception.

Practice tips

- Enquire about the patient's previous health, in addition to illness. 'Well-person' and insurance health checks and family planning clinic visits have probably recorded measurements, e.g. blood pressure, and performed blood tests that might be helpful for comparison with present findings.
- Enquire specifically about attendance to, and treatments received from, chiropractors, osteopaths, and other practitioners outside mainstream medicine.

- Information from the PHx considered to impact on the presenting complaint should be placed in the 'history of the presenting complaint' (see ⬚ HxPC p.28) section when the history is being written or presented—e.g. a previous history of deep vein thrombosis in a patient presenting with leg pain.
- Remember to be tactful when addressing sensitive issues in the past medical history, particularly relating to the psychiatric, sexual and obstetric elements of it.

Pitfalls

- Accepting patients' 'ready-made' diagnoses without further questioning. If there are no medical records available to back them up, ask the patient about symptoms, circumstances, and treatments. 'Diagnoses' made by other practitioners in the past might not always be correct, e.g. patients may have been told that they had 'an ulcer' on the basis of epigastric pain and never had an endoscopy to confirm it. Always question such diagnoses.
- Failing to record accurately the names of treating physicians, surgeons, and alternative practitioners and the locations and timing of the treatments. This information can be important for retrieval of information or for onward referral.

Drug history/allergies

Background

The drug (DHx) and allergy history is an extremely important part of the medical history. The presenting symptom might be owing to the side-effect of a drug. Current medications and previous allergies may influence further prescriptions.

Procedure

- Ask the patient to list all the medications that they are taking on medical advice or otherwise.
- Ask the patient for a recent prescription. Ideally, you should also see their medications.
- Note the name, dose, route, and frequency of use of all medications. Note the indications for each one, unless they are self-evident.
- List non-prescription drugs, vitamin and mineral supplements, and herbal and alternative remedies.
- Ask about illicit drug use.
- Enquire about allergies or adverse reactions to medications, foods, animals, pollen, or other environmental factors.
- If the patient gives a history of allergy, record the exact nature and circumstances of the reaction and the treatment given.

Practice tips

- If the patient cannot supply information about their medications because of illness, mental disturbance, dementia or young age, try to obtain accurate information from their relatives, friends, General Practitioner or medical notes.
- The oral contraceptive pill is often not perceived as a medication. Ask specifically about it in ♀ of the appropriate age.
- Patients might omit to mention medications that are not tablets (e.g. inhalers, home oxygen therapy, creams, eye or ear drops, pessaries, or suppositories). Ask specifically about such agents.
- Information about drugs and allergies considered to impact on the presenting complaint should be placed in the 'history of the presenting complaint' section when the history is being written or presented— e.g. warfarin in a patient with a head injury.
- Beware of abbreviations when recording, prescribing or administering drug dosages, e.g. 5IU (5 international units) looks very similar to 51U (fifty-one units) with potentially fatal consequences if the wrong dose is given. Also μg for micrograms can look like mg or ng if not written clearly or read carefully.

Pitfalls

- Failing to record accurately the names, dosages, or frequency of drugs. Use the *British National Formulary*, or equivalent drug formulary, to check names and doses.
- Recording the medication list from an out-of-date prescription or past medical notes (although these sources might be helpful for identification of drugs, they are not necessarily up to date).
- Accepting the patient's word that they are 'allergic' to a drug. It might simply be a side-effect—e.g. nausea with an antibiotic.
- Not asking about over-the-counter preparations or herbal and other alternative remedies. Patients are often slow to volunteer information about self-medication and medications given to them by relatives. Enquire specifically.
- Poorly legible written records, which have the potential to lead to serious drug errors.
- Failing to record dosage units such as mg or mL accurately or clearly. Beware of abbreviations (see final practice tip above).

Family history

Background

Information regarding the age and health or cause of death of the patient's relatives can be invaluable and provide vital clues in the diagnostic process. In many conditions, there is a well-defined mode of inheritance. In other conditions, there is a genetic or environmental component. The family history (FHx) might also explain some of the patient's ideas, fears, and expectations.

Procedure

Taking the FHx from the patient

- Enquire about any illnesses that run in the family as a screening question.
- If more detailed information is required, enquire about the age and health or cause of death of immediate relatives, including brothers and sisters, parents, grandparents, blood aunts and uncles, children, and grandchildren.
- Enquire specifically about the following common conditions that have a hereditary or familial element:
  - Hypertension.
  - Coronary artery disease.
  - High cholesterol.
  - Diabetes mellitus.
  - Kidney disease
  - Thyroid disease.
  - Cancer (specify type).
  - Gout.
  - Arthritis.
  - Asthma or other lung disease.
  - Infectious diseases (e.g. tuberculosis).
  - Headache.
  - Epilepsy.
  - Mental illness.
  - Alcohol or drug addiction.
- Enquire about allergies present in family members.

Presenting or recording the FHx

If any part of the FHx is directly relevant to the presenting complaint, present it in the 'history of the presenting complaint' (□ see HxPC on p.28) section—e.g. a FHx of ischaemic heart disease in a patient presenting with chest pain.

Practice tips

- A useful way to record the FHx is on a diagrammatic representation of the family tree (see Box 3.1 for an example).
- Be tactful if asking about problems such as alcoholism or mental illness in a close relative. A display of interest in the welfare of the family might help to secure rapport.
- Remember some people are adopted and unaware of their FHx.

Box 3.1 A family tree

Drawing up a family tree begins with the patient that you are concerned with, called a propositus if male or proposita if female—indicated by a small arrow (↗). Males are represented by a square (□) and females by a circle (○).

Horizontal lines are relationships resulting in children. Vertical lines descend from these to a horizontal line, from which children of the relationship 'hang'. Members of the family who have died have a diagonal line through their symbol (⊠ ⊘) and should have the age and cause of death added beside it. The ages and any relevant conditions should also be added beside the symbols of relatives who are alive.

The family tree should extend upwards as far as grandparents and downwards to include children. (If drawing up a family tree to identify a genetic disease, for example colon cancer, shade in the symbols of family members affected by the disease in question. (■ ●))

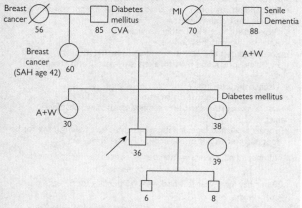

CVA — Cerebrovascular accident
MI — Myocardial infarction
SAH — Subarachnoid haemorrhage
A+W — Alive and well

Fig. 3.1 Example of a family tree recording family history for a 36-year-old male married with two sons. He has two sisters. Both parents and two grandparents are still alive.

Personal and social history

Background
The personal and social history (SHx) is a crucial aspect of the comprehensive health care history. All illnesses, treatments, and rehabilitation must be seen in the context of the patient's personality, spirituality, and personal and social circumstances. Occupation and lifestyle habits can have a profound impact on health and disease. Not all the elements of the social history outlined will be relevant in every encounter and the experienced health care worker will tailor the history appropriately.

Procedure
Enquire about the following:
- Occupation/education:
  - Title(s) and nature of current and previous occupations.
  - Economic situation—e.g. whether the patient has financial difficulties.
  - Educational level.
- The home:
  - Home situation and significant others.
  - Number of rooms and occupants.
  - State of repair.
  - Sanitary and heating arrangements.
  - Number of steps leading up to and within the home.
  - Aids and adaptations—stair lift, commode or other toileting aids, walk-in bath, grab rails etc.
  - Proximity of shops and other services.
  - Relationship with neighbours.
- Personal interests and activities of daily living (ADLs).
  - Hobbies, sports, and physical exercise—nature and quantity.
- Diet:
  - Usual daily food intake.
  - Dietary supplements or restrictions.
  - Use of coffee, tea and other caffeine-containing substances.
- Habits:
  - Tobacco use and type. If patient has given up smoking, note for how long. Cigarettes are often recorded in 'pack years':

  Number of pack years = (number of cigarettes smoked per day × number of years)/20

  20 per day for a year is 1 pack year. 10 per day for 8 years = 4 pack years.
  - Alcohol—usually recorded in units/week. One unit is roughly equivalent to half a pint of beer, one standard glass of wine, or a standard measure of spirits.
  - Illicit drugs—e.g. cannabis, cocaine, and heroin.

- Risk awareness and use of safety measures:
  - Safety belts, bicycle helmets, sun block, cupboard and window locks, fire alarms, and carbon monoxide detectors.
  - Attendance to alternative health care practitioners: osteopaths, chiropractors, faith healers, homeopaths, and herbalists.
- Religious affiliation and spiritual beliefs.

Practice tips

- Personal and social questions should be mixed in with other elements of the history to make the patient feel more at ease.
- It is informative to get the patient to talk about their normal working and leisure days.
- A full dietary history should be obtained if there is obvious nutritional deformity.
- The 'Habits' section is often recorded in the history as a section on its own following the medication history. This underlines the important effects of smoking, drinking alcohol and illicit drug use on a patient's health.
- Patients are often reluctant to reveal the full extent of their drinking following direct questioning. Suggesting a very large amount to heavy drinkers might lessen their embarrassment and lead to the truth. The question 'would you drink three bottles of whisky per day?' might provoke the response 'oh no, not at all—I would only drink one to one-and-a-half bottles'.
- Elicit the strength of the alcohol and sizes of bottles, measures, and glasses.
- It might be necessary to retake the alcohol history if the physical examination or investigations reveal the possibility of concealed alcohol abuse.

Pitfalls

- Failing to ask pertinent questions about the patient's occupation that might aid diagnosis—e.g. repetitive movements at work might be the cause of a patient presenting with wrist pain.
- Failing to ask relevant questions about the home environment that will impact on the patient if they are sent home—e.g. an elderly person who cannot climb steps following a knee injury and only has an upstairs toilet.
- Not appreciating that many people underestimate or deliberately conceal the amount of alcohol that they drink.
- Not enquiring about previous smoking. A patient might say that they don't smoke and omit to mention that they smoked 40 cigarettes/day until the previous week!

Systems review

Background

The systems review (SR)—or systems enquiry, which is undertaken at the end of the history, involves a series of screening questions that systematically cover all the body systems. It is usually performed in a head-to-toe sequence and its purpose is to elicit any further information that might be relevant to the current illness or uncover present or past problems that the patient has overlooked. The SR might provide information that leads the health care worker (HCW) to suspect a multi-system disease process, e.g. systemic lupus erythematosus (SLE), or demonstrate associated symptoms in another system, e.g. arthritis associated with inflammatory bowel disease.

Procedure

Explain to the patient that you are going to finish the interview by asking a number of questions about different parts of the body, to be completely thorough. The following is a standard list of SR questions:

- General:
  - Usual weight, appetite, recent weight loss or gain, energy levels, any fevers or sweats.
- Central nervous system (CNS):
  - Headache, dizziness, vertigo, fainting, blackouts, seizures, weakness, paralysis, numbness, tingling, 'pins and needles', incoordination, tremors, involuntary movements, memory loss, mood changes, problems with concentration, or problems with speech.
- Ear, nose, and throat (ENT):
  - Ear—hearing, tinnitus, earache, discharge, ear infection, wax, or use of a hearing aid.
  - Nose—nasal stuffiness, blockage, discharge, itching, nose bleeds, sinus problems, or frequent colds/runny nose.
  - Throat and mouth—sore throat, hoarseness, sore tongue, blisters, cold sores, dry mouth, or problems with teeth or gums.
- Eyes:
  - Vision, glasses/contact lenses, double vision, blurred vision, pain, redness, floaters, spots, specks, flashing lights, dry eyes, or excessive tearing.
- Neck:
  - Swollen glands, lumps, goitre, pain, or stiffness.
- Cardiovascular system (CVS):
  - Chest pain, dyspnoea (breathlessness), palpitations, paroxysmal nocturnal dyspnoea (PND—waking at night short of breath), orthopnoea (breathlessness lying flat), or ankle swelling.
- Respiratory:
  - Cough chest pain, sputum, haemoptysis (coughing blood), dyspnoea, or wheeze.
- Breasts:
  - Lumps, pain, nipple discharge or bleeding, or nipple inversion.

- Gastrointestinal (GIT):
  - Abdominal pain, bloating, appetite, food intolerance, excessive belching or passing of flatus, nausea, vomiting, haematemesis (vomiting blood), dysphagia (trouble swallowing), odynphagia (pain on swallowing), heartburn, acid reflux, weight loss or gain, stool colour and size, change in bowel habit, diarrhoea, constipation, pain on defaecation, tenesmus (sensation of incomplete evacuation of stool), rectal bleeding, melaena (black tarry stools), or haemorrhoids.
- Genito-urinary tract (GUT):
  - Urinary—frequency, polyuria (↑ volume of urine), dysuria (pain or burning on micturition), haematuria (blood in the urine), nocturia (rising at night to pass urine), eneurisis (bed wetting), abdominal pain (in particular, suprapubic, kidney, or flank pain), incontinence, ↓ calibre and flow of urinary stream, or terminal dribbling.
  - ♂ genital—hernias, penile sores, discharge, sexual history, orientation, number of partners, safe sex in particular use of condoms, or impotence (erectile or ejaculatory dysfunction).
  - ♀ genital—age at menarche, last menstrual period, characteristics of periods (regularity, frequency, and duration), amount of bleeding (how many pads/tampons used), intermenstrual bleeding, postcoital bleeding, dysmenorrhoea (painful periods), Premenstrual Syndrome (PMS) symptoms, age at menopause, menopausal symptoms, postmenopausal bleeding, vaginal discharge, itching, sores lumps, dyspareunia (pain during intercourse), sexual history, orientation, number of partners, use of contraception, safe sex, number of pregnancies, miscarriages, induced abortions, or complications of pregnancy.
- Musculoskeletal:
  - Joint or muscle pain, stiffness, limitation of mobility and/or function, redness of joints, or neck or low back pain.
- Skin:
  - Rashes, lumps, sores, dryness, swelling, itching, colour changes, or changes in hair or nails.
- Peripheral vascular:
  - Leg pain or cramps, intermittent claudication (pain in legs on exercise), varicose veins, swelling in calves legs or feet, ulcers on limbs, or changes in colour of the digits in cold weather.
- Haematologic:
  - Easy bruising, excessive bleeding, spontaneous joint effusions, anaemia, or transfusion history.
- Endocrine—many of the symptoms characteristic of endocrine abnormalities will have been covered in other systems (e.g. weight loss or tremor):
  - Thyroid—heat or cold intolerance, weight loss or gain, tremor, or excessive sweating.
  - Diabetes mellitus—polyuria, polydipsia (excessive thirst), or excessive hunger.
  - Pituitary—↑ in hand or foot size or coarsening of features.

- Psychiatric:
  - Mood changes, anxiety, panic attacks, loss of interest, loss of appetite, poor concentration, altered sleeping pattern, waking in the early morning, paranoia, or auditory or visual hallucinations.

Practice tips
- The SR can be performed in combination with the physical examination (e.g. asking about cardiovascular and respiratory symptoms while examining the chest). If there are multiple symptoms, however, this can interfere with the flow of the examination.
- Specific questions about diseases, e.g. angina and tuberculosis, can be asked about in the SR if it is felt that they were not adequately covered in the past medical history (PHx) (📖 on p. 30).
- Relevant major symptoms or events uncovered by the SR should be moved to the history of the presenting complaint (HxPC) or the PHx when writing up and presenting the history e.g. rectal bleeding ascertained in the SR of a patient presenting with back pain and weight loss would raise the possibility of a bowel malignancy with bony metastases. This symptom should therefore be highlighted in the HxPC.

Vital signs

Background

The vital signs are measures of crucial physiological functions. They consist of the pulse rate, respiratory rate, temperature, and blood pressure. The term 'observations' is also used, although this usually implies a broader range of measures. Vital signs are essential for a complete assessment of a patient. They enable prompt detection of adverse events or a delayed recovery. Pain has been called 'the fifth vital sign'. Oxygen saturation is also measured during the assessment of vital signs in many clinical settings.

Equipment

- Clock or watch with a second hand.
- Thermometer.
- Sphygmomanometer.
- Stethoscope.

Procedure

- The procedures for measurement of individual vital signs are outlined on p.44–59.

Practice tips

- Vital signs should always be considered in the general context of the patient's age, medications, and clinical presentation.
- When recording the vital signs, it is useful to comment if the patient was anxious or in pain.

Pitfalls

- Being falsely reassured by 'normal vital signs' in a patient who otherwise appears unwell—other factors (e.g. general appearance, colour, mental state, capillary refill, and urinary output) should be considered.
- Ignoring or failing to report abnormal vital signs, particularly in a patient who does not appear unwell—an explanation should always be sought for abnormal vital signs.
- Failing to measure the patient's temperature because of a misguided perception that it is not required—e.g. in an elderly patient presenting following a fall. The fall might be the result of an underlying infection and a pyrexia might suggest this.
- Failing to record respiratory rate or not assessing it accurately. It is as important as the other vital signs.
- Not recording the rhythm of a pulse, in addition to the rate. Arrhythmias, in particular atrial fibrillation are frequently missed.
- Recording abnormal vital signs and not reporting them to senior personnel.
- Not advocating for a more senior opinion if concerned that another health care worker (HCW) is not managing a patient's abnormal vital signs appropriately.
- Not using a rectal thermometer in suspected hypothermia or hyperthermia.
- Using faulty or inappropriately sized equipment—e.g. a sphygmomanometer cuff that is too big or small.

- Using equipment incorrectly—e.g. not positioning the sphygmomanometer correctly or not sealing the external auditory meatus with a tympanic thermometer.
- Not recording oxygen treatment concentrations when recording oxygen saturations with the vital signs.
- Failing to recognize spurious pyrexias in patients with Munchausen's syndrome (or Munchausen's by proxy). Although not commonly seen, these patients simulate high temperatures by various methods, including dipping the thermometer in a hot drink or placing it against a radiator. Suspect if the temperature is out of sync with the patient's general condition.

Measurement of the oral temperature

Background

The oral temperature is measured by means of a glass or an electronic digital thermometer placed in the sublingual pocket. It is used if the patient's temperature is not likely to be outside the range 34.5–40.0°C.

Equipment

- Gloves.
- Glass thermometer with an oral bulb or electrical digital thermometer.
- Disposable single-use thermometer cover.
- Paper/electronic observation record chart.

Procedure

- Explain the procedure and gain consent.
- Decontaminate your hands.
- Put on the gloves.
- Cover the tip and shaft of the thermometer with a single-use disposable cover.
- If using an electronic digital device, activate the thermometer.
- Place the tip of the thermometer in the sublingual pocket by gently inserting under the tongue as far back as possible on either side of the frenulum (the vertical fold of mucous membrane under the tongue attaching it to the floor of the mouth).
- Ask the patient to close their lips gently to hold the thermometer in place.
- Leave the thermometer in this position for at least 3min or, if using an electronic thermometer, until the alarm sounds.
- Remove the thermometer and dispose of the single-use cover and gloves in clinical waste disposal.
- Decontaminate your hands.
- Record the time, recording method, and temperature reading.
- Report abnormalities to senior nursing or medical staff.

Practice tips

- Oxygen therapy does not affect oral temperature readings. The presence of an oxygen mask, however, might interfere with placing the thermometer safely in the patient's mouth. The use of nasal oxygen cannulae might facilitate this.
- Wait at least 15min before taking the recording if the patient has recently eaten or had a drink. Chewing gum and smoking might also affect the reading.
- A patient whose respiratory rate is >18breaths/minute is likely to have a ↓ oral recording.
- Use the same thermometer, if possible, to record consecutive readings.
- Multiple recordings are needed to detect trends in the patient's temperature.
- The most sensitive time for detection of pyrexia is the early morning, between 07.00 and 08.00 hours.

Pitfalls

- Not leaving the thermometer *in situ* for the recommended time, resulting in an inaccurate temperature reading.
- Positioning the thermometer incorrectly so that it rests behind the lower incisors and not in the sublingual pocket. This can ↓ the reading by up to 1.7°C.
- Not supervising or instructing the patient sufficiently and being unaware that they have removed the thermometer to speak, cough, or reposition it.
- Recording the oral temperature shortly after a patient has eaten or had a drink.
- Attempting to take an oral temperature in patients who are agitated or confused or have a ↓ level of consciousness for any reason.
- Attempting to take an oral temperature from a patient who is markedly breathless.
- Taking an oral temperature in a patient at high risk of a seizure.

Measurement of the aural temperature

Background

The aural temperature is taken in the ear canal, using a tympanic thermometer. This site offers a reasonably precise measurement of the core body temperature.

Equipment

• Aural temperature probe.
• Disposable probe cover.

Procedure

• Explain the procedure and gain consent.
• Decontaminate your hands.
• If the patient wears a hearing aid, remove it carefully.
• Inspect the external ear canal for excess wax. Wipe any visible wax with a warm, moist cloth.
• Ensure the probe lens is clean.
• Attach a new probe cover.
• Turn the thermometer on and wait until the 'reading' sign appears on the display screen.
• Stand slightly to the front of, and facing, the patient.
• Stabilize the patient's head.
• Gently pull the pinna of the ear backwards and slightly upwards (straight backwards in young children).
• Insert the covered probe into the patient's ear.
• Point the probe downwards and towards the front of the ear canal until the canal is sealed.
• Press the activation button to take the temperature. Keep the button depressed and probe in place until the instrument blinks or bleeps to indicate that the temperature recording is complete (usually ~1sec).
• Remove the probe and note the temperature on the display screen.
• Remove the probe cover from the probe by pushing the button on the side of the instrument.
• Discard the probe cover in clinical waste disposal.
• Turn the thermometer off and replace it in its charger.
• Document the episode of care and record the reading, noting the method of recording (aural/tympanic) used.

Practice tips

• If possible wait at least 20min from the time the patient has been exposed to an ambient temperature before taking the temperature.
• Once a reading has been taken, that ear should not be used again for taking another reading for at least 20min.
• If the patient has been lying on a pillow, the ear on that side should not be used to take the reading for at least 20min.

Pitfalls

- Not pushing the probe in far enough or pushing it too far can lead to inaccurate readings.
- Placing the thermometer back in the charger before taking the reading, because this clears the display screen.
- Reusing probe covers, which can cause inaccurate readings and is an infection risk.
- Not using a probe cover can damage the probe and give an inaccurate reading. The thermometer is calibrated to account for the presence of a cover. It is also an infection risk.
- Taking a reading if the patient has just come in from outdoors.
- Prescribing antipyretics and making diagnoses on the basis of a tympanic recording in the normal range—a tympanic reading is generally 0.5–1.0°C higher than an oral temperature.

Measurement of the rectal temperature

Background

The rectal temperature is used to measure the core body temperature and is more accurate than oral or axillary readings. It is used in severely ill patients and should be taken in cases of suspected hypothermia or hyperthermia. The technique is contraindicated if the patient has diarrhoea, severe haemorrhoids or has had recent rectal surgery. It is relatively contraindicated in patients with cardiac disease because vagal stimulation can cause cardiac arrhythmias.

Equipment

- Rectal thermometer.
- Disposable rectal thermometer cover.
- Lubricant.
- Gauze pad.
- Gloves.
- Tissues.
- Apron.

Procedure

- Explain the procedure and gain consent.
- Have a chaperone present. If this is not possible ask the patient whether they are happy for you to proceed without a chaperone and record this in the notes.
- Ensure privacy by drawing the bedside curtains and shutting doors.
- Have the patient lie on their side, with the uppermost knee flexed— Sims' position.
- Arrange the patient's clothing and bed sheet so that the rectal area is exposed but dignity is maintained as much as possible.
- Put on the gloves and an apron.
- Put a disposable cover on the thermometer.
- Squirt a small amount of lubricant onto a gauze pad and lubricate ~4cm of the thermometer shaft with it.
- Lift the patient's upper buttock with your free hand until the anus is clearly exposed.
- Insert the thermometer gently into the rectum and along the rectal wall towards the umbilicus (~4cms in an adult).
- Release your hold on the patient's upper buttock but do not let go of the thermometer.
- Hold the thermometer in place for 2min or until the alarm sounds.
- When you are ready to remove thermometer, lift the upper buttock again with your free hand and gently remove the thermometer.
- Wipe the thermometer clean with a gauze swab and remove the disposable cover, being careful not to contaminate the thermometer.
- Wipe the patient's anal area to remove excess lubricant or faeces.
- Discard clinical waste in the clinical waste disposal.
- Remove the gloves and clean your hands.
- Document the episode of care and record the temperature reading, stating the method used.

Practice tips

- Provide adequate privacy and dignity, and make sure that the patient is positioned comfortably. If there is a possibility that someone might barge through the cubicle curtains or into the room, put up a warning sign or have somebody 'stand guard'.
- Be aware that some patients might find this method of taking their temperature unacceptable. This might be for cultural reasons or there might be a history of sexual abuse.
- Allow the patient to empty their rectum, if necessary, before undertaking the procedure. Be aware that soiling might occur and prepare for this.
- Continuous rectal temperature monitoring can be performed using a rectal probe left in situ and connected to a monitor.

Pitfalls

- Failing to hold the thermometer securely. The thermometer can be pushed out if it is not held securely. A more serious consequence is losing the thermometer in the rectum if it is advanced too far and not held securely.
- Failing to reassure and relax the patient, with resultant failure to insert the thermometer because the patient is too tense.
- Causing damage to, and in extreme instances perforation of, the rectal wall owing to rough insertion and poor technique.
- Failing to evacuate the rectum, if necessary, before the procedure.

Measurement of the skin temperature

Background

The body temperature can be calculated from the skin with liquid-crystal/chemical-dot thermometers. These possess heat-sensitive liquid crystals in a plastic strip that change colour to indicate different temperatures. Chemical-dot thermometers are particularly useful in young children, although they are not as accurate as other methods of measuring the temperature. For this reason, they are not recommended in critically ill patients or if a very accurate recording is required. They are not reliable in hypothermia or hyperthermia.

Equipment

- Liquid-crystal/chemical-dot thermometer.

Procedure

- Explain the procedure and gain consent.
- Decontaminate your hands.
- Remove the thermometer from its protective packaging, according to the manufacturer's instructions.
- Place the thermometer on a clean, exposed area of the patient's skin—usually the forehead.
- Leave in position for the recommended time—usually 45secs.
- Record the reading, reporting any abnormalities.
- Document the episode of care.

Practice tip

- Take the colour reading in a well-lit area to avoid misinterpretation.

Pitfalls

- Not incorporating the temperature reading into an overall assessment of the patient's condition and being falsely reassured.
- Attempting to use a chemical-dot thermometer on an agitated patient because it is not likely to remain attached to the skin if they are moving excessively.

Assessment of the peripheral pulse

Background

When the ventricles of the heart contract, the output of blood into the aorta causes a surge in the flow of blood around the body, producing a pressure wave or pulse. The pulse can be detected in arteries lying close to the body surface. The radial artery at the wrist is the site most commonly used for the assessment of the pulse. The rate/minute, regularity, and strength of the pulse are measured. These parameters give information about the patient's cardiac function and circulatory status. The pulse might also give clues to pathology in other systems of the body.

Equipment

• Watch or clock with a second hand.

Procedure

• Explain the procedure and gain consent.
• Decontaminate your hands.
• Position the patient in a comfortable sitting or supine position, with their arms at their side.
• Locate the radial artery on the thumb side of the palmar aspect of the wrist.
• Count the rate (number of pulse beats) in 1 minute, noting the regularity.
• Record the pulse rate and report abnormalities.
• Document the episode of care.

Practice tips

• Anxiety, exercise, and pain can affect the pulse rate. If possible, take the reading when the patient is relaxed.
• To locate the radial pulse, turn the patient's hand palm downwards and clasp the wrist over the top with your hand, encircling the wrist with your fingers, which should then rest over the radial pulse.
• Ask the patient politely not to speak to you during the procedure, unless it is urgent. It is easy to get distracted and lose count.
• Plan the most effective time to record the pulse rate—e.g. while the patient is trying to eat their lunch is not an appropriate time.
• Patients sometimes hold their breath when having their pulse taken, which might make them uncomfortable and affect their pulse rate. Advise them to relax and breathe normally before and during the procedure.
• If there are concerns about the accuracy of a pulse rate, ask a colleague to check it. You can also take an apical rate by palpating or auscultating at the apex of the heart.

Pitfalls
- Only feeling the pulse for 10 or 15secs, which can lead to an irregular rhythm being undetected. Ideally, the pulse should be felt for a full 1 minute.
- Exerting excessive pressure when palpating the radial pulse, which might make it difficult to detect or lead to an inaccurate assessment.
- Using the thumb to detect the pulse—the thumb has its own pulse, which might be confused with the patient's pulse.
- Not relating the pulse rate to previous recordings and other observations.

Measurement of the respiratory rate

Background

The respiratory rate is the number of breaths taken in 1 minute. The normal rate in adults is between 12 and 20 breaths/minute. It can be measured by observation or by non-invasive mechanical methods such as capnography or pulse oximetry. Normal breathing at rest should be regular, effortless, and virtually silent. The respiratory rate can give vital information about a patient's respiratory, cardiovascular, neurological or metabolic status. It should be considered in association with the other vital signs and patient's general condition. When the respiratory rate is being recorded, the rhythm, effort, depth, and additional noises (e.g. gurgling) should also be noted.

Equipment

• Watch or clock with a second hand.

Procedure

• Explain the procedure and gain consent.
• Ensure, if possible, that the patient is in a comfortable, upright position.
• Maintain the patient's privacy and dignity.
• Expose the patient's chest if necessary so that it can be observed easily.
• Look and listen for any signs of respiratory distress—e.g. use of the accessory muscles of respiration (e.g. neck muscles), intercostal recession, nasal flaring, or grunting.
• Count the number of breaths taken over a period of 1 minute by watching the patient's chest and abdomen rise.
• Note the rhythm and depth of the breathing.
• Record the rate, rhythm, effort, and depth of breathing, in addition to the presence of any additional noises.
• Document the episode of care and report any significant changes or abnormalities.

Practice tips

• Patients might alter their breathing pattern if they feel that they are being observed. Pretending to take the pulse while covertly watching the chest or abdomen rise might overcome this.
• If you have difficulty seeing the patient's chest or abdomen rise, move closer to the patient and observe more closely. A last resort is to place your hand lightly on the patient's abdomen or chest—be aware, however, that this might alter their breathing pattern.
• If the patient is distressed, anxious, or in pain, record this when documenting the episode of care, because these factors might influence the respiratory rate.
• Remember that an ↑ respiratory rate might be a manifestation of metabolic acidosis.

Pitfalls

- Not exposing the patient's chest and/or abdomen sufficiently to assess accurately the rate, depth, and pattern of respiration.
- Underestimating the importance of an accurate respiratory rate and taking it in a hurried, inaccurate manner.
- Failing to record the respiratory rate when doing vital signs.
- Not recording the respiratory rate for a full minute. Abnormalities in the pattern of breathing might be missed if measured over shorter time periods.

Manual measurement of blood pressure

Background

Blood pressure is the pressure of the blood against the walls of the arteries. The systolic pressure is the pressure in the arterial system when the ventricles are contracting and the diastolic pressure is the pressure when the ventricles are at rest. Adequate blood pressure is essential to maintain the blood supply and function of vital organs. High blood pressure ↑ the risk of stroke and ischaemic heart disease. It also causes damage to the kidneys and eyes. Blood pressure can be measured by non-invasive manual or automatic or invasive techniques (🕮 on p. 58 and 256).

Korotkoff sounds

The auscultatory (Korotkoff) sounds, heard as the blood pressure cuff is slowly deflated when measuring blood pressure manually, are divided into five phases:
- Phase 1—the first appearance of faint, repetitive, clear tapping sounds.
- Phase 2—the sounds soften and acquire a 'swishing' quality.
- Auscultatory gap—the sounds might disappear for a while.
- Phase 3—the return of sharper sounds.
- Phase 4—distinct muffling sounds, soft and blowing in quality.
- Phase 5—the point at which all sounds disappear completely.

Equipment
- Sphygmomanometer.
- Stethoscope.

Procedure
- Explain the procedure and gain consent.
- Decontaminate your hands.
- Allow the patient to settle or rest before taking the measurement.
- Remove any constrictive clothing from the patient's arm.
- Position the patient's arm at the level of the heart (midsternum), with the palm of the hand facing upwards.
- Apply a cuff that covers 80% of the length of the upper arm.
- Ensure that the identified mark is over the brachial artery.
- Position the column of the manometer vertical, at eye level within 1m of the patient.
- Palpate the radial pulse and inflate the cuff until it can no longer be felt—this measurement represents the estimated systolic pressure.
- Deflate the cuff and wait 15–30secs.
- Locate the brachial artery, just medial to the midline in the cubital fossa.
- Ensure the diaphragm of the stethoscope is warm and place it over the brachial artery.
- Inflate the cuff to 30mmHg higher than the systolic pressure, as estimated by palpation.
- Allow the cuff to deflate at a rate of 2–3mmHg/second—the systolic reading is the point in phase 1 at which two repetitive tapping sounds can be heard and the diastolic reading is the point at which sounds can no longer be heard (phase 5).

- Remove the cuff and replace the patient's clothing.
- Document the episode of care. Record the readings and report any abnormalities or changes in the trend. The arm in which the blood pressure has been recorded and position of the patient should also be noted (e.g. left arm and supine). If the patient was in pain, anxious, or distressed during the procedure, record this because these factors might affect the reading.

Practice tips
- Ensure that the patient is relaxed because this will give a more accurate reading.
- Limit the amount of external noise to facilitate use of the stethoscope and taking the reading.
- Position the cuff on the arm with the tubing at the upper end. This will stop it banging against the stethoscope and interfering with auscultation by causing artefactual sounds.
- In some patients, sounds persist greatly below the muffling to very low readings. This can be indicated by recording both phases 4 and 5 of the Korotkoff sounds when recording the blood pressure, e.g. 162/72/10 where 72 is the phase 4 reading and 10 the phase 5 reading.
- The blood pressure in patients on antihypertensive drugs might vary, depending on the time of the day at which the readings are taken. Note the time the drugs were taken in relation to the time of the measurement.
- Changes in drug treatment should not be made on the basis of one blood pressure reading.

Pitfalls
- Recording sequential blood pressures on different arms and in different positions will affect the reliability of the readings.
- Not removing restrictive clothing on the patient's arm or using inappropriate cuff sizes—e.g. a cuff that is too large in a thin person.
- Not positioning the patient's arm at the level of the heart—the reading will be higher below the heart and lower above it.
- Placing the diaphragm of the stethoscope under the cuff, causing excessive pressure and distortion of the sounds heard.
- Not calculating the systolic pressure by palpation first. This might lead to underestimation of the systolic blood pressure because of the 'auscultatory gap'.
- Digit preference—observers round up the blood pressure to record a favourite number, commonly 0 or 5mmHg. The systolic and diastolic pressures should be recorded to the nearest 2mmHg.

Electronic measurement of blood pressure

Blood pressure (📖 on p. 56 for definition and effects of hypertension)—can be measured by non-invasive manual or automatic techniques or invasive techniques (📖 on p. 256). Electronic automated sphygmomanometers have replaced manual devices in most clinical settings.

Equipment

- Electronic sphygmomanometer.

Procedure

- Explain the procedure and obtain consent.
- Decontaminate your hands.
- Allow the patient to settle or rest before taking the measurement.
- Remove any constrictive clothing from the patient's arm.
- Position the patient's arm at the level of the heart (midsternum), with the palm of the hand facing upwards.
- Apply a cuff that covers 80% of the length of the upper arm.
- Ensure that the identified mark is over the brachial artery.
- Press the start button.
- Record the reading.
- Remove the cuff and replace the patient's clothing.
- Document the episode of care. The arm in which the blood pressure has been recorded and position of the subject should also be noted (e.g. left arm and supine). If the patient was in pain, anxious, or distressed during the procedure, record this. Report any abnormalities or changes in the trend.

Practice tips

- Ensure that the patient is relaxed because this will give a more accurate reading.
- The blood pressure in patients on antihypertensive drugs might vary, depending on the time of the day at which the readings are taken. Note the time the drugs were taken in relation to the time of the measurement.
- Changes in drug treatment should not be made on the basis of one blood pressure reading.
- It can sometimes take a few attempts to record a reading in patients with a very high or low blood pressure and severely ill or traumatized patients. This can prove uncomfortable on the limb if the cuff is left on the same arm. The other limb should be used after 2 attempts.

Pitfalls

- Recording sequential blood pressures on different arms and in different positions.
- Using inappropriate cuff sizes, e.g. a cuff that is too large in a thin person, or not removing constrictive clothing.
- Not positioning the patient's arm at the level of the heart—the reading will be higher below the heart and lower above it.
- Allowing the patient to talk while recording the electronic blood pressure. This can interfere with the reading.

Systematic examination

Background

The physical examination usually follows the history in the assessment of a patient. The vital signs are an integral part of it. A comprehensive examination covers all the body systems. In many situations, the examination will be focused on one system or anatomical area. The definitive techniques for examination of the different systems are outlined in the relevant chapters. In addition, specific assessments for the skin (📖 on p. 62), nutritional status (📖 on p. 416), hydration (📖 on p. 68), and height and weight (📖 on p. 70) are described. The general principles of the physical examination are outlined below.

Equipment

- Stethoscope.
- Patella hammer.
- Tuning fork.
- Cotton wool/needle.
- Ophthalmoscope/auroscope.

Procedure

- Explain the procedure and gain consent.
- Wash your hands.
- Ensure that the patient is comfortable and their privacy/dignity is maintained.
- Make any adjustments necessary to the light and surrounding environment.
- Have a chaperone present for intimate examinations.
- Examine the patient from the right-hand side of the bed.
- Perform a systematic examination using the 'look, feel, move, listen, and special tests' technique, as appropriate for the system being examined:
  - Look for discolouration, scars, wounds, swellings, rashes, erythema, muscle wasting, and symmetry.
  - Feel for skin temperature, tenderness, crepitus, fluctuance, pulses, and thrills (palpable murmurs).
  - Move—assess the active and passive range of movements of joints.
  - Listen—auscultate for breath sounds, heart sounds, added sounds, murmurs, bowel sounds, and bruits.
  - Special tests—e.g. stress testing of ligaments and tendon reflexes.
- In general, commence the examination with the patient's hands and then move from 'head to toe'. The following is a suggested sequence of examination:
  - General survey/vital signs.
  - Hands.
  - Head and neck, including the thyroid, trachea, oropharynx, and lymph nodes, and relevant elements of the cardiovascular/respiratory and gastrointestinal systems.
  - Eyes and ears.
  - Thorax and lungs/heart/breasts.

- Abdomen/rectal and vaginal examinations.
- Lower and upper limbs—musculoskeletal, neurological, and peripheral vascular.
- Mental status and cranial nerves.
- Back.
- Document the episode of care.

Practice tips

- Wash your hands in the presence of the patient, because this is reassuring for them—patients are concerned about hospital-acquired infections.
- Although convention mandates examination from the right side of the bed, this is often not possible in community practice or at the roadside. It is therefore worth also practising examination from the left side.

Assessment of the skin

Background

Inspection and palpation of the skin for localized or diffuse pathology is an important part of the patient assessment. It should be performed in a well-lit area. Remember to include the mucosal surfaces of the mouth, the nails, hair and scalp. The colour and condition of the skin might give an indication of cardiorespiratory status, hydration, or systemic illness. Always assess the patient's general status and treat any urgent problems before performing an in-depth assessment of the skin.

Procedure

- Explain the procedure and gain consent.
- Consider the need for a chaperone.
- Decontaminate your hands.
- Ensure that the patient is comfortable and their privacy/dignity is maintained.

Inspect the skin

- Colour:
  - Jaundice—a yellow discolouration often seen best in the sclera of the eye or on the undersurface of the tongue.
  - Cyanosis—a blue discolouration of the skin or mucous membranes. Central cyanosis is best identified in the oral mucosa, tongue, and lips. Cyanosis of the nails, hands, and feet might be central or peripheral in origin.
  - Pallor—which might be owing to anaemia or ↓ blood flow after a faint. Localized pallor could be owing to arterial insufficiency.
  - Generalized or localized erythema—a flushed appearance might be the result of embarrassment, pyrexia or a disease such as systemic lupus erythematosus (SLE). Localized redness might be due to infection.
  - ↓ pigmentation— as in vitiligo.
  - ↑ pigmentation (browness)—might be caused by Addison's disease or pituitary tumours amongst other causes.
- Lesions/rashes—note the colour, anatomical location, pattern, and shape, in addition to the type.
- Swellings or ulcers.

Palpate the skin

- Temperature—use the backs of your fingers to feel temperature. Note generalized warmth or coolness and pay particular attention to areas of redness.
- Moisture—is the skin dry, oily, sweaty or clammy (moist, sticky and cold)?
- Texture—is the skin excessively roughened or smoothened?
- Tenderness of any lesions present.
- Capillary refill—press the thumb over the sternum or an extremity (usually over a nail bed) or 5secs and then release. Count how many seconds it takes for the blanched skin to return to its previous colour (normally <2secs).

- Mobility and turgor—lift a fold of skin and feel how mobile it is. The skin is tight in oedema or connective tissue diseases, e.g. scleroderma. The speed with which pinched skin returns to normal is its turgor. Skin turgor is ↓ in dehydration, in which it takes longer to return to normal.
- Character of rashes/lesions—are they elevated or depressed, or blanching or non-blanching? To ascertain whether a lesion or rash is blanching or non-blanching, run your thumb firmly over it. If it disappears transiently as a result of the pressure, it is blanching. See 📖 p.64 for methods of describing a lesion or rash.
- Document the findings and report abnormalities.

Practice tips

- Remember to inspect concealed areas e.g. undersurface of female breasts, axillae, inner thighs, external genitalia and natal cleft (between the buttocks).
- Take protective measures if there is a suspicion that the skin changes might be infective.
- Always consider changes in the patient's skin in association with the general condition of the patient. For example, an unwell patient who is pale with bluish extremities will require an urgent primary survey and possible interventions.
- Older patients have decreased skin turgor due to loss of inherent elasticity with ageing. Skin turgor in the elderly is best tested in the forehead as this is the last area to lose elasticity.
- What you perceive as being abnormal might be a peculiarity for that patient. If unsure about a lesion check with the patient or their relatives whether it has been present for years and is 'normal' for them.

Pitfalls

- Assessing skin colouration in inadequate or false light, particularly at night. Turn on the full lights on a ward at night to assess a sick patient.
- Inaccurate assessment of capillary refill time as a result of not pressing for long enough or pressing on an extremity that is cold.
- Not being aware of the normal skin pigmentation in different ethnic groups.
- Mistaking dyes from clothing as a pathological skin change (one of the authors was called in the middle of the night to assess 'severe cyanosis of the hands' that turned out to be due to the blue dye from the patient's new pyjamas).

Describing a lesion or rash

Background

- It is important to have a system for assessing and describing lesions (localised areas of abnormal tissue) and rashes. Describing rashes from the outset in terms that suggest a diagnosis e.g. 'a meningitis rash' or 'chickenpox rash' should be avoided. It might be misleading, cause unnecessary anxiety to the patient or relatives, and bias a subsequent assessment. It is better to use the rash descriptors outlined below until a definitive diagnosis is made.

Description

- Describe a lesion or rash using the following descriptors and terminology:
  - **Site**—generalized or localized? Does it involve specific areas, e.g. exposed areas, the extensor or flexor surfaces, the skin folds, or areas adjacent to potential allergens or irritants, e.g. bracelets or earrings?
  - **Pattern**—are the lesions linear, clustered, annular (in a ring shape), arciform (in the shape of an arc), or serpiginous (in a snake like pattern)? Are they dermatomal (in the distribution of a dermatome) as in shingles? Is there evidence of the koebner phenomenon which refers to skin lesions appearing in lines of trauma, seen in a number of conditions including lichen planus, molluscum contagiosum and psoriasis?
  - **Type**—are the lesions
    - Macular— a macule is any non-raised lesion <0.5cm in diameter.
    - Papular— a papule is any raised lesion <0.5cm in diameter.
    - Patchy—a patch is a flat lesion >0.5cm in diameter (i.e. a large macule).
    - Maculopapular—contains both macules and papules.
    - Nodular—a nodule is a raised area >0.5cm and <2cm in diameter.
    - A plaque is a raised area >2cm (i.e. a large papule).
    - Vesicular—a vesicle is a fluid-filled collection beneath the epidermis < 0.5cm.
    - Blistering—a blister is a fluid-filled collection beneath the epidermis > 0.5cm.
    - Pustular—a pustule is a visible collection of pus in the subcutis.
    - Petechial—petechiae are pinpoint, flat, rounded, red haemorrhagic spots <3mm in diameter. They do not blanch when pressed.
    - Purpuric—purpura is a haemaorrhagic area >3mm in diameter. Early purpura is red. It becomes darker, then purple and yellow brown as it fades. It does not blanch when pressed. 'Palpable purpura' is the result of vasculitis.
    - Bruising (ecchymosis or contusion)—a bruise results from trauma and bleeding into the tissues. It is a type of purpura. In its early stages it is usually a red or blue purple colour and doesn't blanch. Older bruises have a yellow/green appearance.
    - Telangiectasia are small dilated blood vessels near the surface of the skin. Because they are vascular lesions, they blanch. Spider naevi are a form of telangiectasia.

- Urticarial—urticaria (wheals) are elevated irregular patches, due to dermal oedema, e.g. nettle stings.
- Callus—hyperplastic epidermis, often found on the soles or palms.
- Mottled—patchy discolouration of the skin usually bluish purple.
- Target or iris lesions have concentric rings with a dark petechial spot in the centre, e.g. in erythema multiforme.
- Burrows—linear lesions produced by infestation of the skin and formation of tunnels, e.g. with infestation by the scabies mite.
- Melanocytic naevi (moles)—flat or protruding skin lesions varying in colour from pink flesh tones to dark brown or black. The majority are benign. Assessment tools are available to assist diagnosis of malignant melanoma e.g. the 'Glasgow 7-point checklist'.
- Erosions are partial epidermal loss and heal without scarring.
- Ulcers involve full thickness skin loss.
- Atrophy is thinning of the epidermis.
- Lichenification is thickening of the epidermis.

Measurement of the capillary blood glucose level

Background

Capillary blood glucose recordings are performed to monitor the glucose levels of diabetic patients. They are also used in the hospital setting as part of the assessment of severely ill, confused, or unconscious patients, to look for hypoglycaemia or hyperglycaemia.

Equipment

- Blood glucose meter.
- Testing strips.
- Lancet.
- Non-sterile gloves.

Procedure

- Explain the procedure and gain consent.
- Decontaminate your hands.
- Ensure that the blood glucose meter is calibrated and the strip codes correspond to it.
- Select an appropriate lancet and put the non-sterile gloves on.
- Select a digit (or the outer aspect of the heel in infants) and wash it.
- If possible avoid using the thumb or index finger.
- Pierce the skin and allow a drop of blood to form without squeezing the digit.
- Approximate the glucose strip to collect the required sample of blood.
- Apply pressure to the digit to stop any further bleeding.
- Discard the sharp in the sharps box.
- Insert the strip into the blood glucose meter, according to the manufacturer's instructions.
- Record the reading and report any abnormality.
- Discard the strip in clinical waste disposal.
- Document the episode of care.

Practice tips

- Hanging the patient's hand downwards will assist in the production of the blood required. Ensuring the hand is warm also helps.
- Using the side of the digit is considered to be less painful than the centre.
- If performing repeated tests on a patient, rotate through different digits.
- In a clinical environment, a knowledgeable patient might prepare and pierce the skin with their own equipment, but the test should be recorded using the blood glucose meter and strips used in that clinical area.
- Assess the patient's knowledge before explaining the procedure. There is a danger of patronizing patients with diabetes, who might know more about the test than you.

Pitfalls

- Not washing the digit before obtaining the sample. Sweet substances on the digit might alter the reading, with serious consequences e.g. false high reading in hypoglycemia.
- Squeezing the digit to produce a drop of blood can damage the blood cells and alter the result.
- Failing to recalibrate the blood glucose meter, as recommended, when using a new pack of testing strips.
- Failing to perform the procedure in all patients presenting with new altered conscious levels.

Assessment of hydration

Background

Hydration should be assessed as part of the overall systematic assessment of a patient. The purpose is to identify patients who are dehydrated or overloaded with fluid. Fluid loss and dehydration can occur in vomiting, diarrhoea, sweating, polyuria, blood loss, burns, and the use of diuretic medications. Fluid overload can result from problems with the heart, kidneys, or lungs. It might also be iatrogenic owing to overzealous administration of intravenous fluid.

Equipment

- Fluid-balance chart.
- Weighing scales.

Procedure

- Explain the procedure and gain consent.

Take a history

- Take a detailed history, questioning about fluid intake and loss and looking for symptoms of dehydration or overload, many of which are nonspecific.
  - *Symptoms of dehydration* —thirst; dry mouth; ↓ urinary output (no urinary output in moderate-to-severe dehydyration); dark, concentrated urine; headache; lethargy; dizziness; fainting; lack of tears when crying; rapid weight loss; and dry skin. In severe cases, sunken eyes, progressing to seizures and progressive loss of consciousness.
  - *Symptoms of overload*—fatigue; shortness of breath; oedema; rapid weight gain; swelling or pain in the abdomen; breathlessness lying flat (orthopnoea); palpitations; persistent wheeze or cough, sometimes with pink frothy sputum.

Examine the patient

- Look for clues in the vital signs.
  - Tachycardia and tachypnoea might be the result of dehydration or fluid overload.
  - Hypotension and/or pyrexia might be present in severe dehydration.
- Look for signs of dehydration:
  - Dry mouth and lips.
  - Dry skin, which might be loose and wrinkled in severe cases.
  - ↓ skin turgor.
  - Sunken eyes and soft eyeballs—owing to the loss of intra-ocular pressure.
- Look for signs of overload:
  - Oedema—best seen in lower limbs and around the sacrum.
  - ↑ jugular venous pulse.
  - Hepatomegaly—enlarged liver.
  - Tachycardia and gallop rhythm on auscultation of the heart.

Fluid-balance chart
- Maintain an accurate fluid-balance chart.
- Study the fluid-balance chart and calculate fluid deficits or overload.

Weigh
- Weigh the patient daily (📖 on p. 70).

Urinary catheterization
- Consider urinary catheterization if moderate-to-severe dehydration or overload.

Haematological indices
- Consider bloods for measurement of full blood count/haematocrit, urea and electrolytes, and plasma osmolality.

Practice tips
- Individual symptoms and signs of dehydration can be unreliable or non-specific—consider them in a holistic review of all the parameters outlined above.
- The change in elasticity of the skin with age and difficulty in manually assessing intra-ocular pressure make these unsatisfactory physical signs.
- To check for oedema, press firmly but gently with your thumb for at least 5secs over the dorsum of each foot, behind each medial malleolus, and over the shins. Look for 'pitting', a depression caused by the thumb. Normally, there is none.
- A postural ↓ in blood pressure is a useful physical sign, indicating intravascular volume depletion.
- If the patient's usual weight is known, weighing the patient is the most satisfactory physical assessment of hydration. It can also be used to monitor the response to treatment.
- Haematological indices are generally more helpful than physical signs in the assessment of hydration.

Pitfalls
- Assuming a dry tongue is owing to dehydration in the absence of other signs—it might be caused by mouth breathing alone.
- Underestimating fluid loss if there is profuse diarrhoea or severe vomiting.
- Not filling in fluid-balance charts accurately or at all.
- Failing to consider insensible fluid loss in the calculation of fluid balance. Insensible loss occurs from the skin and respiratory tract and is ~800mL/day in an unstressed adult.

Measurement of height and weight

Background

Height and weight are measured in the assessment of the nutritional and fluid status. These values can be used to determine the body mass index and serve as a guide for prescribing drug doses. There are a wide variety of scales and measures available. The method chosen will depend on the patient's size, mobility, understanding, and general condition.

Measuring weight

Equipment

- Standing, chair, or bed weighing scales.

Procedure

- Explain the procedure and gain consent.
- Identify which scales are appropriate to use.
- Ensure that the scales are calibrated and read 'zero'.
- Plan so that the location of the procedure maintains the patient's safety and dignity.
- Decontaminate your hands.
- Decontaminate the scales.
- Ensure the patient's shoes and heavy articles of clothing are removed.
- Ask the patient to stand on the weighing scales or transfer them to the scales, if necessary.
- When the reading has stabilized, record the weight measurement.
- Ask the patient to get off the weighing scales or transfer them, as appropriate.
- Decontaminate the scales.
- Decontaminate your hands.
- Document the episode of care.

Practice tips

- Assess the patient carefully before the procedure, to ensure that they are fit to undergo the chosen method.
- Ensure that there is an adequate number of staff available if help is likely to be required to transfer the patient from a chair or bed to the scales.
- Carry out a pain assessment and, if necessary, give analgesia before moving a dependent patient.
- Patients are often embarrassed about their weight so sensitivity is required.
- If a patient refuses to be weighed, provide counselling and health promotion. Document the refusal and patient education in the notes.

Pitfalls

- Not ensuring that the scales are calibrated and zeroed before use.
- Attempting to stand an unwell patient on scales. Use a chair or bed weighing scales.
- Accepting the patient's estimate of their weight and not formally weighing them if an accurate reading is required.

Measuring height

Equipment

- Standing-height scale, measuring tape, or stick.

Procedure

- Explain the procedure and gain consent.
- Decontaminate your hands.
- Ask the patient to remove their shoes, heavy clothing, and hats and undo any hairstyle that might interfere with the measurement.
- Ask the patient to stand against the wall on a flat surface, looking straight ahead. Their weight should be evenly distributed, with their legs straight, heels together, and arms at their sides. Their buttocks and shoulders should be touching the wall.
- Measure their height from the floor to the top of their head.
- For a bed-bound patient, measure from the heel to the top of their head.
- Record your measurement.
- Decontaminate your hands.
- Document the episode of care.

Practice tips

- An easier measurement for the bed- or chair-bound patient is the 'knee height'. This measurement, from the bottom of the foot to the patella, is obtained with a knee-height calliper (a device that resembles a T-square). The patient must be able to flex the knee to 90°. The knee height is then entered into a mathematical formula to estimate the patient's height.
- The height of bed-bound patients can also be assessed by measuring the body in sections (from head to knee, knee to hip, hip to shoulder, and shoulder to the top of the head) and totalling these measurements to determine the height.
- The arm-span measurement (from the sternal notch to the fingertips) correlates closely to half of the patient's height.

Pitfalls

- Not asking the patient to remove footwear.
- Accepting the patient's estimate of their height and not formally measuring them, if accuracy is required.

Monitoring

Background

Electronic monitoring is used most commonly in Emergency Departments and Critical Care Areas. The cardiac monitor is a device that displays the electrical and pressure waveforms of the cardiovascular system for measurement and treatment. Electrical connections are made between the monitor and the patient. Parameters of respiratory function, e.g. oxygen saturation and the respiratory rate can also be monitored. There are numerous different brands of electronic monitor. It is important to have had training on the one in use in the area where you are working. The machines must be calibrated regularly.

Equipment

- Monitor.
- Monitor leads.
- Electrodes.
- Blood pressure cuff.
- Oxygen saturation probe.

Procedure

Establishing monitoring

- Explain the procedure and gain consent.
- Decontaminate your hands.
- Set up the monitoring equipment, ensuring the patient's safety and dignity are maintained.
- Clean and dry the sites at which the electrodes will be applied (Fig. 3.2).
- If the application site is hairy, clip or shave the hair.
- Check the expiry date of the electrodes.
- Attach the leads to the electrodes.
- Remove the backings from the electrodes before applying them to the patient.
- Place each electrode in its recommended site, applying firm pressure.
- Attach the blood pressure cuff—📖 on p. 58.
- Place the oxygen saturation probe on a digit—📖 on p. 302.
- Set the alarm limits, as appropriate for the patient.
- Record baseline observations.

Ongoing monitoring

- Check regularly that the electrodes and other attachments remain in place.
- Ensure that the patient's skin is protected from pressure injury from repeated blood pressure measurements.
- Record readings at a frequency appropriate to the severity and stability of the patient's condition.
- Record the time and nature of any interventions or treatments that might impact on readings.

Practice tips

- Keep the patient warm and relaxed—this will help to minimize muscle and movement artefact.

- Ensure the electrodes are firmly attached—this ↓ artefact and prevents the conductive gel from drying out.
- Place the electrodes over bone rather than muscle to minimize interference from muscle artefact in the electrocardiogram (ECG) signal.
- If the patient is sweaty or clammy, it might be necessary to dry the area and change the electrodes.
- Don't apply electrodes over injured areas, scar tissue, burns, rashes, or other lesions—different positions might be used, as necessary.
- Most leads are colour coded to aid correct connection. The usual scheme (except in the United States) is red for right arm lead, yellow for the left arm and green for the leg lead (usually placed on the abdomen or lower left chest wall).
- Medical equipment might provoke anxiety in the patient and relatives—explain its purpose and reassure them.
- Ensure that the monitor is plugged into the mains if possible—this will ensure that the battery is fully charged if transfer is required.
- If the monitor is dropped or damaged, always have it serviced, even if it seems to be functioning correctly.

Pitfalls
- Using electrodes that are out of date or for which the conductive gel has liquefied or dried out.
- Applying electrodes in fatty areas or over major muscles, large breasts, or bony prominences.
- Treating the monitor rather than the patient. It has been known for the cardiac arrest team to be called to a patient with 'ventricular fibrillation' on the monitor when in fact it was an artefact caused by the patient cleaning their teeth.

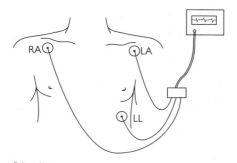

RA right arm
LA left arm
LL left leg (positioned left lower chest)

Fig. 3.2 Positions of the chest leads.

Infection control

Jacqueline Randle
Associate Professor, Clinical Skills Lead for Masters of Nursing
Science, School of Nursing, Midwifery & Physiotherapy,
University of Nottingham, UK

Natalie Vaughan
Senior Nurse, Infection Prevention and Control, Nottingham
University Hospitals NHS Trust, Nottingham, UK

Mitch Clarke
Infection Prevention and Control Nurse Specialist, Nottingham
University Hospitals NHS Trust, UK

Standard precautions

Background

Standard precautions (formerly known as 'universal precautions') must be adopted at all times, to promote the safe practice of prevention and control of infection. The aim is to minimize the risk of infection to health care workers (HCWs), patients, and visitors. Standard precautions are as follows:

- Effective hand hygiene.
- Correct use of personal protective equipment.
- Safe handling and disposal of sharps.
- Safe handling and disposal of clinical waste.
- Appropriate management of blood and other body fluids.
- Effective decontamination of equipment.
- Achieving and maintaining a clean clinical environment.
- Appropriate use of medical devices.
- Managing accidents and adverse incidents.

Practice tips

- Prevention and control of infection is everyone's responsibility and this includes all HCWs, patients, and visitors.
- Good prevention and control of infection must be an integral part of all clinical practice.
- A high standard of practice must be implemented routinely at all times.
- A risk assessment should be conducted as part of the implementation of standard precautions for prevention and control of infection.
- HCWs must be familiar with and consistently apply local policies, procedures, and guidelines for prevention and control of infection.
- Any breach of practice must be reported according to the local reporting system.
- Effective communication with other HCWs, patients, visitors, and the Infection Prevention and Control Team.
- Ongoing training and education is required.

Risk assessment

Background

Risk assessment is a structured approach to ↓ or eliminate the transmission of infection.

Assessment

Ask:

- What is the source of infection?
- How is the infection transmitted?
- Are additional risk factors involved?
- What are the individual patient risk factors?
- Who are the individuals at risk: health care workers (HCWs), patients, or visitors?
- What facilities are available or unavailable?
- Is the staffing mix appropriate?
- What are the contamination risks?

Planning

Account for the following issues:

- The primary aim is to ↓ or eliminate the risk of transmission of a pathogen, in addition to taking measures to avoid compromising patient care.
- Implementation of the standard precautions for prevention and control of infection.
- Local policies, procedures, and guidelines for prevention and control of infection must be followed.
- Advice, support, and guidance should be obtained from the Infection Prevention and Control Team.

Implementation

When implementing care consider the following issues:

- Ensure care is up to date and both evidence-based and research-based.
- Implement the standard precautions for prevention and control of infection in a timely, consistent, and appropriate manner.
- Documentation must be undertaken according to local policy.
- Care must be reassessed at regular intervals and the necessary changes made to practice and the documentation.

Evaluation

Ask:

- Is the patient still symptomatic?
- Is the pathogen that caused the infection still present?
- Has the pathogen spread to others or other clinical areas?
- Do the standard precautions for prevention and control of infection still need to be in place?
- Should further advice, support, and guidance be obtained from the Infection Prevention and Control Team?

Hand hygiene

Background

Hand hygiene is the single most important factor in ↓ the spread of health-care-associated infection. Hand hygiene refers to the practices of both hand washing and hand disinfection using products such as alcohol hand rubs. Both methods decrease the colonization of transient bacteria on the hands.

Procedure (Fig. 4.1)

- Remove all wrist jewellery (including wrist watches).
- Remove stoned rings.
- Turn on taps to a comfortable temperature and wet hands and wrists.
- Apply enough cleaning product to cover surface of the hands.
- Vigorously rub hands together (palm to palm).
- Vigorously rub the back of each hand.
- Interlace and interlock fingers to cover all surfaces.
- Rotationally rub each thumb and wrist.
- Ensure that all the cleaning product is effectively rinsed off.
- Turn off taps with disposable paper towel.
- Dry all parts of the hands and wrists thoroughly using disposable paper towel, paying particular attention to the inter-digital surfaces of the fingers and thumbs.
- Dispose of the paper towel in a bin without re-contaminating your hands.

If decontaminating your hands using alcohol hand rubs, follow the above procedure using the alcohol hand rub in place of the soap, water, and paper towel. Allow to dry naturally for 30sec.

Practice tips

- Hands must be decontaminated immediately before and after every episode of direct patient contact or care and after any activity or contact that potentially results in your hands becoming contaminated.
- Hands that are visibly soiled or contaminated by dirt or organic material must be washed using liquid soap and water.
- An alcohol hand rub can be used between caring for patients or different care activities, if your hands are not soiled.
- When caring for a patient who has *Clostridium Difficile* use soap and water between caring for patients and between different care activities.
- Cover any cuts and abrasions with waterproof dressings.
- Avoid hot water as this can increase the risk of dermatitis.
- Use running water whenever possible.
- Nails must be kept short. Artificial nails and nail polish must not be worn.
- Emollient hand creams can be used to protect hands from drying. If hand problems develop, advice should be sought from the Occupational Health Department.

Pitfalls

- Gloves are often seen as a replacement for good hand hygiene. However, hands must be decontaminated before and after the removal of gloves.
- Alcohol hand rub is often seen as a replacement for soap and water, however it is ineffective in reducing *Clostridium Difficile* spores.

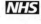

Hand-washing technique with soap and water

Wet hands with water

Apply enough soap to cover all hand surfaces

Rub hands palm to palm

Rub back of each hand with palm of other hand with fingers interlaced

Rub palm to palm with fingers interlaced

Rub with back of fingers to opposing palms with fingers interlocked

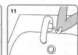

Rub each thumb clasped in opposite hand using a rotational movement

Rub tips of fingers in opposite palm in a circular motion

Rub each wrist with opposite hand

Rinse hands with water

Use elbow to turn off tap

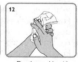

Dry thoroughly with a single-use towel

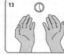

Hand washing should take 15–30 seconds

clean**your**hands®
campaign

NHS
National Patient
Safety Agency

© Crown copyright 2007 283373 1p 1k Sep07

Adapted from World Health Organization *Guidelines on Hand Hygiene in Health Care*

Fig. 4.1 Hand decontamination. Technique based on procedure described by G.A.J Aycliffe *et al.* in *Journal of Clinical pathology* 1978; 31; 928. Reproduced with permission from the British Medical Journal Publishing Group.

Aseptic non-touch technique (ANTT)

Background

The aim of the ANTT is to prevent micro-organisms on hands, surfaces, or equipment from being introduced to body sites, such as surgical wounds or equipment (e.g. catheters or central venous lines). It is not necessary to use sterile gloves and a sterile dressing pack for all procedures requiring ANTT, for example when changing an intravenous infusion bag, but the aim of ANTT should still be adhered to. The following procedure relates to a wound dressing.

Equipment

- Dressing trolley.
- Alcohol hand rub.
- Sterile dressing pack.
- 2% chlorhexidine gluconate in 70% isopropyl alcohol application.
- Sachets of 0.9% saline solution.
- Dry dressing.
- Sterile gloves.
- Apron.
- Additional dressings and equipment, as required for a specific procedure.

Procedure

Ideally this should be performed by two healthcare workers (HCWs).
HCW1/HCW2

- Refer to the care plan or assessment so that the type of dressing and equipment can be prepared and added to the trolley.
- Explain the procedure and gain consent.
- Wash and dry their hands.
- Ensure the dressing trolley is clean—if visibly dirty, clean using detergent and water.
- Assemble equipment and put it on the bottom shelf of the trolley.
- Put on a clean, disposable apron.
- Decontaminate your hands.
- Check the expiry date and that packaging is intact on sterile equipment.
- HCW1 open a sterile dressing pack on the top shelf of the dressing trolley, touching only the corners of the paper.
- HCW1 take the clinical waste bag, without touching other equipment, and pass it to HCW2 to adhere it to the side of the trolley.
- HCW1 decontaminate your hands.
- HCW2 place any other sterile equipment onto the sterile field.
- HCW1 wipe a sachet of 0.9% saline solution along the opening strip using 2% chlorhexidine gluconate in 70% isopropyl alcohol application and allow to dry.
- HCW1 put on sterile gloves, ensuring they are put on by only touching the wrist end.
- HCW2 remove the patient's dressing.
- HCW1/HCW2 visually assess the wound.

- HCW1 commence the ANTT using the following principles:
  - Only sterile items should come into contact with susceptible sites.
  - Sterile items should not come into contact with non-sterile items.
- HCW1 clean the wound, if appropriate.
- HCW1 cover the wound with sterile dressing.

HCW1/HCW2

- Dispose of clinical waste and any sharps correctly.
- Decontaminate their hands.
- Ensure the patient is comfortable.
- Clean the trolley using detergent and water.
- Document the care episode.

Practice tips

- Effective hand decontamination is the most significant procedure in preventing cross-infection and should be used following contamination.
- Although it is possible to perform this technique independently, consideration should be given to having an assistant, wherever possible, to place the equipment onto the sterile field and remove dressings. This enables the procedure to be completed more quickly and provide more support for the patient.
- Forceps can be used during an ANTT in preference to sterile gloves, but they could damage tissue. If appropriate, irrigation may be preferred when cleaning the wound. Whichever method is used, a light, delicate touch should be used. The assessment that determines which method to use is dependent on the experience of the HCW and procedure to be undertaken.
- Administer-prescribed analgesia before the procedure, if required.

Pitfall

- Taking 'short-cuts' can result in contamination.

Care of the isolated patient— source isolation

Background

- Source isolation aims to prevent infected patients from infecting others.

Procedure: underlying principles

- Decontaminate your hands before and after any contact with the patient.
- Wear the correct personal protective equipment. The choice of personal protective clothing should be determined by a risk assessment of the anticipated contact with the patient.
- Explain the need for isolation and gain consent.
- Isolate the organism, not the patient, and consider the psychological needs of the patient.
- Maintain confidentiality of a patient's diagnosis while ensuring that health care workers (HCWs) and visitors are aware of the appropriate precautions for prevention and control of infection.
- Review the need for isolation regularly.
- The most appropriate type of isolation room should be selected— ideally a room with en-suite facility or a designated isolation ward.
- If isolation is not possible, patients can be cohorted in a bay, with appropriate precautions for prevention and control of infection.
- Furniture and equipment should be kept to a minimum in an isolation room.
- Equipment should, where possible, be single-use only, designated for single-patient use, or easily decontaminated.
- A dedicated team of HCWs should be allocated to caring for the patient/s.
- A trolley or dispenser for protective clothing must be allocated to an isolation room, to provide equipment relevant to the type of special precautions for prevention and control of infection.
- The patient's documents and charts should be kept outside the room.
- Visitors should be encouraged to decontaminate their hands. They do not, generally, need to wear protective clothing, unless they are involved in the practice of care.
- Avoid visits or transfers to other departments, where possible. The department should be notified in advance and the patient should follow other patients.
- Regularly and thoroughly clean, complying with local guidance for cleaning and decontamination. Detergent and hot water are usually recommended.
- Damp-dusting, normally using detergent and hot water, should be undertaken daily using a disposable cloth.
- The floor must be mopped daily.
- Soiled linen and clinical waste must be treated as infectious and bagged correctly and stored in a secure collection area.
- Spillages must be dealt with promptly, according to local policy.

- On discharge or death of the patient, ensure terminal cleaning of the room.
- Change curtains if they are soiled or the room has been occupied by a patient with an airborne infection.
- The room can be occupied by another patient after thorough cleaning has taken place.

Practice tips

- Adhere to local guidance that designates specific responsibilities for enhanced and terminal cleaning of the room and equipment.
- HCWs should use the correct colour-coded cleaning equipment.

Pitfalls

- HCWs not fully understanding the procedures and policies relating to isolation.
- Not considering the psychological needs of the patient with the result that they feel isolated and vulnerable.

Source isolation for airborne spread

Procedure

- Use single/negative pressure room, with the door kept closed.
- Decontaminate your hands using soap and water followed by an alcohol hand rub.
- Use gloves and an apron for contact with respiratory secretions
- Wear High Efficiency Particulate Air (HEPA) masks for close facial contact.
- Use a soluble bag for all linen.
- Refer to the Infection Prevention and Control Team for advice and to alert them of a case.
- Inform the appropriate hotel services staff.
- Ensure equipment is damp dusted daily with detergent and hot water but ensure floors are not buffed.
- Use single-use equipment or decontaminate equipment after use with 1% sodium hypochlorite.
- Change curtains on discharge.
- Only stop precautions following consultation with the Infection Prevention and Control Team.
- Inform relatives and visitors for the need for isolation.
- Encourage relatives and visitors to wash/clean their hands.

Source isolation for contact and/or air-borne route of spread

Procedure
- Use single room, with the door kept closed.
- Decontaminate your hands using soap and water followed by an alcohol hand rub.
- Use gloves and an apron during all patient contact.
- Use a soluble bag for all linen.
- Refer to the Infection Prevention and Control Team for advice and to alert them of a case.
- Inform the appropriate hotel services staff.
- Ensure equipment is damp-dusted daily with detergent and hot water but ensure floors are not buffed.
- Use single-use equipment or decontaminate equipment after use with 1% sodium hypochlorite.
- Change curtains on discharge.
- Only stop precautions following consultation with the Infection Prevention and Control Team.
- Inform relatives and visitors for the need for isolation.
- Encourage relatives and visitors to wash/clean their hands.

Practice tip
- Health care workers with hand lesions should avoid contact with the patient.

Source isolation for faecal–oral spread

Procedure

- Use a single room if possible.
- The patient must have their own toilet facilities—e.g. en-suite or designated toilet or commode.
- Decontaminate your hands using soap and water followed by an alcohol hand rub.
- Use gloves and an apron during contact with faeces.
- Use a soluble bag for soiled linen.
- Refer to the Infection Prevention and Control Team for advice and to alert them of a case.
- Inform the appropriate hotel services staff.
- Ensure equipment is damp-dusted daily with detergent and hot water but ensure floors are not buffed.
- Use single-use equipment or decontaminate equipment after use with 1% sodium hypochlorite.
- The patient must be free of diarrhoea for 48 hours before discontinuation of precautions and 72 hours if being transferred to another healthcare facility or a nursing home.
- Only stop precautions following consultation with the Infection Prevention and Control Team.
- Inform relatives and visitors for the need for isolation.
- Encourage relatives and visitors to wash their hands.

Practice tip

- Alcohol hand rub alone is not effective against all enteric organisms: hand washing with soap and water followed by the use of alcohol hand rub should be used.

Care of the isolated patient— protective isolation

Background
- Protective isolation aims to protect a susceptible patient from acquiring an infection, either directly or indirectly, from an infectious source.

Procedure: underlying principles
- The most appropriate type of isolation room should be selected—e.g. accommodation that has an en-suite facility. In some cases, the patient may be accommodated in a positive-pressure room.
- Before the patient is admitted, the room should be thoroughly cleaned using detergent and hot water, and curtains changed.
- Damp-dusting, using detergent and hot water, should be undertaken according to local policy.
- No-one with a cough, cold, or any other transmissible infection should enter the room.
- Hand hygiene is of the utmost importance for all those entering the room.
- Health care workers should wear the appropriate personal protective equipment.

Sharps management

Background

Sharps include any item that has the potential to cause a penetration injury, as follows:

- Needles.
- Lancets.
- Scalpel blades.
- Syringes.
- Glass vials.
- Broken glass.
- Slides.
- Biopsy needles.
- Disposable razors.
- Intravascular guide wires.
- Intravenous giving sets.
- Cannulae.
- Arterial blood sample packs.
- Other disposable sharps.

Procedure: underlying principles

- Avoid the use of sharps wherever possible.
- It is the responsibility of the sharps user to ensure that sharps are correctly used and disposed of.
- Dispose of sharps immediately after use.
- Dispose of the entire needle and syringe—the needle should not be bent, broken, or disconnected.
- Ensure that the sharps containers are available in close proximity to where the sharp is to be used.
- Sharps containers must conform to approved standards and be correctly assembled.
- Sharps containers should be emptied when three-quarters full or once weekly, labelled with the ward, department, or location, and securely closed for removal.
- Containers must be removed by designated staff wearing appropriate personal protective equipment.
- Do not re-sheath used needles under any circumstances.
- Do not re-sheath clean needles, unless there is safe means— e.g. a capping device.

Practice tips

- If performing an invasive procedure, gloves should be worn for some protection.

Pitfalls

- Resheathing needles
- Attempting to put sharps into nearly full containers.
- Sharps being trapped in the entrance to containers with flaps and injuring subsequent users.

Action to be taken following a sharps injury

Procedure

- Encourage the wound to bleed, but do not suck.
- Wash the wound under running water and apply a dry waterproof dressing.
- Obtain advice from the Occupational Health or Emergency Departments, depending on local policy. Further advice can be obtained from the Infection Prevention and Control Team.
- Report to line manager and complete an adverse incident form.
- If the injury is from a used sharp, medical advice should be sought to assess the potential risk of transmission of blood-borne viruses.
- Retain the sharp item, if known, and identify the source patient, if possible.
- Blood samples can be collected from the patient and healthcare worker if they consent.

Waste management

Background

'Waste' refers to substances or objects that are no longer part of a cycle or chain. The disposal of waste is regulated by statutory regulations, and health care workers (HCWs) have legal and moral duties to dispose of waste properly.

Procedure: underlying principles

- Household waste (e.g. packaging, paper towels, flowers, and other waste uncontaminated by potentially infectious substances) is disposed of in black plastic bags.
- Clinical waste (e.g. body fluids and human tissue) is disposed of in an orange plastic bag.
- Infectious or grossly contaminated waste is disposed of in a red plastic bag, with hazard warning tape.
- All bags should only be filled to two-thirds full, to protect colleagues from over-spillages.

Practice tips

- In the community, the responsibility for waste disposal is the householder's, but clinical waste can be collected, on request, by the local authority.
- If the householder is treated by a HCW, the clinical waste produced as a result of the treatment is the responsibility of the HCW.
- Sharps bins are provided to patients who are required to use sharps as part of their treatment. These must be returned for disposal to the patient's doctor, who will need to be registered with the local environment agency.
- Alternatively, householders can request that their local authority collect and dispose of clinical waste and/or sharps. The local authority might charge householders for this service.
- Advise patients and householders using sharps in the community not to dispose of sharps in soft drink cans, plastic bottles, or similar containers, because this can present serious hazards to staff disposing of domestic waste.

Pitfall

- Disposing of clinical waste and sharps in domestic waste.

Management of peripheral intravenous cannulae

Background

Peripheral intravenous cannulae (PICs) are used to administer fluids, blood products, and nutritional support. 📖 p.162–170 for insertion, changing and removal of PICs

Procedure: underlying principles

- Decontaminate your hands before and after touching PICs and any PIC insertion site.
- Use a strict aseptic technique when handling PICs.
- Use a phlebitis grading chart to observe for signs of tenderness, erythema, swelling, or palpable cord at the insertion site during every shift and document your observations.
- Routinely replace PICs every 72–96 hours.
- If inserted in an emergency, replace PICs within 24 hours.
- Document the insertion date and time in the prescription chart and medical and nursing notes.
- Cover the insertion site with a transparent sterile dressing.
- Replace the dressing using an aseptic non-touch technique ANTT 78 when the PIC is removed or replaced, or when the dressing becomes damp, loosened, or soiled, and at least every 72–96 hours.

Practice tips

- Avoid shaving at the insertion site because this causes micro-abrasions. This ↑ risk of bacterial colonization, which ↑ the risk of infection.
- If a patient has extermely poor venous access and there is a need for continuing IV theraphy, the cannula can be left in situ for more than 72 hours (this should be disscussed with the treating medical team).

Management of fluid administration sets

Procedure: underlying principles (📖 preparation for IV therapy, p. 172)

- Decontaminate your hands before and after using administration sets.
- Check the expiry date and packaging of the administration set. Dispose of the administration set if the date has expired or the packaging is not intact.
- Use an ANTT (📖 on p. 80) when handling the catheter hub, connections ports, and sterile parts of the administration set.
- Avoid contact with non-sterile surfaces.
- Label peripheral lines with the date and time.
- Change the administration set every 72–96 hours and document the change.
- Change the administration set after the administration of blood products.
- Clean access points using an isopropyl-impregnated swab or povidone–iodine solution before accessing the system.
- Administer intravenous drugs through the latex membrane on peripheral lines and avoid the use of ports.

Practice tips

- If administration sets are accessed frequently, they will need changing every 24–48 hours.
- Keep the number of access points to a minimum. If they are not in use, remove them.

Specimen collection

Background

The correct collection of specimens for investigations is essential to accurate diagnosis.

Procedure: underpinning principles

- Explain the procedure and gain consent.
- Inform the patient when the results will be available.
- Decontaminate your hands before and after the procedure.
- Personal protective clothing might be required following a risk assessment.
- Specimens should be collected at the appropriate time, using the correct technique and equipment.
- Transport the specimens to the laboratory without delay or store them in a fridge or incubator.
- To ↑ the chance of isolating an organism, gain a sufficient specimen, wherever possible, before antibiotic therapy.
- Different specimens require different media and methods of sampling. If unsure, contact the receiving laboratory for advice before proceeding.
- Before taking a specimen, ensure any corresponding specimen documentation, request form, and container label is fully completed, including the patient's details, date, specimen taken, and what investigations are required.
- Do not contaminate specimens during transfer to the container.

Midstream urine

Background

A urine culture is a test to find and identify micro-organisms (usually bacteria) that may be causing a urinary tract infection (UTI). A urine specimen is kept under conditions that allow bacteria and other organisms to grow. If few organisms grow, the test is negative. If organisms grow in numbers large enough to indicate an infection (100,000 or more bacteria per millilitre), the culture is positive. The type of organism causing the infection is identified with a microscope or by chemical tests. A midstream urine (MSU) sample is used to confirm the diagnosis of an urine infection and/or to decide the most appropriate antibiotic to be used. Urine is sterile so the presence of bacteria is indicative of an infection. The midstream is used as the first stream of urine may be contaminated with bacteria from the skin.

Procedure

- Explain the procedure and gain consent.
- Decontaminate your hands.
- If possible obtain sample immediately after the patient has showered or bathed, asking the patient to clean:
  - The vulva,(if female) from front to back.
  - Glans penis and behind the prepuce (if male).
  - Ask patient to decontaminate their hands.
  - If the patient is unable to perform this activity ensure the vulva or the glans penis and behind the prepuce is cleaned.
- Ask the patient to void an initial stream into the toilet or bedpan.
  The MSU sample should then be collected in a sterile receiver, allowing the final stream into the toilet or bedpan.
- Place the specimen directly into a sterile container.
- Decontaminate your hands.
- Label the sample and send to the laboratory immediately or store in refrigerator until ready to send.
- Document the episode of care.

Practice tips

- 5–10mL of urine is sufficient for microbiological examination.
- If the patient is unable to control the flow, collect the whole specimen and advise the laboratory that the specimen is a 'clean catch'.
- Always use soap and water and not disinfectants for cleaning the vulva or glans penis.
- In the female, cleaning of the vulva is very important.

Pitfall

- Failing to document if the patient is on antibiotics when the sample was taken.

Catheter specimen of urine collection

Background

A urine culture is a test to find and identify micro-organisms (usually bacteria) that may be causing a urinary tract infection (UTI). A urine specimen is kept under conditions that allow bacteria and other organisms to grow. If few organisms grow, the test is negative. If organisms grow in numbers large enough to indicate an infection, the culture is positive. The type of organism causing the infection is identified with a microscope or by chemical tests. A catheter specimen of urine (CSU) is used to confirm the diagnosis of an urine infection and/or to decide the most appropriate antibiotic to be used. Urine is sterile so the presence of bacteria is indicative of an infection. Using a catheter to collect a urine specimen reduces the chance of getting bacteria from the skin or genital area in the urine specimen, but catheter use sometimes causes a UTI.

Procedure

- Explain procedure and gain consent.
- Clamp the urinary drainage tube, if necessary, just below the sampling point and wait 15min.
- Wipe the sample point with an 2% chlorhexidine gluconate in 70% isopropyl alcohol application.
- Aspirate the required amount of urine.
- Release the clamp, if used.
- Transfer the urine to a sterile container and label as 'CSU'.
- Document the episode of care.

Practice tips

- Patients who have a urinary catheter in place for a long time are at a high risk of UTI.

24-hour urine specimen collection

Background
This collection measures the amount of urine produced in a day.

Equipment
- 24-hour urine collection container.
- Disposable bedpans or urinals.

Procedure
- Explain the procedure and gain consent.
- At the allocated time to start collection, ask the patient to empty their bladder into a toilet—this specimen must be discarded.
- Collect all subsequent voided urine into the 24-hour specimen container.
- At the start label the container with the date, time and patient's details.
- Discontinue collection after 24 hours and label the container.

Faecal specimen collection

Background

Many intestinal disorders are due to intestinal parasites, bacteria, viruses and toxins which require laboratory investigation.

Procedure

- Explain the procedure and gain consent.
- Ask the patient to defecate in a bedpan.
- Decontaminate your hands.
- Wear gloves and an apron.
- Observe the stool for colour, consistency, and volume.
- Using a spatula, spoon a portion of faeces into a container. In the case of liquid faeces, a syringe might be required to obtain a specimen.
- Decontaminate your hands.
- Label the sample and send it to the laboratory with an appropriate request form.
- Offer patient hand cleaning facilities.
- Document the episode of care.

Wound specimen collection

Background

- Wound swabs should only be taken if:
  - there is clinical evidence of infection;
  - there is unexplained deterioration of the wound
  - the wound fails to heal.

Procedure

- Explain the procedure and gain consent.
- Decontaminate your hands.
- Wearing gloves or using a dressing bag, remove the wound dressing.
- Rotate the swab in the wound, working from the middle outwards or zig-zag across to cover the full expanse of the wound. Do not touch the surrounding skin. For large wounds, swab the most contaminated area.
- Place the swab in the appropriate transport medium.
- If copious pus is present, aspirate a quantity using a syringe and transfer into a sterile container.
- Decontaminate your hands.
- Label the sample and send it to the laboratory with an appropriate request form.
- Document the episode of care.

Practice tips

- If the site being swabbed is dry, the swab can be moistened using 0.9% saline solution.
- Swabs should be taken before wound cleaning at which time the maximum number of bacteria is present; however, the dressing residue should be removed.

Nasal specimen collection

Background

A nasal swab may be helpful in indicating the causes of any infection, and is of particular assistance in guiding appropriate antibiotic therapy. They can also be taken for surveillance purposes in order to prevent transmission and to identify individuals who are at risk for developing infection e.g. meticillin-resistant *Staphylococcus aureus* (MRSA).

Procedure

- Explain the procedure and gain consent.
- Decontaminate your hands.
- Ask the patient to blow their nose and tilt their head slightly back.
- Swab the anterior nares of the nostrils by gently rotating and directing the swab upwards into the nostril.
- One swab can be used for both nostrils.
- Place the swab in the appropriate transport medium.
- Decontaminate your hands.
- Label the sample and send it to the laboratory with an appropriate request form.
- Document the episode of care.

Practice tip

- If the site being swabbed is dry, the swab can be moistened using 0.9% saline solution.

Throat specimen collection

Background
Throat (oropharynx) swabs are taken in order to isolate organisms known to cause upper respiratory tract infections.

Equipment
- Strong light.
- Tongue depressor.
- Tissues.
- Sealed plastic container.

Procedure
- Explain the procedure and gain consent.
- Ask the patient to sit in such a position that they are facing a strong light source.
- Decontaminate your hands.
- Explain to the patient that the procedure might cause a gagging reaction.
- Obtain a good view of the oropharynx before swabbing.
- Depress the tongue with a tongue depressor or ask the patient to stick their tongue out.
- Gently slide the swab down the side of the throat until you make contact with the tonsil/posterior pharynx.
- Gently but firmly rotate the swab in any exudates from the tonsillar area and/or posterior pharynx.
- Avoid touching the lips, cheeks, tongue, or teeth.
- Place the swab in the appropriate plastic container.
- Label the container and send it to the laboratory with an appropriate request form.
- Decontaminate your hands.
- Document the episode of care.

Practice tips
- Specimens should be transported and processed as soon as possible.
- If process is delayed, refrigeration may be suitable.
- Ensure specimens are processed within 48 hours.

Pitfall
- If the patient gags they can contaminate the swab.

Aural specimen collection

Background

Swabs are taken to see if infection is present in the ear canal.

Procedure

- Explain the procedure and gain consent.
- Decontaminate your hands.
- Direct a light into the patient's ear.
- Gently grasp the pinna of the ear, lifting it upwards and backwards.
- Gently rotate the swab into the external auditory canal.
- Place the swab in the appropriate transport medium.
- Label the container and send it to the laboratory with an appropriate request form.
- Decontaminate your hands.
- Document the episode of care.

Practice tip

- Do not push the swab any further into the external auditory canal beyond what you can see.

Conjunctival specimen collection

Background
Conjunctival swabs are taken in an attempt to identify the causative organism in infective conjunctivitis and determine the most effective treatment after organisms are cultured.

Equipment
- Appropriate swabs.
- Culture medium.

Procedure
- Explain the procedure and gain consent.
- Decontaminate your hands.
- Ask the patient to sit down and tilt their head slightly backwards.
- Pull the lower lid down so that the conjunctiva is exposed and ask the patient to look upwards.
- Run the swab firmly along the surface of the exposed conjunctiva, from the medial canthus towards the lateral canthus (Fig. 4.2).
- On completion, remove the swab from the lid and ask the patient to blink or close their eyes briefly, to help dispel any discomfort.
- Place the swab securely in the appropriate media and send it off to the laboratory.
- Decontaminate your hands.
- Document the episode of care.

Practice tips
- Advise the patient that the procedure could feel a little uncomfortable.
- Take swabs before the use of eye drops for examination purposes and the commencement of any treatment.
- Twisting the swab will help ensure that epithelial cells are picked up.
- If you are unable to send the swab to the laboratory immediately, it can be refrigerated.

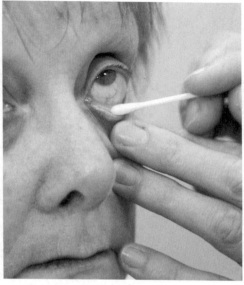

Fig. 4.2 Taking a conjunctival swab for culture.

Pain management and 'last offices'

Jennifer Walker
Clinical Educator, Trauma and Orthopaedics Department,
Nottingham University Hospitals NHS Trust, UK

Alison Whitfield
Emergency Nurse Practitioner, Clinical Educator in Emergency
Medicine, Trauma and Orthapaedics Emergency Department,
Nottingham University Hospitals NHS Trust, UK

Classifying pain

Background

Pain is the commonest reason for patients to seek medical attention. The International Association for the Study of Pain has defined pain as 'an unpleasant sensory and emotional experience associated with actual or potential tissue damage or described in terms of such damage'. It is a subjective experience that is influenced by physiological, psychological, social and cultural factors. The management of pain often requires a multi-professional and multifaceted approach, involving both pharmacological and non-pharmacological measures. It is important to identify and treat the underlying pathology, if possible.

Classification of pain

- Pain can be classified according its site, cause, type and chronicity.
- There are 2 main types of pain: *nociceptive* and *neuropathic*.
- Nociceptive pain is the reaction of the body to injury, such as trauma, surgery, or the inflammatory response. It can be classified as follows:
  - Somatic—which involves skin, muscle, or bone and is described as 'aching', 'throbbing', 'pressure', or 'stabbing'.
  - Visceral—which involves organs, is more difficult to pinpoint, and might be described as 'gnawing', 'cramping', 'aching', or 'sharp'.
- Neuropathic pain is the result of injury to or malfunction of the peripheral or central nervous system.
- The term *functional pain* is used when there is no obvious injury or pathological condition to account for the pain experienced.
- *'Acute'* pain follows an injury to the body and usually dissipates when the injury heals.
- Pain persisting for >3 months is categorized as *'chronic'*. It can be owing to a multitude of causes, including cancer and arthritis. Psychological factors can play a major role in chronic pain.

Assessing pain

Background

- The effective assessment of the patient with pain is essential for choosing the most appropriate intervention(s) to treat it. The system of assessment is similar for acute and chronic pain (🕮 on p. 106 for definitions) although the urgency to initiate treatment is greater in acute pain. The assessment should be systematic and holistic, taking into account biological, psychological, cultural and social factors.

Equipment

- Pain scale.
- Usual equipment required for assessment of a patient including pen torch, thermometer, stethoscope and sphygmomanometer.

Procedure

- Take a history from the patient, including allergies, medications and the previous response to analgesia.
- Characterize the pain using the following headings:
  - Onset
  - Location
  - Character
  - Duration
  - Frequency
  - Periodicity
  - Severity
  - Aggravating or relieving factors
  - Radiation
- Use a pain scale to assess the severity of pain (🕮 on p. 108). Review the patient's medical records.
- Ask about associated symptoms, e.g. sweating.
- Evaluate how the pain impacts on the patient's lifestyle.
- Observe the patient—how are they moving? How are they holding the affected area? Are they guarding (protecting the affected area by holding it still)? Is there facial grimacing or wincing?
- Perform a full or focused examination, as appropriate, to try and elicit the cause of the pain.

Practice tips

- Questionnaires can be useful for assessment of the impact of pain on the patient's life and activities of daily living.
- Reassure the patient that taking analgesia will not interfere with your assessment of their pain. Patients often think that analgesia will mask their symptoms or signs and prevent the health care worker (HCW) elucidating the cause.

Pitfalls

- Not providing pain relief to a patient in severe pain before assessing them in depth.

Use of pain scales

Background
The severity of pain can be assessed using verbal, visual, or numerical scales, which can be adapted to the patient's age or understanding. There are numerous pain scales, so it is important to choose one that is suitable for your area of work. A representative sample of rating scales for assessment of the intensity of pain is described below.

Equipment
- Pain scale.

Procedure
- Choose a pain scale appropriate to the patient's age and level of understanding.
- Explain the procedure and gain consent.

Types of pain scale
- The Categorical Pain Scale has four categories (none, mild, moderate, and severe). Ask the patient to select the category that best describes their pain.
  - The Numerical Rating Scale (Fig. 5.1) assigns a number to grades of pain, with 0 usually representing no pain and 10 representing the worst pain imaginable. Explain to the patient the meaning of the numbers and ask them to identify how much pain they are having by choosing a number from 0 to 10.
  - The Visual Analogue Scale (Fig. 5.2) is a straight line, with the left end of the line representing no pain and the right end representing the worst pain imaginable. Ask the patient to mark a point on the line where they think their pain is in relation to the two extremes.
  - The Pain Faces Scale (Fig. 5.3) uses four to six faces with different expressions, ranging from a happy face (representing no pain) to increasingly sad faces (representing pain of worsening severity). This scale can be used by people aged 3 years and older. Ask the patient to point to the face that best describes how they are feeling.
  - The Face, Legs, Activity, Cry, Consolability (FLACC) Scale (Fig. 5.4) is derived from observation of pre-verbal children. Numerical values are assigned to permutations of the various elements, which are then added up to give a severity score for pain.
  - The Pain Ladder Scale (Fig. 5.5) combines pain severity with the effect of pain on function. Ask the patient about the severity of the pain and what the pain prevents them from doing.
- Document the episode of care, recording the level of pain and method of assessment used.
- Repeat the procedure after administering analgesia, to assess its effect.

Practice tips
- Ensure that the patient is as relaxed as possible. Anxiety ↑ the patient's perception of pain.
- One-off assessments of pain are performed most easily using the Categorical Pain Scale. A numerical value of pain is of little use as a one-off measurement. Numerical values or Visual Analogue Scales are

useful, however, for sequential assessment (e.g. evaluation of the effects of treatments).
- Ask the patient about pain at rest and on movement. A patient with a hip fracture might be pain-free while sitting on a trolley and then experience severe pain if moved for radiography or transfer.
- Elderly people tend to be stoical and understate their pain.

Pitfalls
- Using pain scales in isolation from observation of the patient as a whole. It is unlikely that a person who self-scores 10 out of 10 for the severity of their pain and is sitting comfortably and chatting is truly experiencing pain of the worst severity. The reverse is also true, and patients can understate their pain when they are obviously in distress.
- Not believing the patient's chosen place on the scale. It is easy to dismiss a patient's description of their pain intensity, particularly if no diagnosis has been found to explain it. All too often, patients with conditions such as cancer, fracture and compartment syndrome have been fobbed off as 'hysterical'.

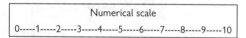

Numerical scale

0-----1-----2-----3-----4-----5-----6-----7-----8-----9-----10

Fig. 5.1 Numerical pain scale. Reproduced from Castledine G and Close A (2007) *Oxford handbook of general and adult nursing*. With permission from Oxford University Press.

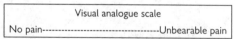

Visual analogue scale

No pain-------------------------------------Unbearable pain

Fig. 5.2 Visual analogue pain scale. Reproduced from Castledine G and Close A (2007) *Oxford handbook of general and adult nursing*. With permission from Oxford University Press.

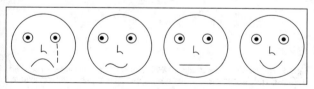

Fig. 5.3 Face rating. Reproduced from Castledine G and Close A (2007) *Oxford handbook of general and adult nursing*. With permission from Oxford University Press.

Categories	Scoring		
	0	1	2
Face	No particular expression or smile	Occasional grimace or frown, withdrawn, uninterested	Frequent to constant quivering chin, clenched jaw
Legs	Normal position or relaxed	Uneasy, restless, tense	Kicking, or legs drawn up
Activity	Lying quietly, normal position moves easily	Squirming, shifting back and forth, tense	Arched, rigid or jerking
Cry	No cry, (awake or asleep)	Moans or whimpers; occasional complaint	Crying steadily, screams or sobs, frequent complaints
Consilability	Content, relaxed	Reassured by occasional touching hugging or being talked to, distractable	Difficulty to console or comfort

Fig. 5.4 FLACC Scale. Merkel S., Voepel-Lewis T., Shayevitz J., & Malviya S., (1997) The FLACC. A behavioural scale for scoring postoperative pain in young children. *Pediatric Nursing*, **23**:293–297.© 2002, The Regents of the university of Michigan.

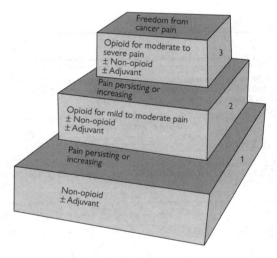

Fig. 5.5 The WHO pain relief ladder. *Palliative Care: symptom management and end of life care*, p.12. Reproduced with permission from the World Health Organisation.

Treatment of pain

Background

- The alleviation of pain is one of the most important roles of health care professionals. There is a wide range of pharmacological and non-pharmacological interventions available. The effective assessment of the patient with pain is essential for choosing the most appropriate intervention(s) to treat it. The system of assessment is similar for acute and chronic pain (🕮 on p. 107) although the urgency to initiate treatment is greater in acute pain.

Equipment

- Analgesics and other drugs required for pharmacological interventions.
- Syringes, needles, pumps and other equipment required for delivery of various pharmacological interventions.
- Equipment associated with various non-pharmacological interventions, e.g. splints, transcutaneous electrical nerve stimulation (TENS) machine, acupuncture needles, heat pad.

Procedure

Acute pain

- Ensure adequate analgesia is provided—use a step-wise approach starting with simple analgesia (e.g. paracetamol ± a non-steroidal anti-inflammatory drug (NSAID) (e.g. ibuprofen), moving on to weak opioids (e.g. dihydrocodeine) and then stronger opioids (e.g. morphine).
- Administer intravenous injections of analgesia if immediate relief of severe pain is required—e.g. administer morphine to a patient having a myocardial infarction.
- Splint fractures as soon as possible—this eases painful muscle spasm and prevents movement at the fracture site.
- Elevate the painful site if possible—this aids circulation and ↓ swelling, which eases pain.
- Inject local anaesthetic into peripheral nerves (e.g. digital or ulnar nerve blocks) or the spine, if appropriate and the expertise is available.
- Consider patient-controlled analgesia (PCA) through an infusion pump (🕮 on p. 118).
- Consider the use of a TENS machine (🕮 on p. 114), which can be effective for rib fractures, postoperative wound pain, or labour pain, for example.

Chronic pain

- The management of chronic pain is more problematic and more likely to involve a multidisciplinary team, including doctors, nurses, physiotherapists, chiropractors, clinical psychologists, and occupational therapists. Management of the underlying pathology is important.
- Ensure adequate analgesia is provided using the same step-wise approach outlined above. It is not ideal, however, for the patient to take regular doses of drugs such as NSAIDs over prolonged periods.
- Educate the patient regarding a healthy lifestyle, including advice about weight and stress management.

- Consider the use of tricyclic antidepressants (e.g. amitriptyline) or anticonvulsant (e.g. gabapentin), which can be effective in neuropathic pain.
- Consider the use of a TENS machine(📖 on p.114).
- Consider PCA (📖 on p. 116). This is common in palliative care settings.
- Injections of steroids or local anaesthetic directly into joints might ↓ pain and enable ↑ function.
- Consider therapies such as acupuncture, relaxation techniques, massage, aromatherapy, reflexology, homeopathy and hypnotherapy.
- Treat any underlying or accompanying depression.
- Reassess pain following any intervention and adjust therapy, as appropriate.

Practice tips

- Be aware of the side effects of analgesics and prescribe and administer them with care—NSAIDs are often poorly tolerated and opioids can cause nausea, dizziness and constipation, particularly in the elderly.
- Talk to and comfort your patient—a smile and kind words can be potent analgesics.
- Give written analgesia guidelines—information given in the medical setting might not be retained by the patient.
- Identify something the patient wants to do and allow them to be the key decision-maker—this empowerment might help them to develop/ maintain a positive attitude.
- Patients are often reluctant to take opioids for fear of becoming addicted. This is often not volunteered and only discovered when the patient is non-compliant. Be aware of this fear and reassure patients where appropriate.

Pitfalls

- Leaving patients in pain. It is distressing to see health care workers (HCWs) ignoring or fobbing off patients in pain while they carry on with other activities. If you cannot provide pain relief, ensure that someone who can is summoned as soon as possible.
- Prescribing 'as required' (prn) analgesia when regular analgesia might be more appropriate and effective (the reverse is also true i.e. prn analgesia might be more appropriate in some circumstances).
- Not involving the patient in decision-making, particularly those in chronic pain. Empowering the patient can help to foster a positive attitude and improve the outcome.
- Giving the patient unrealistic expectations of pain relief—this can lead to frustration if things aren't improving or, worse, the patient is experiencing ↑ levels of pain.
- Underestimating the effect of chronic pain on the patient. The impact on their life can lead to depression and isolation.

Transcutaneous electrical nerve stimulation (TENS)

Background

A TENS machine is a portable, battery-operated device that emits a painless electrical current to peripheral nerves or directly to a painful source. This alters the patient's perception of the pain by blocking the painful stimuli. Electrodes can be placed on the patient to cover a painful area (e.g. muscle tenderness or rib fracture), capture a painful area between electrodes (e.g. an incision site), or stimulate dermatomes in peripheral nerve injury. TENS interventions are characterized by the amplitude, duration (width) and frequency of the pulse produced by the stimulators during treatment.

Equipment

- TENS machine.
- TENS leads.
- Electrodes.
- Electrode gel.
- Hypoallergenic tape

Procedure

- Explain the procedure and gain consent.
- Ensure that there are no contraindications to the use of TENS, in particular the presence of a cardiac pacemaker.
- Ensure that the skin on which electrodes are to be placed is clean and dry. If necessary, clean the skin with soap and water and dry thoroughly.
- If electrodes do not have gel already applied, apply electrode gel to the bottom of each electrode.
- Place the electrodes on to the skin close to the site of pain, leaving at least 5cm between them. The sites of placement depend on the individual machine. Refer to the manufacturer's guidelines.
- Secure the electrodes with adhesive patches or hypoallergenic tape, ensuring that all the electrodes are firmly attached to the skin. Stimulation should never be applied over the eyes, laryngeal or pharyngeal muscles, or carotid sinus nerves.
- Plug the pin connections of the lead wires into the connectors on the electrodes.
- Ensure that the TENS controls are in the 'off' position or as directed by the manufacturer's guidelines.
- Plug the lead wires into the control box.
- Turn the amplitude and rate dials slowly, according to the manufacturer's manual, adjusting the settings to the prescribed settings or those that are most comfortable for the patient. The patient should feel a tingling sensation.
- Attach the TENS box to the patient's clothing (e.g. a belt, bra, or pocket) to enable the patient to mobilize, if they wish.
- Monitor the patient for signs of excessive stimulation (e.g. muscular twitches) or inadequate stimulation (the patient doesn't feel the tingling sensation).
- Document the application of TENS and note its effectiveness.

After TENS treatment is complete
- Turn off the controls, peel off the electrodes, and clean the skin underneath.
- Unplug the lead wires from the TENS unit and disconnect the lead wires from the electrodes.
- Wipe the gel from electrodes.

Practice tips
- Check that the pads or tape do not irritate the patient's skin. If the skin is red, you might need to use a different type of pad, contact gel, or tape.
- The machine should be used for at least 45min for best effect.
- The machine can be left on for up to 12 hours before re-siting of the electrodes is required.

Pitfalls
- Incorrect placement of the electrodes, resulting in poor pain control.
- Setting the controls too high, causing pain.

Setting up patient-controlled analgesia (PCA)

Background
A PCA infusion pump enables patients to self-administer opioid analgesia within limits prescribed by a practitioner. Small boluses can be delivered, maintaining levels within a narrow therapeutic range. This provides good analgesia and helps to avoid side-effects (e.g. nausea) associated with larger boluses. PCA is commonly used to manage acute pain, typically in postoperative or trauma patients. It also has a major role in palliative care.

Equipment
- PCA pump.
- Syringe—consult the manufacturer's guidelines for the size.
- Prescription.
- Documentation.
- Intravenous (IV) tubing.
- Labels.

Procedure
- Explain the procedure and gain consent.
- Check the prescription, which should include the following details:
  - Name of the drug and concentration to be used in PCA.
  - Loading dose.
  - Lock-out duration—the prescribed period of time during which the patient cannot deliver another dose.
  - Background/maintenance infusion (basal rate).
  - Bolus dose—the amount of drug the patient receives on pushing the button.
- Draw up the prescribed analgesia in the syringe.
- Label the syringe with the patient's name, drug, dose, concentration, date and time.
- Attach the IV tubing to the syringe.
- Prime the giving set.
- Attach the syringe to the pump, making sure that the flange of the syringe is aligned with the flange slot on the pump. The body of the syringe should be parallel to the pump, with the markings facing outwards.
- Move the driver so that it presses firmly against the syringe plunger.
- Close and lock the cover of the device.
- Attach the IV set to the vascular access (flush the venous access with 0.9% sodium chloride solution before connection, to ensure patency).
- Programme and check the PCA device. The loading dose, lock-out duration, background infusion, and bolus dose should be programmed, according to the prescription.
- Undo the safety clamp on the IV set.
- Give the patient the handset and explain how it works.
- Allow the patient to practice on a spare handset and observe them, to ensure that they can use it correctly.

- Label the IV lines with the date and time.
- Document the episode of care, making sure to include the syringe volume.

Practice tips

- If a patient is going to use PCA for postoperative analgesia, explain how it works before their operation.
- Check venous access is available before drawing up the syringe.

Pitfalls

- Not assembling the PCA pump, syringe, or IV lines properly.
- Failing to explain adequately to patients how the device works and not checking their understanding.
- Not ensuring that patients are physically able to control the device. Patients might not be able to press the button owing to arthritis, weakness in the upper extremities or lowered level of consciousness.

Care of the patient on patient-controlled analgesia (PCA)

Background
PCA enables patients to self-administer a preset dose of analgesia (usually an opioid). This gives patients the autonomy to manage their pain without being dependent on staff. The administration of frequent small boluses maintains drug levels within a narrow therapeutic range and minimizes side effects.

Equipment
- Prescription.
- PCA.
- Pulse oximeter.
- Stethoscope.
- Sphygmomanometer.

Procedure
- Explain the procedure and gain consent.
- Check the prescription for PCA.
- Check that the label on the syringe has the correct patient's name, drug, dose, concentration, date and time.
- Check the PCA programme—the loading dose, lock-out duration, background/maintenance infusion (basal rate), and bolus dose (the amount of drug the patient receives on pushing the button).
- Press 'history' on the PCA device to display the number of requests for analgesia and doses delivered.
- Measure the volume in the syringe and check that this correlates to the amount used.
- Check the integrity of the venous access, looking for signs of infiltration, swelling, or erythema.
- Check the patency of the IV lines and ensure that they are correctly labelled with dates for change.

Assessment of the patient
- Measure and document the patient's vital signs—pulse, blood pressure, respiratory rate and depth and oxygen saturation.
- Assess the patient's level of consciousness.
- Determine the patient's assessment of pain relief. If it is unsatisfactory, offer guidance on how PCA might be used more effectively or, if appropriate, inform a more senior member of staff.
- Document the episode of care, including any patient education given.

Practice tips
- Encourage patients to press the button if they feel they need analgesia, even if this is within the 'lock-out' period. This will provide a more accurate picture of analgesic requirements and enable modification of the dosage.
- Collate observations and other documentation in a central location, so that documentation does not become fragmented. This facilitates a quicker and easier assessment of pain management and ↓ the risk of omission or error.

Pitfalls
- Patients not using PCA to its maximum effect because of misconceptions about it, e.g. fears of overdosing or becoming addicted—patient education is important.
- Respiratory depression, if PCA is used with opioids.

Last offices

Background

'Last offices' is the care given to the deceased patient following certification of death in the medical setting. It involves washing the body and laying it out in an appropriate manner for transfer to the mortuary. It should be undertaken with respect and dignity. The wishes of the family should be taken into consideration. Procedures may vary with religious beliefs (📖 on p. 122).

Equipment

- Non-sterile gloves and apron.
- Shroud—usually made of cloth, paper, or plastic.
- Sheet.
- Water, wipes, and towels, if required.
- Ribbon gauze/bandage.
- Two identification labels, property book, and death-notification forms.

Procedure

- Explain the procedure to next of kin, if present.
- Check the patient's religion, to conform to religious customs. Ask the relatives or close friends about any special requests.
- Screen off the bed area to maintain privacy.
- Put on gloves and apron.
- Close the patient's eyelids, insert dentures (if applicable), close the mouth, and position the limbs in a natural position as soon as possible after death. This helps to prevent the disfiguring effects of rigor mortis.
- Remove any drips, placing a spiggot on any cannulae.
- Leave any lines, drains, or tubes *in situ* if there is a possibility that a post mortem is required. Otherwise, remove them.
- Apply pressure above the symphysis pubis to empty the bladder. Use a suitable container to collect any urine.
- Apply dressings to any wounds or sores.
- Remove jewellery—in the presence of another health care worker (HCW), unless relatives have requested that it remains on the body. Jewellery not removed should be covered with tape and the site and item type documented in patient notes.
- Gently wash and dry any heavily soiled areas.
- Place an incontinence pad under the buttocks.
- Attach two identification labels, containing the patient's name, dates of birth and death, hospital number and general practitioner details onto the body—the usual positions are the wrist and ankle.
- Tie the lower limbs together at the knees and ankles using ribbon gauze or a narrow bandage. This is not done at all institutions. Follow local policy.
- Dress the body in a shroud.
- Place a clean sheet under the body.
- Fold the top of the sheet to cover the head and bottom of the sheet to cover the feet. Then, fold in each side of the sheet to cover the rest of the body and secure with tape.

- Place the completed mortuary form on the chest and secure with tape.
- Use an impermeable and sealable body bag if the body poses an infection risk or there is continuing fluid loss following trauma.
- Arrange for transfer to the mortuary.
- Document the episode of care.

Children
- HCWs involved in laying out children should be aware of differences in procedures. Children are often laid out in their own clothes and have special toys or blankets, which remain with them. These should be labelled. The parents are encouraged to be involved in the process. They are offered keepsakes, e.g. a lock of hair, photographs, or foot or hand prints.

Practice tips
- Noises might emanate from the body as air escapes while you move it. It might sound like the body sighs or breathes—do not be alarmed by this.
- Carry out last offices as soon as possible. Rigor mortis sets in after 2–4 hours making repositioning more difficult.
- Early rigor mortis can be broken down by gentle massage and flexing of joints, e.g. the fingers, wrists, elbows, and shoulders.
- Elevate the head to ↓ discolouration from pooling of blood.
- A pillow might be placed under the chin to support the jaw.
- Use caution when removing tape from the body because the skin becomes less elastic as the temperature ↓, making it easier to damage.
- Removal of rings might be difficult—use lubricating gel or a moisturiser to aid removal.
- Recognize the impact a death might have on other patients in a ward.
- Ensure any relatives who are in the hospital are given the option to view the body before wrapping it.
- Ensure the body has been formally certified as dead before transfer to the mortuary.

Pitfalls
- Not showing respect—it is inappropriate to gossip or laugh over the body.
- Treat the body with care—it should not be moved roughly.
- Not providing adequate privacy—curtains should be drawn and the private parts kept covered, as for a living person.
- Removing lines or tubes if a post mortem is to be carried out.

Common cultural and religious customs around death and dying

Background

Health care workers (HCWs) should recognize the need for relatives and friends of dying and recently deceased patients to complete rituals surrounding death. Those with different or no religious beliefs may find it difficult to understand these practices but should respect them as they are important in the grieving process. Different cultures have different attitudes to external signs of emotion, such as crying and wailing, e.g. in Chinese culture crying is encouraged and seen as a tribute to the deceased, whereas it is frowned upon in other cultures, particularly for men. The following outlines some of the common procedures and rituals surrounding death in different ethnic groups.

Procedure

- Always consult the family of a dying or recently deceased patient regarding specific rituals they wish to observe.
- Discuss the procedure for 'last offices' with the relatives.

Christians

- Christians may like to have a minister present at the time of death or as soon as possible afterwards. Practising Roman Catholics in particular will want a priest to be present.
- Christians are happy for HCWs to prepare the body. Some may want to participate in this preparation.
- Religious symbols such as the crucifix may be placed on or near the body.

Muslims

- Muslims prefer non-Muslims not to touch the body. If necessary, family consent should be sought and gloves worn.
- Do not wash the body. Clothing is removed and ritual washing is performed by family members or close friends of the same sex.
- The head should be turned to the right so that it may face Mecca when buried. The body is then covered with a sheet.
- Prayers from the Qu'ran may be read out to a dying patient but should not be recited near the deceased.
- Burial should ideally be within 24 hours of death.

Hindus

- Hindus are not offended if non-Hindus touch the body but prefer to wash the body at home. If a child dies the elders of the same sex wash them.
- Do not remove jewellery or religious objects.
- It is preferred that the eldest son is present at the time of death.
- Care of the dying patient may involve holy water being sprinkled over the body and laying them on the floor, symbolizing closeness to mother Earth.
- Post-mortem examinations are felt to be disrespectful.

Sikhs

- Sikhs are generally happy for non-Sikhs to attend to the body but, similar to Muslims, the tradition is that family members perform ceremonies and rites, e.g. washing the body.
- Respect the five 'K's of Sikhism: Kesh (uncut hair), Khanga (comb), Karra (bracelet), Kachha (shorts), and Kirpan (sword), which have deep spiritual significance. Wash your hands before touching these objects and keep them with the body. Do not trim the hair or beard.
- The dying patient may be given holy water to drink or have it sprinkled around the bed.
- Cremation ideally within 24 hours of death.

Jews

- Jews prefer the body to be handled as little as possible.
- If feasible, a child of the deceased should close the eyes.
- Straighten the limbs with the hands open.
- Cover the body with a white sheet.
- Contact the Rabbi as soon as possible after death if they are not present at the time.
- Post mortems are disliked by Jews.
- Burial should ideally be within 24 hours of death.

Buddhists

- Buddhists needs vary depending on the particular lineage they follow.
- Buddhists believe that entering death in a positive state of mind surrounded by monks and family helps the deceased to become reborn on a higher level.
- Disturb the deceased as little as possible immediately following death as it is believed that it can take some time for the consciousness to leave the body. The body is then considered an empty shell. No special rites are required although the body should be handled in a worthy and respectful way.

Practice tips

- Discuss the death with relatives and give time for questions.
- Involve the appropriate religious representative. They will be able to answer questions and give advice if the relatives are unavailable or too distressed to talk.
- Consider referring relatives to a counselling service.

Pitfall

- Not asking about religious beliefs and causing distress to the relatives by not following procedures relating to their culture or religion.

Drug administration

Martyn Bradbury
Clinical Skills Network Lead, School of Nursing and
Community Studies, Faculty of Health and Social Work,
University of Plymouth, UK

Related topics
Rectal (PR) administration 📖 on p.448
Inhalers 📖 on p.322
Nebulizers 📖 on p. 330

Prescribing choices

Background

Having established a diagnosis, it is essential to involve the patient in a negotiation of the clinical management plan/plan of care and the decision on the most appropriate treatment.

Prescribing choices should be made with regard to the following:

- The desired therapeutic outcome.
- Alternative treatment options.
- Age.
- Ethnicity.
- Previous medical history.
- Comorbidities.
- Previous medication history.
- Polypharmacy.
- Is the patient in a high-risk group?
- Any contraindications.
- Any side-effects.
- The most suitable route of administration.
- The most suitable formulation.
- The lifestyle of the patient.
- Factors likely to affect concordance.

Medication history

- Any allergies/sensitivities.
- Any previous adverse drug reactions (ADRs).
- Nature of previous allergic reactions/ADRs.
- Is the patient taking any other prescribed medication?
- Is the patient taking any other over-the-counter medication?
- Is the patient taking any home remedies?
- Has the patient used any other 'borrowed' medications from friends or relatives?

Selecting the correct drug: a mnemonic (EASE)

- E—is the proposed medicine effective and its use supported by accepted practice, national guidelines and a strong evidence base?
- A—is the proposed medicine appropriate and acceptable to the patient?
- S—is it safe?
- E—is it cost-effective?

The prescription

All prescriptions must be:
- Written in indelible ink.
- Signed by the prescriber.
- Dated.
- In addition, the prescription should contain clear instruction regarding the drug and:
  - Clear instruction regarding the dose.
  - Clear instruction regarding the frequency of administration.
  - Clear instruction regarding the formulation.
  - The generic drug name, whenever possible/clinically appropriate.
  - The Patient's name and address.
  - The address of the prescriber—(this is pre-printed on NHS prescription forms).
  - The age of the patient—this is a legal requirement if the patient is <12 years.
  - Any special instructions—e.g. 'to be taken with food'.

The drug
- The generic name should be used, whenever possible/clinically appropriate.
- Abbreviations for drug names should not be used—e.g. state 'isosorbide mononitrate' rather than 'ISMN'.

The frequency
- Instructions should be written so that they are clear and not open to misinterpretation—e.g. state 'every 6 hours' rather than '6-hourly'.

The dose
- Doses of <1g should be written in milligrams (mg)—e.g. 750mg rather than 0.75g or .75g.
- Doses of <1mg should be written in micrograms—e.g. 250 micrograms rather than 0.25 milligrams or .25 milligrams.
- If prescribing in micrograms, the full unit name should be used— i.e. micrograms rather than *mcg or µg*.
- Doses prescribed in 'units' (e.g. insulin) should be written in full— i.e. 10 units rather than 10u.

Principles of drug administration

Background

The aim of drug administration is to ensure the right medicine is given to the right patient at the right time, in the right formulation, and at the right dose.

Local policies and procedures will be in place to achieve this and reference must be made to these. However, general principles will apply to all health care workers (HCWs) who administer medications to patients.

Importantly, the HCW should be aware of the patient's treatment plan and:

- Understand the indications for use of the prescribed drugs.
- Be aware of any potential precautions, contraindications, side-effects, and drug interactions—refer to the drug formulary, as required.
- Ensure that the prescription is signed, dated, and unambiguous.
- Ensure that the route, timing, formulation, and administration instructions are appropriate—refer to the drug formulary, as required.
- Involve and educate the patient so that they can self-administer, as appropriate.

If there is a concern regarding any of the above, the HCW should contact the prescriber before proceeding with administration.

Procedure

- Decontaminate hands.
- Check the start and end dates of the prescription, as appropriate.
- Check that the medication has not already been given.
- Check the expiry date of the medication.
- Check the integrity of the packaging.
- Calculate the volume of drug required.
- Follow any medication-specific or manufacturer's instructions—e.g. shake the bottle before administration.
- Check the patient's level of understanding regarding the prescribed treatment and educate the patient, as appropriate.
- Gain consent for administration.
- Confirm the patient's identity against the prescription—procedures for checking the patient's identity will vary according to the healthcare setting and local policy should be followed.

Post-administration, the HCW should:

- Ensure that the medication has been taken.
- Make a record of all drugs administered.
- Decontaminate hands.
- Monitor the patient's response to treatment.
- Follow the manufacturer's instructions regarding safe storage of the medication.
- If an adverse drug reaction (ADR) is noted, this should be reported using local procedures and the national yellow card system.

If administration is not possible, e.g. owing to patient refusal or the drug being withheld for clinical reasons, this should be recorded and the prescriber informed.

Resources

British National Formulary http://www.bnf.org.uk
National Prescribing Centre http://www.npc.co.uk
Clinical Knowledge Summaries Service (CKS)
http://www.cks.library.nhs.uk

Oral administration

Background

Administration via the oral route is the most common form of drug administration. It is easily accessible and socially acceptable. Drugs taken via the oral route are subject to individual variation in absorption and the hepatic first-pass effect before entering the systemic circulation.

Equipment
- Prescription chart.
- Drug formulary.
- Medication to be administered.
- Medication pot.
- Drinking water or other fluid.

Procedure
- Decontaminate your hands.
- Explain the procedure and gain consent.
- Check and confirm the prescription. See principles of drug administration 🔲 on p.128.
- Empty the required medication into the medicine pot.
- Check and confirm the patient's identity.
- Position the patient, preferably sitting or standing.
- Ensure drink/fluid is available, if appropriate, to aid swallowing.
- Assist the patient to take the drug(s), as required.
- Clean the medicine pot/equipment.
- Decontaminate your hands.
- Record the administration.
- Monitor the effect of treatment.

Practice tips
- Drugs from blister packs can be placed directly into the medicine pot, whereas tablets and capsules in medicines bottles should first be emptied into the cap to prevent handling of the drug.
- Drugs should not be left unattended at the patient's bedside.
- The patient should swallow tablets and capsules whole unless the prescription indicates otherwise.
- Liquid should be measured to the base of the meniscus or alternatively drawn up with a syringe.
- Fluid or mouth care should be given to clear orally administered syrup/liquid-based medications. This is particularly important following the administration of antibiotics.

Pitfalls
- Altering the formulation of the drug prior to administration, e.g. crushing a slow-release medication.
- Covertly administering a medicine, e.g. by disguising in food without the patient's consent.

Sublingual (S/L) administration

Background
S/L administration is useful because it is easily accessible, drugs are well absorbed, and the first-pass effect associated with enteral absorption is reduced. Drugs administered via the S/L route can be given as a spray or dissolvable tablet.

Equipment
- Prescription chart.
- Drug formulary.
- Medication to be administered.
- Non-sterile gloves.

Procedure
- Decontaminate your hands.
- Explain the procedure and gain consent.
- Check and confirm the prescription. See principles of drug administration 💷 on p.128.
- Check and confirm the patient's identity.
- Ensure the patient is in a comfortable position—usually sitting.
- Put on the non-sterile gloves.
- Ask the patient to open their mouth and lift their tongue.
- Place the tablet under the tongue in the posterior lingual pocket.
- Make the patient comfortable.
- Discard the equipment using clinical waste disposal.
- Remove gloves and wash hands.
- Record the administration.
- Monitor the effect of treatment.

Practice tips
- When administering S/L spray under the tongue, ask the patient to close their mouth immediately following administration.
- Instruct the patient not to swallow for at least 10sec following administration of the S/L spray.
- The patient should avoid eating or drinking until the drug is dissolved.
- The patient should avoid smoking/nicotine because this causes vasoconstriction and alters absorption of the drug.
- Encourage the patient to self-administer medication as appropriate.

Nasogastric (N/G) administration

Background
A nasogastric tube can be used to administer a wide range of medications that are absorbed via the enteral route.

Equipment
- Prescription chart.
- Drug formulary.
- Medication to be administered.
- Diluent.
- 50mL syringe (non-Luer lock).
- pH paper.
- Non-sterile gloves.

Procedure
- Decontaminate your hands.
- Explain the procedure and gain consent.
- Check and confirm the prescription. See principles of drug administration 📖 on p.128.
- Position the patient (ideally in a semi-recumbent position with their head up so that the drug drains quickly into the stomach).
- Check and confirm the patient's identity.
- Put on the non-sterile gloves.
- Verify the position of the nasogastric tube using pH paper (📖 on p. 424).
- Draw up and prepare the medication, as required.
- Remove the plunger from the syringe.
- Clamp/kink the nasogastric tube and attach the barrel of the syringe.
- Pour the measured volume of drug into the syringe.
- Unkink/unclamp the nasogastric tube and allow the drug to flow into the patient under gravity.
- Administer 50mL of water or other diluent to clear the tube.
- Spigot the tube or reconnect feed, as appropriate.
- Make the patient comfortable.
- Discard the equipment using clinical waste disposal.
- Wash your hands.
- Record the administration.
- Monitor the effect of treatment.

Practice tips
- Medication for nasogastric administration should, if possible, be prescribed in a formulation suitable for this route—e.g. dispersible tablet, liquid, or syrup.
- Seek advice from a pharmacist where the patient is prescribed a non-dispersible tablet or capsule. Ensure it is suitable for crushing and that this will not alter the formulation—e.g. slow-release and enteric-coated drugs should not be crushed.
- Observe the patient throughout for signs of discomfort and respiratory embarrassment.

- Raising the height of the syringe above the patient will increase the speed of drug delivery.
- If more than one drug has to be administered, the nasogastric tube should be flushed with water between drugs.

Pitfalls
- Failing to verify the position of the nasogastric tube prior to administration of the drug.
- Verifying the position of the tube by using blue litmus paper or pushing air down the NG tube and listening for this over the stomach (whoosh test).
- Altering the formulation of the drug prior to administration, e.g. crushing slow-release tablets.

Eye drops

Background

Usually given for a local effect, e.g. to dilate the pupil (mydriatics) or constrict the pupil (miotics). Anaesthetics, anti-inflammatories/steroids, antibacterials, and antivirals can also be given by this route.

Equipment

- Prescription chart.
- Drug formulary.
- Medication to be administered.
- Tissue.

Procedure

- Decontaminate your hands.
- Explain the procedure and gain consent.
- Check and confirm the prescription. See principles of drug administration 📖 on p.128.
- Check and confirm the patient's identity.
- Position the patient (the patient's head should be supported, with their head tilted back and turned slightly to the affected side).
- Apply gentle downwards traction on the skin overlying the lower orbit, and form a pocket in the lower eyelid (conjunctival sac).
- Instil a drop of the drug into the formed pocket.
- Ask the patient to gently close their eye for 30sec.
- Make the patient comfortable and offer a tissue.
- Discard the equipment using clinical waste disposal.
- Decontaminate your hands.
- Record the administration.
- Monitor the effect of treatment.

Practice tips

- Apply medication into the pocket formed in the lower eyelid and avoid applying the drug directly onto the eyeball.
- Ensure you have the correct eye because different drugs might be administered to each eye.
- Asking the patient to apply finger pressure to the puncta post instillation will decrease enteral absorption of the drug.

Pitfall

- Failing to remember that the patient's right eye will be on your left when facing the patient.

Eye ointment

Background

Usually given for a local topical effect—e.g. anaesthetics, anti-inflammatories/steroids, antibacterials or antivirals.

Equipment

- Prescription chart.
- Drug formulary.
- Medication to be administered.
- Tissue.

Procedure

- Decontaminate your hands.
- Explain the procedure and gain consent.
- Check and confirm the prescription. See principles of drug administration ⧠ on p.128.
- Check and confirm the patient's identity.
- Position the patient (the patient's head should be supported, with their head tilted back and turned slightly to the affected side).
- Apply gentle downwards traction on the skin overlying the lower orbit so that you retract the lower eyelid and form a conjunctival pocket into which the medication will be placed.
- Gently squeeze the prescribed measure of medication into the formed pocket, starting at the inner aspect and working outwards.
- Ask the patient to gently close their eye and move their eyeball behind the closed eyelid.
- Make the patient comfortable and offer a tissue.
- Discard the equipment using clinical waste disposal.
- Decontaminate your hands.
- Record the administration.
- Monitor the effect of treatment.

Practice tips

- The dose of ointment is measured on the basis of the length of drug ribbon extruded from the tube.
- If administering more than one ointment, wait 10–15min after administration of the first medication before applying a second medication.
- Apply the medication into the pocket formed and avoid applying drug directly onto the eyeball.
- Avoid contact between the ointment tube and eye/conjunctiva. Warn the patient that blurred vision after administration is normal until the medication has melted/dispersed. They should avoid driving while their vision is blurred.

Pitfall

- Failing to remember that the patient's right eye will be on your left when facing the patient.

Subcutaneous injection (S/C)

Background
Injection into subcutaneous (S/C) fat is beneficial because systemic distribution is gradual. As such, this route is usually used for drugs that are required to have a prolonged period of action e.g. insulin and heparin.

Equipment
- Prescription chart.
- Drug formulary.
- Medication to be administered.
- 25g or 26g needle and syringe.
- Sharps bin and injection tray.
- Non-sterile gloves.
- Alcohol-impregnated swab, according to local policy.

Procedure
- Decontaminate your hands.
- Explain the procedure and gain consent.
- Check and confirm the prescription. See principles of drug administration 🕮 on p.128.
- Check and confirm the patient's identity.
- Position the patient and expose the preferred site for injection.
- Decontaminate hands and put on gloves.
- Draw up and prepare the injection, as required.
- Label the syringe with the name of the drug it contains.
- With your non-dominant hand, gently pinch the skin between thumb and index/middle finger to form a skin fold. Introduce the needle at the apex of the skin fold. (If a short, ≤16 mm, or ultrafine needle is used then the needle should enter the skin at 90°. If a longer needle is used (>16mm), or there is minimal subcutaneous fat, it may be necessary to introduce the needle into the skin at 45° and aspirate prior to administration to ensure subcutaneous administration has been achieved).
- Slowly inject the drug.
- Wait 5sec and then withdraw the needle.
- Apply gentle pressure to the injection site, as required.
- Do not resheath the needle and immediately dispose of it into the sharps bin.
- Make the patient comfortable.
- Discard the equipment using clinical waste disposal.
- Remove gloves and wash your hands.
- Record the administration.
- Monitor the effect of treatment.

Practice tips
- Assess the patient before administration to determine that there is adequate subcutaneous fat.
- Avoid rubbing the injection site post-injection.
- When drawing up from multi dose vial ensure that the rubber bung is cleaned with an alcohol swab and allowed to dry before drawing up drug.

Pitfalls

- Failing to rotate the site of injection.
- When administering low molecular weight heparin, such as enoxaparin sodium, from a prefilled syringe, do not remove the air bubble adjacent to the plunger before administration.

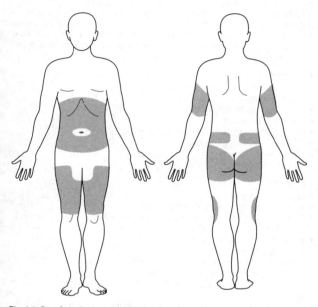

Fig. 6.1 Sites for subcutaneous injection.

Intramuscular injection (I/M)

Background

With the increasing use of intravenous injection, the intramuscular route is not as extensively used as it once was. However, it is still an appropriate route for the administration of a wide variety of drugs, including analgesics, anti-emetics, antibiotics, and vaccines. Depot injection into the larger muscle groups is also used if sustained release of the medicine is required—e.g. antipsychotic preparations, such as flupentixol decanoate. In addition to the standard intramuscular injection, the Z-track technique is also available and is the preferred technique for many health care workers (HCWs).

Equipment

- Prescription chart.
- Drug formulary.
- Medication to be administered.
- Needle and syringe.
- Alcohol-impregnated swab, according to local policy.
- Sharps bin and injection tray.
- Gauze swab.
- Non-sterile gloves.

Procedure

- Decontaminate your hands.
- Explain the procedure and gain consent.
- Check and confirm the prescription. See principles of drug administration 📖 on p.128.
- Put on the non-sterile gloves.
- Draw up and prepare the injection.
- Label the syringe with the name of the drug it contains.
- Check and confirm the patient's identity.
- Position the patient and expose the preferred site for injection (see Fig. 6.2).
- If indicated clean the skin using an alcohol-impregnated swab and allow to dry for a minimum of 30sec.
- Use your non-dominant hand to support the skin over the selected injection site.
- Introduce the needle into the muscle at 90° to the skin.
- Support the hub of the needle/lower part of the syringe with your non-dominant hand.
- Gently withdraw the plunger and observe for any blood entering the syringe. (If blood is observed, withdraw needle and recommence procedure.)
- Slowly inject the drug and wait 10sec for it to disperse.
- Withdraw the needle.
- Do not resheath the needle and immediately dispose of it into the sharps bin.
- Use a gauze swab to apply gentle pressure to the injection site, as required.
- Make the patient comfortable.
- Dispose of clinical waste.

- Remove gloves and wash hands.
- Record the administration.
- Monitor the effect of treatment.

Practice tips

- When selecting an appropriate needle size, assess the patient before administration to determine their muscle mass and depth of subcutaneous tissue.
- The advice regarding skin cleaning with alcohol-impregnated swabs before intramuscular injection is varied and your local policy should be followed.
- When introducing the needle, ensure that part of the needle remains proud of the skin before injection.
- Slow injection enables gradual expansion of muscle fibres and reduces discomfort.
- Selecting a larger-gauge needle reduces the pressure required for injection and can be less painful than a smaller-gauge needle.

Table 6.1 Sites for intramuscular injection

Injection site	Typical volume	Notes
• Deltoid	0.5–1mL	Easily accessible. Only suitable for small-volume drugs, such as vaccination.
• Ventrogluteal	1–3mL	Free from major blood vessels and nerves. Predictable depth of subcutaneous fat.
• Dorsogluteal	1–4mL	Slowest rate of absorption, some risk of causing sciatic nerve damage and risk of subcutaneous injection because the fat layer can be deep.
• Vastus lateralis	1–4mL	Easily accessible and free from major blood vessels and nerves. Inject into the middle one-third.
• Rectus femoris	1–3mL	Easily accessible and free from major blood vessels and nerves. Inject into the middle one-third. The site might be more painful.

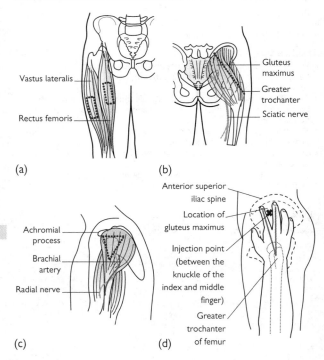

Fig. 6.2 Intramusuclar injection sites: (a) vastus lateralis and rectus femoris; (b) gluteus medius; (c) deltoid, (d) ventrogluteal.

Intramuscular injection 2

Z-track technique

A technique that helps to prevent the leakage of injected medicine into the superficial tissues. It is particularly useful when injecting irritant drugs or medications that might cause skin discolouration. The procedure is similar to that for intramuscular injection.

Procedure

- Decontaminate your hands.
- Explain the procedure and gain consent.
- Check and confirm the prescription. See principles of drug administration 📖 on p.128.
- Put on the non-sterile gloves.
- Draw up and prepare the injection.
- Label the syringe with the name of the drug it contains.
- Check and confirm the patient's identity.
- Position the patient and expose the preferred site for injection.
- If indicated clean the skin using an alcohol-impregnated swab and allow to dry for a minimum of 30sec.
- Use your little finger and the ulnar surface of your non-dominant hand to retract the skin over the injection site.
- While maintaining traction, introduce the needle into the muscle at 90° to the skin.
- Support the hub of the needle/lower part of the syringe with your non-dominant hand.
- Gently withdraw the plunger and observe for any blood entering the syringe. (If blood is observed, withdraw needle and recommence procedure.)
- Slowly inject the drug and wait 10sec for it to disperse.
- Withdraw the needle.
- Release the traction and the skin will return to its pre-injection position, thereby causing a kink (Z-track) in the injection–needle track.
- Do not resheath the needle and immediately dispose of it into the sharps bin.
- Use a gauze swab to apply gentle pressure to the injection site, as required.
- Make the patient comfortable.
- Dispose of clinical waste.
- Remove gloves and wash your hands.
- Record the administration.
- Monitor the effect of treatment.

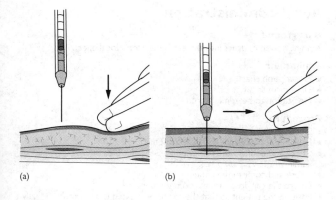

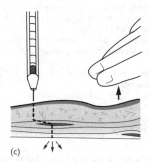

Fig. 6.3 Z-track intramuscular injection technique.

Aural administration

Background

Administration of drugs into the ear is used for a local effect.

Equipment

- Prescription chart.
- Drug formulary.
- Medication to be administered.

Procedure

- Decontaminate your hands.
- Explain the procedure and gain consent.
- Check and confirm the prescription. See principles of drug administration 📖 on p.128.
- Check and confirm the patient's identity.
- Ensure the ear drops are at room temperature.
- Position the patient so that the ear to be treated is uppermost. (Ideally with the patient lying on their side with the head resting on a pillow).
- Gently pull on the pinna to open up the ear canal. (Apply traction in an upwards and backwards direction for an adult and downwards and backwards direction for a child.)
- Administer the prescribed number of drops.
- Maintain traction on the pinna until the medication is seen to run into the ear.
- Ask the patient to remain on their side for a minimum of 2min.
- Make the patient comfortable.
- Discard the equipment using clinical waste disposal.
- Decontaminate your hands.
- Record the administration.
- Monitor the effect of treatment.

Practice tips

- Avoid touching the ear with the medication bottle/dropper.
- Cotton wool might be needed to prevent leakage of the drug from the ear canal.

Nasal administration

Background

Drugs are usually administered into the nose for a local topical effect, e.g. decongestants and topical steroids. However, the intranasal route is also used for systemic drug absorption in a limited number of conditions, e.g. desmopressin for the treatment of diabetes insipidus. Nasal medication is normally administered as drops or a spray.

Equipment (Nasal drops)

- Prescription chart.
- Drug formulary.
- Medication to be administered.
- Tissues.

Procedure

- Decontaminate your hands.
- Explain the procedure and gain consent.
- Unless contraindicated, ask the patient to blow their nose.
- Check and confirm the prescription. See principles of drug administration 📖 on p.128.
- Check and confirm the patient's identity.
- Position the patient supine, with their head extended over the end of the bed and tilted back.
- Support the patient's head and administer the prescribed number of drops to the nose.
- Ask the patient to remain in position for 2min and breathe through their mouth.
- Make the patient comfortable and offer a tissue.
- Discard the equipment using clinical waste disposal.
- Clean the dispenser.
- Decontaminate your hands.
- Record the administration.
- Monitor the effect of treatment.

Practice tips

- Avoid contaminating the dropper by touching the external nares.
- Pushing gently upwards on the tip of the nose might aid administration.
- Nasal drops should not be instilled with the patient in a sitting/standing position with the head simply tilted back.
- Alternative positions for instilling nasal drops include kneeling with head downwards and supported on the floor or standing and bending forwards with the head low.

Nasal spray

Equipment
- Prescription chart.
- Drug formulary.
- Medication to be administered.
- Tissues.

Procedure
- Decontaminate your hands.
- Explain the procedure and gain consent.
- Unless contraindicated, ask the patient to blow their nose.
- Check and confirm the prescription. See principles of drug administration 📖 on p.128.
- Check and confirm the patient's identity.
- Shake the medication bottle (if the spray is new or hasn't been used for more than 7 days then it will be necessary to clear the jet mechanism by spraying into the air while pointing the spray away from the body and face).
- Position the patient by getting them to tilt the head forward such that the patient is looking at their toes.
- Occlude the other nostril by pressing on the side of the nose with a finger.
- Position fingers with index and middle finger at top and thumb at base of spray (see Fig 6.4).
- Keep the bottle vertical and insert the tip (approx 1cm) of the nasal spray into the nostril.
- Ask the patient to breathe in slowly through their nose and as they do so deliver the spray ensuring that it is not sprayed directly onto the nasal septum.
- Patient should then exhale through their mouth.
- Tilt the head backward such that the medication drains toward the back of the nose.
- Repeat if a second dose is required or if administration is indicated for second nostril.
- Clean nozzle using a clean tissue and replace dust cap.
- Make the patient comfortable and offer a tissue.
- Dispose of clinical waste and clean the dispenser.
- Decontaminate your hands.
- Record the administration.

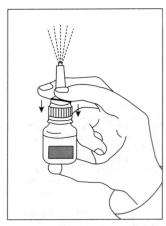

Fig. 6.4 Nasal spray showing finger position. From patient information leaflet for Beconase® Aqueous Nasal spray. Reproduced with permission of GlaxoSmithkline.

Practice tips

- Advise the patient to avoid blowing their nose after using the spray.
- Dismantle and clean the applicator and nozzle at least once a week in warm water. The applicator should then be allowed to air dry.

Pitfall

- Trying to clear a blocked applicator nozzle with a pin or similar object. This can change the aperture size and the dose administered.

Topical and transdermal administration

Background

Topical medications are absorbed through the epidermal layer into the dermis. The rate of absorption is largely determined by the vascularity of the area and condition of the epidermis. Topical administration of creams, pastes and ointment is commonly used for a local effect—e.g. hydrocortisone for treatment of eczema. Alternatively, dermal patches can be used to ensure a slow release of the drug into the systemic circulation—e.g. glyceryl trinitrate for angina management.

Topical, cream, paste, and ointment
Equipment

- Prescription chart.
- Drug formulary.
- Medication to be administered.
- Applicator, as appropriate.
- Sterile gauze.
- Non-sterile gloves (sterile if applying to an open wound).
- Dressing, as required.

Procedure

- Decontaminate your hands.
- Before administering new medication, the previous medication should be removed, as appropriate.
- Explain the procedure and gain consent.
- Check and confirm the prescription. See principles of drug administration ⬚ on p.128.
- Check and confirm the patient's identity.
- Position the patient and expose the site for application.
- Measure the required volume of drug onto a gloved finger or gauze swab.
- Apply the medication.
- Apply a covering dressing, if required.
- Make the patient comfortable.
- Discard the equipment using clinical waste disposal.
- Decontaminate your hands.
- Record the administration.
- Monitor the effect of treatment.

Practice tips

- Apply the cream in the direction of hair growth.
- If the medication is applied to an open wound, for example a burn, the application should be performed aseptically.

Transdermal patch
Equipment
- Prescription chart.
- Drug formulary.
- Medication to be administered.

Procedure
- Decontaminate your hands.
- Explain the procedure and gain consent.
- Check and confirm the prescription. See principles of drug administration 🕮 on p.128.
- Check and confirm the patient's identity.
- Position the patient and assess the site for application.
- Remove body hair, by clipping, as required.
- Remove the previous patch, as required.
- Clean and dry the skin.
- Apply the new patch using firm pressure.
- Discard the equipment using clinical waste disposal.
- Decontaminate your hands.
- Record the administration.
- Monitor the effect of treatment.

Practice tips
- Avoid application of patches below the knee or elbow.
- Rotate the site of application.
- Remove transdermal nitrate patches prior to defibrillation.

Pitfall
- Applying transdermal patches to areas of broken skin or sites of high movement, e.g. joints.

Vaginal (PV) administration

Background

Drugs are administered through the PV route for a local topical effect—e.g. the application of topical hormone replacement therapy (estriol), antifungals (clotrimazole), or antibacterials (metronidazole). Vaginal drugs must be placed high within the vagina to ensure that the whole vaginal mucosa is coated. Drugs administered via the PV route are usually administered as a cream or pessary and supplied with an applicator to facilitate administration.

Equipment

- Prescription chart.
- Drug formulary.
- Medication to be administered and applicator.
- Water-soluble lubricant.
- Non-sterile gloves.
- Gauze.
- Sanitary pad/panty liner.

Procedure

- Decontaminate your hands.
- Explain the procedure and gain consent.
- Ask the patient to void urine.
- Check and confirm the prescription. See principles of drug administration 📖 on p.128.
- Check and confirm the patient's identity.
- Position the patient supine, with their legs flexed and extended apart.
- Decontaminate hands and put on gloves.
- Prepare the medication and applicator by following manufacturer's instructions.
- Use the gauze to lubricate the applicator with water-soluble gel, as appropriate.
- Expose as little of the perineum as possible.
- Insert the applicator into the vagina and release the drug.
- Remove the applicator.
- Remove any excess drug and make the patient comfortable.
- Discard the equipment using clinical waste disposal.
- Remove gloves and wash your hands.
- Record the administration.
- Monitor the effect of treatment.

Practice tips

- Drugs administered PV should ideally be administered at night when the patient will be lying flat.
- Initially insert the applicator downwards and towards the back wall of the vagina, before tilting it forwards and towards the cervix.
- The aim should be to apply the medication as high within the vagina as is comfortable.
- If the medication is not administered at night, the patient should lie flat for at least 20–30min post administration. A panty liner might also be required.
- If appropriate, encourage the patient to self-administer medication.

Pitfall

- The use of tampons immediately following PV drug administration.

Entonox

Background

Entonox is a 50% oxygen and 50% nitrous oxide mixture. Nitrous oxide is a powerful analgesic, with euphoriant and anxiolytic properties. Its use is indicated in the management of acute trauma, labour, and in procedures in which pain is predicted—e.g. burns, wound-dressing changes, suturing, and wound debridement. It is also useful if short-term pain relief is required to facilitate comprehensive physical assessment. Entonox is self-administered through a mouthpiece or face mask.

Equipment

- Prescription chart.
- Drug formulary.
- Gas cylinder and breathing circuit.
- Mouthpiece or face mask, as appropriate.
- Antibacterial filter.

Procedure

- Decontaminate your hands.
- Explain the procedure and gain consent.
- Check and confirm the prescription. See principles of drug administration 📖 on p.128.
- Turn on the cylinder and check the volume gauge.
- Assemble the circuit with the antibacterial filter and mouthpiece or face mask.
- Test the function of the equipment and prime the circuit—press the demand/test button.
- Check and confirm the patient's identity.
- Demonstrate the technique for use.
- Allow the patient to self-administer.
- Encourage the patient to breath normally.
- Ensure an airtight seal around the mask/mouthpiece.
- Monitor the effects.
- Allow a minimum of 2min before commencing any other procedure.
- Discard the equipment using clinical waste disposal.
- Decontaminate your hands.
- Record the administration.
- Monitor the effect of treatment.

Practice tips

- Ensure the area is well ventilated and that no smoking/naked flame precautions are being observed.
- The patient should not have eaten for 1 hour before administration.
- Monitor oxygen saturation (SpO_2) if there is any underlying or suspected cardiac or respiratory pathology.
- The patient should not walk until any dizziness or disorientation is resolved.
- The patient should not drive or operate machinery for the first 12 hours after administration.
- If use is continued for >24 hours, monitor red blood cells for signs of megaloblastic anaemia and white blood cells for leukopaenia.

Pitfalls

- Using grease or other oil-based products on the cylinder or breathing circuit.
- Using nitrous oxide in the following situations:
  - Head injuries with impairment of consciousness.
  - Artificial, traumatic, or spontaneous pneumothorax.
  - Air embolism.
  - Decompression sickness.
  - Severe bullous emphysema.
  - Gross abdominal distension.
  - Intoxication.
  - Maxillofacial injuries.
  - Following a recent underwater dive.
  - Following air encephelography.
  - During myringoplasty.

Drug calculations

Metric/System Internationale (SI) units
Weight

> 1000 grams (g) = 1 kilogram (kg)
> 1000 milligrams (mg) = 1g
> 1000 micrograms = 1mg
> 1000 nanograms = 1 microgram

Volume

> 1000 millilitres (mL) = 1 litre (L)
> 1000 microlitres = 1mL

Tablets and capsules
Before starting, you must know the following:
- The dose of drug prescribed.
- The dose of drug per individual tablet/capsule.

$$\text{Calculation} = \frac{\text{dose required}}{\text{dose per tablet/capsule}}$$

Example

You must give 250 micrograms of digoxin (dose required) and stock tablets contain 62.5 micrograms (dose per tablet)

$$\frac{250}{62.5} = 4 \text{ tablets}$$

Liquids and syrups
Before starting you must know the following:
- The dose of drug prescribed
- The dose of drug in the stated volume of liquid/syrup

$$\text{Calculation} = \frac{\text{dose required}}{\text{dose of drug in stated volume of liquid}} \times \text{volume of liquid}$$

Example

You must give 75 mg of chloramphenicol syrup (dose required).
The stock solution contains 125 mg (dose of drug) in 5 mL (volume)

$$\frac{75}{125} \times 5 = 3 \text{ mL}$$

Infusion drip rate

Before starting you must know the following
- The type of infusion set and how many drops per 1mL it delivers.
- The total volume to be infused.
- Number of hours the infusion is prescribed over.

$$\frac{\text{total volume in millilitres}}{\text{Number of hours}} \times \frac{\text{number of drops per ml}}{60 \text{ (minutes)}}$$

Example

1000 mL of sodium chloride 0.9% solution (total volume) to be infused over 10 hours (number of hours) using a crystalloid giving set that delivers 15 drops per 1 mL (number of drops per mL).

$$\frac{1000}{10} \times \frac{15}{60} = \frac{15000}{600} = 25 \text{ drops per minute}$$

Percentages

This is most commonly used when dealing with liquids—e.g. intravenous fluids and some injections.

The amount of substance is expressed as the weight in grams (w) per 100mL volume (v). This will be shown as (w/v).

Example

Glucose 5% solution will contain 5g (w) of glucose per 100mL (v). Thus, a 1L (1000mL) bag of glucose 5% solution contains 50g of glucose.

Ratios

These are less common, but are used, for example, when prescribing epinephrine (adrenaline):
- Adrenaline 1:1000.
- Adrenaline 1:10 000.

This means that there is 1g of drug in the given volume in millilitres.

Example

Adrenaline 1:1000 contains 1g of adrenaline in 1000mL (1L) or 1mg/mL.
Adrenaline 1:10 000 contains 1g of adrenaline in 10 000mL (10L), 1mg/10mL or 100 micrograms/mL.

Peripheral intravenous access and care

Bob Tudor
Clinical Nurse Trainer and Senior Staff Nurse, Emergency
Department, Nottingham University Hospitals NHS Trust, UK

Venepuncture

Background

Venepuncture involves taking blood from a peripheral vein. Vacutainer® systems are the most commonly used method. A needle and syringe can also be used.

Equipment

- Disposable apron and non-sterile disposable gloves.
- Alcohol hand rub.
- Tourniquet.
- Isopropyl alcohol-impregnated swab.
- Cotton wool balls.
- Sterile hypoallergenic dressing.
- Needle for venepuncture system (usually 21G for adults).
- Plastic needle holder.
- Specimen bottles/vacutainers®.
- Specimen forms and transport bags.
- Sharps disposal bin.

Procedure

- Explain procedure and gain consent.
- Wash and dry your hands.
- Put on non-sterile gloves.
- Select an appropriate vein.
- Attach the needle to the plastic needle holder.
- Support the patient's arm on a protective pillow, if available.
- Apply tourniquet approximately 10cm proximal to venepuncture site.
- Rotate the limb to visualize and palpate the area.
- Clean the area with an isopropyl impregnated alcohol swab using circular motions outwards from the proposed venepuncture site.
- Allow to dry passively for 30 sec.
- Stretch the skin over the vein with the thumb of one hand.
- Insert the needle, bevel up, into the vessel at an angle of 30–45°.
- Stabilize the needle and specimen holder with the thumb, index finger, and middle finger of one hand.
- Insert the specimen bottle and observe for blood flow.
- When there is sufficient blood in the bottle remove from the needle holder and invert the bottle to ensure mixing with additives.
- Obtain further samples as required.
- When all the samples have been collected, release the tourniquet.
- Cover the needle with cotton wool.
- Withdraw the needle.
- Keep the limb extended and apply firm pressure for 30–60 sec. You can ask the patient to maintain the pressure.
- Check the site—if clotted apply sterile hypoallergenic dressing (if not clotted apply pressure for a further minute. Observe and repeat until clotted).
- Dispose of the needle and any contaminated waste in the appropriate container.

- Complete the labels on the blood samples before leaving the patient, checking the details with the patient and against the request forms.
- Apply 'high risk' labels if appropriate (e.g. hep B/HIV risk).
- Document episode of care.

Practice tips
- Ask the patient if they have had blood taken previously. They may be aware of the best site available and of particular problems encountered, e.g. fainting.
- Spend time selecting a suitable vein. This is time well spent.
- Clenching and unclenching the patient's fist can help but can cause a minor alteration in test results.
- Palpation is often better than visualization. Veins are firm and bouncy to the touch, tendons are ropey.
- Consider topical anaesthesia in needle phobic and anxious patients.
- Avoid veins that are fibrosed, inflamed, or fragile. Avoid veins in bruised or infected areas. Avoid the same limb as an arteriovenous (AV) shunt.
- A tourniquet should not be applied to an arm that has undergone lymphoid surgery (e.g. axillary clearance for breast cancer). The patient will have been counselled about this and will usually inform you.
- Insert the needle smoothly and rapidly. Slow penetration of skin is very painful. Ask the patient to take a deep breath as you insert the needle to distract them.
- The tourniquet should be applied firmly enough to produce venous distention by impeding venous return but still allowing arterial flow. Check for a pulse.
- If the tourniquet has been on for more than 2 min prior to inserting the needle, release and allow blood to return to the hand before reapplying.
- If a venous valve is entered during the procedure, the patient will feel sudden, acute pain. Observe the patient throughout the procedure for signs of dizziness, fainting, or paraesthesiae.
- If using a syringe the plunger should be pulled back gently to create a steady suction. Pulling the plunger forcefully increases the risk of the vein collapsing.
- When taking blood for drug or hormone levels, or fasting samples, check with the patient the time and dose of last medication or time last food or drink was taken. This information is essential for assessment of drug efficacy and accurate diagnoses.
- Be aware of local policies and guidelines concerning needlestick injuries and contamination with blood.
- A needle and syringe is better for venepuncture in patients with difficult veins as gentle suction will demonstrate blood in the needle when the vein is entered.

Pitfalls
- Puncturing an artery, e.g. the brachial artery in the antecubital fossa—release the tourniquet and apply firm pressure for at least 3–4 min if this occurs. Check pulse and sensation distally. Document the incident.
- Taking blood from a vein on the same limb as an IV infusion, resulting in contaminated results.
- Forgetting to release the tourniquet before removing the needle from the arm resulting in spillage of blood.

Preparing for insertion of a peripheral IV cannula

Background

A peripheral IV cannula allows and maintains IV access. It enables the patient to receive fluids, medication, blood, and blood products. The shortest and smallest gauge cannula appropriate for the indication should be used. Large-gauge cannulae may be required for the administration of viscous fluids/drugs and in shocked patients, particularly in hypovolaemic shock following trauma. It is worth spending time finding a suitable vein and site for insertion of the cannula.

Equipment

- Disposable apron.
- Alcohol hand rub.
- IV cannula of appropriate size.
- Non-sterile disposable gloves.
- Procedure tray.
- Tourniquet.
- Isopropyl alcohol-impregnated swabs.

Procedure

- Choose an appropriately sized IV cannula and have a spare cannula of the same size on the procedure tray.
- Explain procedure and gain consent.
- Wash and dry your hands.
- If possible select the patient's non-dominant arm and the most distal site for initial cannulation (except in a trauma patient where larger proximal veins are used).
- Select an appropriate vein. Ideally the vein should feel soft and bouncy and refill quickly following compression. Metacarpal, cephalic, and basilic veins are best as they are long and straight with large lumens. Avoid bruised, painful, burnt, or infected skin and mobile, tortuous, or thrombosed veins. Limbs with fractures, oedematous extremities and the affected limb in a stroke patient should be avoided if possible. Also avoid an arm that has undergone axillary lymphoid surgery.
- Areas of flexion may compromise flow into the vein and increase catheter movement which adds to the risk of infection.
- Clean visibly dirty skin with soap and water.
- Apply the tourniquet.
- If there is no obvious suitable vein encourage venous distension by stroking veins with your fingertips or gently tapping over them.
- Palpate and assess the selected vein again for its suitability.
- Clean the area of proposed insertion with an isopropyl alcohol impregnated swab moving outwards with circular motions. Allow to dry passively for 30 sec.
- Insert the cannula. (📖 on p. 164)

Practice tips

- Ask the patient if they have had previous venous cannulations. They may be aware of the best site available and of particular problems encountered, e.g. fainting.
- Practise palpating veins wearing gloves to increase the sensitivity of your fingers.
- Removal of hair is only necessary if adhesion of the sterile dressing to the skin is in doubt. Only use scissors.
- Avoid shaving the insertion site because this causes microabsorptions. This is the risk of bacterial colorisation and subsequent infection. Put the patient's limb in warm water if you are having difficulty locating a vein. This will cause vasodilatation and should make it easier to palpate a vein.
- Consider the use of topical anaesthesia for patient comfort.
- For large-bore cannulae (>18G), consider injecting local anesthetic subcutaneously with a 25G needle at the site where you wish to puncture with the cannula.

Pitfalls

- Depending on vision rather than palpation in choosing a vein.
- Choosing a site that will potentially interfere with flow of fluids and/ or cause pain to the patient when other more appropriate sites are accessible.

Insertion of a peripheral IV cannula

Background
(📖 on p. 162)

Equipment
- Appropriately sized IV cannula (see Table 7.1).
- Sterile cannula dressing.
- 5 mL sterile saline and syringe.
- Luer cap ('bung') or prepared IV infusion.
- Cotton wool.
- Sharps bin.

Procedure
- Assemble equipment, choose a vein and prepare the site for insertion of the cannula. (📖 on p. 162)
- Put on gloves.
- For the remainder of the procedure do not repalpate the vein or touch surrounding cleaned skin after disinfection.
- Remove the cannula with its contained trocar (needle) from the packaging and inspect for any faults.
- Remove the luer cap from the cannula and place it in a sterile package ensuring aseptic non-touch technique.
- Stabilize the vein by applying manual traction on the skin.
- Ensure the needle is in the 'bevel up' position and place the device over the vein.
- Insert the cannula and needle at the selected angle (10–45°) according to the depth of the vein.
- Observe for the first flashback of blood into the flashback chamber of the needle. Level the cannula/needle by decreasing the angle between the cannula and the skin.
- After the flashback is observed slowly advance the cannula and needle a few millimetres to ensure entry into the vein.
- Withdraw the needle from the cannula slightly and a second flashback of blood should be seen along the shaft of the cannula. *Never reinsert the needle.*
- Maintaining skin traction, slowly advance the cannula off the needle into the vein, keeping the needle very steady at all times.
- When the cannula is inserted release the tourniquet.
- Apply gentle but firm pressure to the vein at the distal end of the cannula tip and then remove the needle.
- Dispose of the needle in the sharps bin.
- Attach a luer lock hub, extension set, or prepared infusion set.
- Apply an appropriate sterile IV dressing (📖 p.168) ensuring the entry site is visible. If using an infusion set the tubing should be secured in a loop with hypoallergenic adhesive tape.
- Record the date of cannula insertion on the dressing.
- Decontaminate your hands.
- Flush cannula with 5 mL 0.9% sodium chloride to ensure patency.

- Observe the site for swelling or leakage and ask the patient if any discomfort or pain is felt.
- Under normal circumstances, in order to prevent unnecessary trauma to the patient, only two attempts should be made, using a new cannula at each attempt. However, in an emergency situation where intravenous access is essential and no-one else is available more attempts or alternative access to the circulation (e.g. intraosseus) will be required.
- Document the episode of care including the size of cannula used and the date, time, site, and number of attempts (if more than one).
- The insertion site should be observed for signs of phlebitis or infection twice daily. A 'phlebitis scoring tool' may be used.
- Cannulae should be flushed with 0.9% sodium chloride at least daily to ensure patency and pre- and post-drug administration.
- Contamination through the use of additional connections is common, therefore, as few connections as possible should be connected to the cannulae. 3-way taps should be avoided.
- Cannulae should usually not be left in situ for more than 72 hours because of the risk of infection.

Practice tips

- Palpate the vein before every cannulation, even if the vein looks easy to cannulate. The vein may be thrombosed and impossible to cannulate. Thrombosed veins feel hard.
- If possible enter a vein at the point of bifurcation with another vein. This provides a larger target.
- Avoid the large cephalic vein at the level of the wrist. Insert cannula 10 cm or more proximal to the wrist.
- Insert the cannula smoothly and rapidly. Slow penetration of skin is very painful. Ask the patient to take a deep breath as you insert the cannula to distract them.

Pitfalls

- Forgetting to release the tourniquet before the trocar needle is removed with resultant dribbling of blood.
- Leaving the trocar needle on the floor or in the patient's bed. Always dispose of sharps immediately.
- Breaking asepsis by leaving the luer cap in an unsterile surrounding.
- Reinserting trocar needle causing shearing of plastic cannula sheath and potential embolization.
- Reinserting the same cannula after an aborted attempt, increasing the risk of infection.
- Puncturing an artery. Release tourniquet and apply firm pressure for at least 3–4 min if this occurs.
- Puncturing a nerve. Be aware—nerves are located close to the superficial veins, especially in the wrist and antecubital fossa. Complaints of tingling, pins and needles sensation, or numbness suggest that a nerve may have been damaged. Remove the cannula immediately and choose another site. Document and report the incident.

Table 7.1 Commonly used cannulae in adults

Gauge (G)	Flow rate (mL/hr)	Colour
14	270	Brown
16	230	Grey
18	100	Green
20	65	Pink

Changing a peripheral IV cannula dressing

Background

A sterile, hypoallergenic, transparent, semi-permeable dressing should be used to secure a cannula to prevent it moving around in the vein. If at any time a dressing becomes loose or moist it must be replaced.

Equipment

- Transparent semi-permeable dressing.
- Sterile gloves.
- Sachet of sterile sodium chloride or water.
- Sterile gauze swabs.
- Procedure tray.

Procedure

- Explain procedure and gain consent.
- Wash hands.
- Open all packages after inspecting for damage and checking expiry dates.
- Decontaminate hands and put on sterile gloves.
- Hold the cannula in place with your non-dominant hand.
- Remove the old dressing.
- Assess for infection (pain, redness, pus), infiltration (area cool with blanching, oedema), and thrombophlebitis (vein firm tender with redness along its course, oedema). If any of these are present the cannula should be removed.
- If the site is okay cover it with a transparent semi-permeable dressing.
- Remove gloves.
- Discard equipment and perform hand hygiene.
- Observe function and patency of cannula following dressing change.
- Document episode of care.

Practice tips

- Be careful not to dislodge the cannula when removing the dressing. Peel dressing in the direction that the cannula is inserted.
- In general bandages should not be used to cover peripheral cannulae. They may be a necessity however in paediatric and confused patients who are likely to dislodge the cannula. The bandage should be removed at least once a day, to inspect the insertion site.

Removal of a peripheral IV cannula

Background
Maintenance of IV sites and systems involves regular assessment and systematic rotation of the cannula site. Peripheral cannulae should be re-sited every 72 hours to minimize the risk of phlebitis and infection. They should be removed immediately if the patient has phlebitis or infection or if they are deemed no longer necessary.

Equipment
- Non-sterile gloves.
- Gauze swab.
- Sterile dressing.
- Hypoallergenic tape.

Procedure
- Explain procedure and gain consent.
- Wash hands.
- Put on gloves.
- Hold a piece of sterile gauze over the insertion site.
- Remove the cannula with a slow steady movement to prevent damage to the vein. Keep the hub parallel to the skin.
- Check the cannula and insertion site for signs of infection (erythema, pus). Send the cannula tip for culture if there are any present.
- Apply pressure to the cannula site after its removal to prevent bleeding. Gentle pressure should be applied for at least 1 min, longer if the patient is receiving anticoagulant therapy.
- Elevate the limb if the bleeding persists.
- A sterile dressing should be used to cover the cannula site and secured with hypoallergenic tape.
- Discard the equipment using clinical waste disposal.
- Decontaminate hands.
- Document the episode of care including the time, date, and rationale for intervention.
- If sending a cannula tip for culture, swab the surrounding skin and any pus before removing the cannula. Then clean the skin with an isopropyl alcohol-impregnated swab and allow it to dry to decrease the risk of contaminating the cannula tip as it is removed. After removal of the cannula, snip 1 cm from the tip with a sterile scissors into a sterile container.
- Label the container and send it to the laboratory for culture and sensitivity with an appropriately filled in request form.

Practice tip
- If the patient has extremely poor venous access and there is a need for continuing IV therapy, the cannula can be left *in situ* for more than 72 hours (this should be discussed with the treating medical team).

Pitfall
- Using scissors to cut the dressing. This carries the risk of cutting the cannula and losing it in the circulation.

Preparation for IV therapy

Background

The administration of IV fluids, blood products and medications is one of the most important nursing responsibilities. As the solutions are being introduced directly into the bloodstream, the risk of iatrogenic complications is extremely high.

Equipment

- Drip stand.
- Giving set.
- IV fluid as prescribed.
- Fluid balance chart.
- Label for giving set.
- Sterile hypoallergenic tape.

Procedure

- Prime and attach the IV administration set in a clean utility area where possible.
- Check the expiry date and packaging of the administration set. Dispose of the administration set if the date has expired or the packaging is not intact.
- Check the 'drop factor' of the IV administration set on the packaging (📖 on p. 178).
- Examine the packaging of the prescribed fluid for any defects. Examine bottles for hairline cracks.
- Examine the fluid contents for discolouration and for particles by gently shaking the container.
- Check the IV fluid with the prescription with a second nurse or doctor. Check the expiry date.
- Remove the outer wrapper and hang the IV fluid on the drip stand.
- Move the clamp of the giving set to the top of the tubing by the drip chamber and close.
- Use an aseptic non-touch technique (ANTT) when handling the catheter hub, connections ports, and sterile parts of the administration set.
- Decontaminate your hands with alcohol gel hand rub.
- Remove protective covers from the insertion site of the infusion fluid and from the spike of the giving set.
- Without touching the newly exposed areas hold the IV fluid container with one hand and, using a twisting action, insert the spike of the giving set into the insertion port.
- Prime by gently squeezing the drip chamber until half full, holding the free luer end (with cap in place) above the level of the fluid container. Slowly open the clamp, the tubing will fill with the solution. Slowly lower the free luer end, until the tubing is full.
- Close the clamp and place the free luer end of the tubing into the notch provided on the clamp.
- Avoid contact with non-sterile surfaces.
- Decontaminate hands.
- Proceed to patient to set up infusion (see p.176).

Practice tip
- The inside of the giving set is sterilized by free circulation of ethylene oxide gas. If the clamp is found in a closed position discard the giving set.

Calculation of infusion rates

Background

Infusion rates for IV therapy are calculated as drops per minute. Accurate calculation is essential as miscalculation can cause serious harm and even result in death. IV Fluids are prescribed as the total volume over a defined period of time (e.g. IL of 0.9% saline over 8 hours). Different IV administration sets are calibrated differently and have a different number of drops per milliliter (mL) or gtt/mL (see Table 7.2). These are two basic types of IV administration sets: macrodrip (delivers 10, 15, or 20 drops per min) and microdrip (delivers 60 drops per min). The formula for calculating infusion rate is the same regardless of the type of set you use.

Procedure

Calculation of infusion rate

Infusion rate = Volume of infusion (in mL)/time of infusion (in min)
e.g. for 1L of 0.9% saline over 8 hours
Infusion rate = 1000 mLs / 480 min = 2.08mLs / min

Calculation of infuse rate in drops

The formula for the calculation of infusion rate in drops is
Volume of infusion (mL) ÷ time of infusion (min) x drop factor for the giving set being used
e.g. The infusion rate for 1 Litre of 0.9% Saline over 8 hours in a standard IV giving set with a drop factor of 20 would be
1000 (volume of infusion) ÷ 480 mins (time of infusion) x 20 (drop factor) = 41.66 drops. Therefore 42 drops per minute should be administered.

Practice tips

- Do not rely on mental arithmetic. Use a pen and paper or a calculator to check calculations. Check the calculation with a colleague
- Ask yourself if the figure arrived at seems sensible for the clinical scenario and recheck if it doesn't.

Table 7.2 Drop factors for administration sets

Administration set	gtt/mL
Standard giving set for clear fluids (crystalloid)	20
Blood giving set (colloid)	15
Burette type giving set	60

Connecting an IV infusion to a cannula

Background
The prescribed fluids are connected to the IV cannula via the administration set.

Equipment
- Primed IV infusion.
- Drip stand.
- A saline flush (10mL syringe).
- Hypoallergenic tape.

Procedure
- Explain procedure and gain consent.
- Check the patient's name and hospital number with the prescription card.
- Check the prescription and the rate of infusion.
- Check the patency of the IV cannula using a saline flush.
- Decontaminate hands.
- Clean the access point using an isopropyl-impregnated swab or povidone–iodine solution before accessing the system.
- Using an aseptic technique, remove the cap from the luer end of the giving set, ensuring that the exposed end is not contaminated.
- Elevate the patient's arm and remove the cap from the cannula and attach the luer end of the giving set.
- Open the roller clamp to regulate the flow rate as prescribed. It can be regulated manually or by an infusion controller.
- Secure the giving set to the patient's limb by looping the IV tubing and securing with hypoallergenic tape.
- Label the giving set with the date and time the IV was set up.
- Sign the prescription card and record the batch number and the time that the IV fluid was commenced.
- Record on the fluid balance chart.
- Document episode of care.
- If administering drugs use the latex membrane on peripheral lines and avoid the use of ports.

Practice tips
- The inside of the giving set is sterilized by free circulation of ethylene chloride gas. If the clamp is found in a closed position discard the giving set.
- Do not use blood-giving sets to administer other solutions.
- Clean the connections prior to manipulation of the set.
- Keep manipulation of connections to a minimum.
- Ensure that the cannula and line are adequately secured.
- Administer IV drugs through the latex membrane on peripheral lines. Avoid the use of ports.

Pitfalls
- Using solutions to dilute drugs which are incompatible with the infusion fluid.
- Not securing the cannula and line adequately leading to movement which can cause leakage and phlebitis due to irritation.
- Not labelling the giving set with the time and date.

Regulation of IV infusion rates

Background

It is vital to maintain accurate infusion rates for solutions. Infusion rates are maintained using infusion control devices such as clamps or volumetric pumps. A standard IV administration set includes a drip chamber and a roller clamp. It depends on gravity to ensure the flow of solution. The infusion rate is adjusted with the roller clamp. If the fluid runs too fast the patient (particularly the young and old) may develop circulatory overload and pulmonary oedema or adverse drug reactions. Slow infusion can predispose to dehydration, inadequate response to drug therapy, or blockage of the cannula from blood clot. Pumps offer increased accuracy but are not necessary for the majority of infusions. They should be used for the infusion of potentially toxic drugs.

Equipment
- Standard IV administration set with roller clamp.
- IV fluid.

Procedure
- Confirm and check the infusion rate (drops per minute) for the patient.
- Ensure the solution is flowing freely through the giving set into the cannula. Ideally the IV fluid should be approximately 1m above the patient to overcome venous pressure.
- Adjust the clamp slowly to the approximate rate and time the infusion for 1min.
- Continue to adjust the roller clamp until the desired rate had been achieved, measured over 1min.
- Discuss with the patient how positioning of IV site affects the flow rate
- Observe regularly for changes in flow rates that require correction. These can occur as a result of changes in venous pressure, changes in the patient's position, bending or kinking of the tubing, an unreliable clamp, blood clotting in the cannula or tubing, or the addition of other inline devices.
- Maintain a fluid balance chart, monitor and record urine output for all patients receiving IV therapy.
- Monitor and record haemodynamic changes—observe for pyrexia and respiratory distress.

Practice tip
- Consider using a volumetric pump (see p. 182) or syringe driver (see p. 184). These should be used when accurate infusion is essential e.g. for potentially toxic drugs.

Changing an IV solution

Background

IV solutions need to be changed when the bag runs out or when solutions have been hanging for more the recommended period. The administration set should be changed every 72 hours or after the administration of blood products. The administration set should be changed every 24 hours when intermittent therapy is being administered through it.

Equipment

- IV infusion fluid.
- Non-sterile gloves.

Procedure

- Collect and check the IV fluid and rate of infusion against the prescription.
- Explain procedure and gain consent.
- Check the patient's name and hospital number with the prescription card at the patient's bedside.
- Close the roller clamp of the administration set.
- Put on gloves.
- Remove the old IV solution from the drip stand.
- Remove the spike of the administration set from the bag and ensure that it does not become contaminated.
- Remove the protective cover from the port of the new bag.
- Place the spike in the port of the new bag.
- Solutions contained in glass bottles should have the administration set inserted after the top of the bottle has been cleaned with an isopropyl-impregnated swab and allowed to dry passively.
- Hang the IV solution container on the drip stand.
- Inspect the tubing to ensure that it is free of air. The drip chamber should remain a third to a half filled.
- Open the clamp and adjust and adjust the flow rate as appropriate.
- Discard the old solution bag using clinical waste disposal.
- Document the episode of care in the clinical notes and on the fluid balance chart.

Pitfall

- Removing the spike without closing the roller clump allowing air to enter the line.

Use of volumetric pumps

Background

Volumetric IV pumps have mechanisms to move solutions along under pressure to deliver fluids and drugs accurately at the desired rate. They are powered by mains or battery. Volumetric pumps are the preferred choice for medium and high flow-rate and large-volume infusions. The rate is selected in millilitres per hour or micrograms per kilogram per hour. There are a variety of devices on the market. You should attend training sessions on how to use the particular pump(s) used in your unit and follow the instruction manual provided by the manufacturer.

Equipment

- IV fluid ± added drug.
- Non-sterile gloves.
- Gloves.
- Drip stand.
- Volumetric pump.
- IV giving set.
- Manufacturer's instruction manual.

Procedure

- Prepare the IV therapy (📖 p. 172).
- Prime the giving set according to the manufacturer's instructions.
- Label the infusion bag if there is a drug additive. Information on the label should include the patient's identity, the name and dose of the drug, the total quantity of fluid, the final concentration of fluid, the date and time the drug was added, your signature, and the signature of a witness.
- Calculate the infusion rate and check it with another health care worker (HCW) (📖 on p. 174)
- Wash and dry your hands.
- Put on gloves.
- Attach the giving set to the volumetric pump as per manufacture's instructions.
- Check that the volumetric pump is attached to the mains or a charged battery.
- At the bedside check the patient's name and hospital number with the prescription card.
- Explain procedure and gain consent.
- Attach giving set to the cannula.
- Key infusion rate into the pump.
- Commence the infusion.
- Document the episode of care.

Practice tip

- As there is a wide variety in volumetric pumps with different modes of operation it is essential to have training and competence assessment. on the device being used.

Pitfalls
- Not setting up infusion correctly, e.g. miscalculating dosages.
- Turning off the alarm settings.
- Pressing the bolus option by mistake.
- Using the device outside of its maintenance date. Devices should have 'maintenance due date' stickers on them.

Use of syringe drivers

Background

Syringe drivers are small, battery-operated infusion pumps. They drive the plunger of a syringe forward at a controlled rate to deliver the fluid/drug to the patient. The rate can be continuous or in boluses. Syringe drivers are designed for lower-volume and low-rate infusions. They are commonly used in palliative care to deliver opiate analgesia and anti-emetics. Other indications include insulin and vasopressor therapy. There are numerous syringe drivers on the market. You should attend training sessions on any syringe driver you might be expected to use. The manufacturers' instructions should be followed.

Equipment

- Syringe pump.
- Giving set.
- Syringe with luer lock.
- Manufacturer's manual.
- Non-sterile gloves.
- IV fluid/drug as per prescription.

Procedure

- Check IV fluid/drugs to be given from prescription with another registered health care worker (HCW).
- Draw up fluid/medication into a luer lock syringe.
- Ensure that the correct brand of syringe is being used.
- Connect the giving set to the syringe.
- Check that the illuminated size of syringe display corresponds to the syringe size loaded.
- Calculate the flow rate and check the calculation with a registered HCW. (📖 on p. 172)
- Label the syringe with the medication contained, the names of the people who prepared and checked the syringe, the time and date prepared, the name and date of birth of the patient.
- Attach the syringe to the syringe driver according to the manufacturer's instructions and secure.
- Ensure the syringe driver is connected to the mains or a charged battery.
- Purge the giving set using the syringe driver.
- At the bedside check the patient's name and hospital number with the prescription card.
- Explain procedure and gain consent.
- Wash and dry hands.
- Put on gloves.
- Connect the giving set to the cannula.
- Cover the site with a semi-permeable dressing and secure the tubing with a non-allergenic tape.
- Key in the infusion rate checking with a registered practitioner.
- Commence infusion.
- Record the machine number in the patient's notes.
- Document the episode of care.

Practice tips

- The infusion must be purged rather than primed.
- Always manipulate the syringe by the barrel and not by the plunger.
- Do not remove the plunger as this reduces the 'stickiness' and decreases the pressure required to push it. The pump, however, will continue at the same pressure and the patient will receive an over-infusion.
- The lines should be clamped when not in use or when changing equipment.
- To prevent a post-occlusion bolus, the line should be clamped and the plunger clamp opened to release the pressure.
- Connect as few connections as possible to the cannulae as contamination through additional connections is common.
- Ensure that the pump is no higher than 70cm above the IV cannula site to prevent siphoning. Most modern syringe drivers have inbuilt anti-siphon systems.

Pitfalls

- Not setting up the infusion correctly, e.g. miscalculating dosages or rate of delivery.
- Turning off the alarm settings.
- Using device outside of its maintenance date. Devices should have 'maintenance due date' stickers on them.

Care of the theatre patient

Rachel Peto
Lecturer, School of Nursing, Midwifery & Physiotherapy,
University of Nottingham, UK

Preoperative care: overview

Background

Preoperative care involves physical, psychological, emotional, and spiritual preparation and support of the patient before surgery. Care takes place from the time a patient decides to have surgery to the time the patient is transferred to and arrives in the operating theatre department. Surgery is either elective (planned) or an emergency.

Elective surgery

Surgical procedures are increasingly performed on the day of admission in a purpose built day-surgery unit or diagnostic treatment centre. Initial preoperative selection and preparation are undertaken in a preadmission/preassessment clinic days or weeks before surgery.

Emergency surgery

Emergency surgery is non-elective surgery performed if the patient's life or well-being is in direct jeopardy. Preoperative care might need to be completed within a timeframe of between a few minutes and a few hours, depending on the patient's condition.

Preoperative care: patient preparation

All preoperative care is aimed at ensuring patients are fully informed and undergo surgery with all potential risks minimized.

Physical preparation

Equipment
- Theatre gown.
- Preoperative care plan.
- Identification bracelet.
- Hypoallergenic tape.
- Containers for dentures and/or hearing aid, if required.
- Equipment to record blood pressure/temperature.
- Patient's medical notes.
- Signed consent.
- Valuables book.

Procedure
- Check the patient's medical and nursing notes for specific instructions.
- Draw the curtains to maintain privacy, if appropriate.
- Ensure the patient is wearing an identification bracelet, with the patient's hospital number and full name—check against the patient's medical notes.
- Ensure the doctor has fully explained the procedure to the patient and that all preoperative information has been fully understood by the patient.
- Ensure that the consent form has been signed, countersigned, and dated.
- Monitor and record the following:
  - Temperature.
  - Pulse.
  - Respiration.
  - Weight.
  - Urinalysis.
- Check the patient has undergone all necessary preoperative examinations and attach the following results to the front of their case notes:
  - X-ray.
  - Blood group.
  - Cross-matching.
- Check and record any allergies the patient has—ask about the following:
  - Medication allergies.
  - Antibiotic allergies.
  - Plaster or tape allergies.
  - Latex allergies—inform the surgeon and theatre staff immediately because the operating theatre might need to be emptied and cleaned if non-latex items are to be used during the procedure.
- Conduct a risk assessment for the following:
  - Compression stockings.
  - Pressure sores.
- Ensure the patient has undergone the appropriate skin preparation.
- Check the surgical site marking—inform the surgeon if this has not been undertaken.

- Check the patient has fasted—the usual criteria for elective surgery are as follows:
  - Drink unlimited amounts of non-carbonated water up to 3 hours preoperatively.
  - No consumption of milk up to 6 hours preoperatively.
  - A light meal can be consumed only up to 6 hours preoperatively.
  - No alcohol consumption within 12 hours preoperatively.
- Encourage the patient to pass urine and open their bowels before any premedication is administered.
- Help the patient to change into the theatre gown.
- Remove prostheses (if appropriate) and document the removal—check for the following:
  - Dentures.
  - Crowns.
  - Caps.
  - Loose teeth.
- Tape the patient's wedding ring with hypoallergenic tape if appropriate.
- Remove any remaining jewellery and record it in the valuables book.
- Leave hearing aid *in situ*.
- Ask the patient to remove all traces of make-up and nail varnish.
- Administer prescribed medication, according to the doctor's orders.
- Advise the patient to remain in bed after administration of premedication—place a call bell within easy reach.
- Ensure that the following accompany patient to the operating theatre department:
  - Medical notes.
  - Investigation results—bloods, scans, X-rays, and electrocardiogram (ECG).
- Ensure the patient is fully supported on the canvas.
- Document the episode of care.

Practice tips

- Consent—must be gained before the patient leaves the ward and before a premedication sedative is administered.
- Showers, rather than baths, are preferable.
- No chewing gum or sweets should be eaten during the fasting period.
- Jewellery of cultural or religious significance can normally be secured.
- If the patient weighs >130kg, check with the theatre staff that suitable equipment is available.
- Fasting in patients with diabetes—check with the anaesthetist; depends on the surgical procedure, length of surgery, and whether the patient is insulin- or non-insulin-dependent.
- If the patient is considered to be 'at risk' following any type of risk assessment, contact the theatre staff to ensure appropriate resources are available.
- It is the responsibility of the registered practitioner who has prepared the patient for theatre to sign the preoperative care plan/checklist.

Pitfalls

- Not gaining consent before the patient receives a premedication sedative.
- Not checking the surgical site marking with the notes to ensure e.g. correct limb etc.

Preparation for day-case surgery

Day-surgery patients are selected on the basis of the following:
- Procedure suitability.
- A predetermined set of criteria—medical, psychological, and social.
- Patients will have undergone a preoperative assessment by the nursing staff before the day of surgery.
- Information will have been given regarding specific preoperative preparation—e.g. fasting.

Physical care

The type of care will depend on whether the surgery is being performed under general or local anaesthetic. Regardless of the type of surgery the following will have to be taken into account:
- Ask the day-surgery patient to put on clean underwear and clothes following a shower.
- Clothing—check with theatre staff whether the patient is having surgery on areas such as the face, neck, arms, or lower legs, which do not usually require underpants to be removed. Disposable pants might be available.
- Fasting—patients are informed of fasting requirements before the day of surgery, but check with the surgeon because fasting is not usually required if the procedure is performed using a local anaesthetic.
- Dentures—need not be removed if the patient is having a local anaesthetic, but document, if present, in case the local anaesthetic is converted to a general anaesthetic during surgery.
- Circulation—encourage patients to walk around before surgery. Patients in day-surgery units often sit for several hours waiting for their surgery.
- Consent—the surgeon will gain consent before surgery if not already gained during preoperative assessment.

Principles of psychological, emotional and spiritual care

- Ensure the patient is informed of what is happening at all stages.
- Ensure all information is given in non-medical, non-jargon terms.
- Encourage the patient to ask questions.
- Patients undergoing surgery are often anxious and it might be necessary to repeat information if it is not fully understood.
- Patients might be grateful to speak to a member of the chaplaincy team.
- Document any significant points.

Practice tips

- Accompany doctors when they speak to patients—to ensure you have understood, so that when the patient asks you later, you are clear what was being explained.
- In a noisy ward, patients do not always hear everything the doctor says and are often afraid to ask again—give them time to ask.
- Reinforce information—wherever possible, by giving it in writing.
- Emergency patients require the same information, but it might be rushed by the surgeon—be prepared to repeat and re-explain.
- A preprinted document is usually available to record all care given before, during, and immediately following surgery.

Journey to theatre

- A registered practitioner should sign the preoperative checklist before the patient leaves the ward.
- Patients who have received no premedication are often allowed to walk to theatre, but check your local policy.
- Some hospitals have implemented wheelchairs because they are easier to push than a trolley.
- Ensure that the health care worker (HCW) accompanying the patient to theatre is appropriate to the patient's medical needs.
- Ensure bed linen is clean (known infection risk) or provide a pack of clean postoperative bedding to accompany the patient.

Intraoperative care

Care begins when a patient enters the operating theatre department and continues until the patent enters the recovery room.

The local policy, type of surgery (day surgery or in-patient), and size of operating theatre department will usually determine whether the patient waits in a reception area before being collected and taken to the anaesthetic room or directly into the operating theatre.

Local policy will determine whether the ward nurse escorts the patient to the anaesthetic room or whether an operating department practitioner (ODP) or anaesthetic nurse collects and takes the patient to the anaesthetic room.

At the handover of the patient from ward to theatre staff (in reception or the anaesthetic room), check the following:

- Patient's identity—patient notes, hospital number, theatre list, and consent.
- Procedure.
- Consent.
- Prostheses have been removed or, if still *in situ*, have been documented.
- Allergies.
- Fasting times.
- Surgical site marking.
- X-ray and scan results are available.

Anaesthetic room

- The patient will be attached to monitoring devices—electrocardiogram (ECG) and pulse oximetry.
- The surgical site is checked by the operating surgeon.
- Shaving might take place at the surgeon's discretion.
- Anaesthetic will be given before transfer to the operating table.

Operating theatre

Compliance with measures for prevention and control of infection include the following:

- Wearing appropriate theatre clothing—theatre scrubs, caps that cover hair, antistatic rubber-soled shoes, no jewellery, and face masks.

Specific care is required to prevent the following:

- Pressure sores.
- Hypothermia.
- Nerve injury.

Postoperative care

The aims of postoperative care are safe recovery from both the anaesthetic and surgical procedure and prevention of complications or early detection and management of them should they occur.

Postoperative care can be divided into the following two forms:

- Immediate postoperative care—which takes place within a recovery room/ postanaesthetic care unit (PACU).
- Postoperative care—which takes place either in the second-stage recovery area of a day-surgery unit or in the surgical ward.

Immediate postoperative care

The patient is usually taken from the theatre to the recovery area by the anaesthetist and scrub practitioner.

The role of the recovery practitioner is to:

- Receive a verbal handover regarding the following:
  - Anaesthetic—including intravenous infusion (IVI) and analgesia.
  - Surgical procedure.
  - Specific care provided during surgery.
- Observe and support the patient's airway until they are breathing unaided and oxygen saturation levels are within the normal preoperative ranges.
- Monitor and record vital signs—pulse, respiration, blood pressure, and oxygen saturation levels every 10min for a minimum of 20–30min.
- Maintain oxygen therapy, according to the prescription.
- Check and record the patient's temperature.
- Assess and record the level of pain and administer analgesia, according to the prescription—contact the anaesthetist to prescribe an alternative, if required.
- Observe for signs of nausea and/or vomiting—give anti-emetics, as prescribed, or contact the anaesthetist to prescribe them.
- Maintain intravenous fluids and/or blood transfusion as prescribed.
- Observe the wound for signs of haemorrhage.
- Observe and record pressure areas.
- Observe and record urinary catheter output— if the patient has not passed urine after several hours, contact the surgeon.
- Assess circulation and movement of limbs following orthopaedic and vascular surgery and neurosurgery.
- Record Glasgow Coma Scale following neurosurgery.
- Check that IVI lines and catheters are labelled with the start date.
- Explain to the patient that surgery is complete—careful and frequent explanations will be required while the patient recovers from the anaesthetic.

Transfer to secondary postoperative care

- Transfer will be to either a second-stage recovery area (in a day-surgery unit) or a surgical ward.
- Local policy will determine whether a ward nurse collects the patient from the recovery area or the recovery staff take the patient back to the ward.
- The patient could be on a trolley or bed.

Collecting/receiving patients from the recovery room/PACU

- Check local policy to determine whether ward staff collect patients from the recovery room or recovery staff escort patients to the ward—a discharge protocol is normally used by recovery staff.
- Before accepting and leaving the recovery room/PACU it is important that the ward nurse has:
  - Read and understood details regarding the surgical procedure and anaesthetic given.
  - Read the nursing care plan before leaving the recovery room.
  - Checked when analgesia was last given/declined and its effect, to ensure it is adequate for transferring the patient from the trolley to the bed.
  - Read the postoperative instructions for the following:
  - Oxygen.
  - When the patient can start to eat and drink.
  - The type of wound care—drains, sutures, clips, removal of pack, and dressing.
- Check appropriate and sufficient prescriptions are written up for the following:
  - Intravenous fluids.
  - Analgesia.
  - Antiemetics.
  - Antibiotics.
  - Oxygen.
  - Subcutaneous heparin.
  - Insulin—might require a sliding scale until the patient is eating and drinking.
- Check the trolley or bed has all the equipment required, as follows:
  - Tipping mechanism.
  - Guedel airway.
  - Oxygen.
  - Suction.
  - Vomit bowl and tissues.
- Check the settings for patient-controlled analgesia (PCA).

Practice tips

- Patients might seem quite sleepy but should be easily roused when spoken to.
- When discussing the patient, remember they might hear you despite appearing to be asleep.
- Patients who have received postoperative opiates should be given oxygen during transfer to the ward.
- Only agree to escort patients to the ward if you are satisfied with their condition.
- Patients who have had a local anaesthetic normally return to the ward immediately—they might have one set of, or no, postoperative observations.

Secondary postoperative care

Care required will depend on whether this is taking place over a period of a few hours in a day-surgery unit or a few days in a surgical ward.

Surgical ward

Prior to the patient returning from surgery, it is important that both the bed area, and all equipment are prepared, to include:
- Suction.
- Oxygen.
- Intravenous infusion (IVI) stand.
- Vomit bowl and tissues.
- Transfer the patient from the trolley to the bed—encourage the patient to move themselves.
- Observe and record the following:
  - Blood pressure.
  - Pulse.
  - Respiration.
  - Temperature.
- Assess the patient's level of pain and provide analgesia, as prescribed.
- Assess nausea and provide an antiemetic, as prescribed.
- Check the IVI for the following:
  - Cannula—for signs of dislodgement during transfer to the bed.
  - IVI prescription.
  - IVI line is labelled with start date.
- Check the wound dressing and drains—apply an extra dressing pad if the wound is oozing through the original dressing.

Practice tips

- If the patient is escorted to the ward, listen to the recovery staff's handover before being distracted to undertake observations—you might miss several important instructions.
- Relatives are often anxious and might need to be asked to wait in the dayroom while the patient is being settled and observations are completed.
- Patients are often hungry and ready to eat a few hours postoperatively—consider food availability for patients who miss an evening meal.

Day-surgery unit

- Observe and record the patient's vital signs until awake and within preoperative limits.
- Observe and check for pain.
- Provide adequate pain relief for the journey home before discharge.
- Provide a drink and light snack (e.g. biscuits, a sandwich, or toast) before discharge.
- Check before discharge that an adult is escorting the patient home—they should not use public transport.
- Check that appropriate analgesia is provided and/or instructions for using their own painkillers.
- Provide advice on wound care, as appropriate.

- Advise the patient that a letter will be posted to their general practitioner (GP) or give the letter to the patient.
- Provide both verbal and written instructions regarding a telephone number to contact if they have concerns.

Emergency and high-dependency care

Fiona Branch
Nurse Consultant, Critical Care Clinical Lead Specialist Support, Nottingham University Hospitals NHS Trust, UK

Frank Coffey
Consultant in Emergency Medicine, Emergency Department, Nottingham University Hospitals NHS Trust, Associate Professor and Consultant in Advanced Clinical Skills, School of Nursing, Midwifery & Physiotherapy, University of Nottingham, UK

ABCDE assessment of the acutely ill patient

Background

The ABCDE method provides a structured and prioritized approach for the assessment of the acutely unwell patient. It facilitates effective communication and ensures that team members are working towards the same goal. Life-threatening problems should be dealt with as they are identified, before moving on to the next stage of assessment.

Equipment

- Stethoscope.
- Automated blood pressure device.
- Pen torch.
- Glucometer.

Procedure

- The assessment should begin by asking the patient the following question: 'How are you?' A normal response indicates a patent airway, adequate breathing, and satisfactory cerebral perfusion.
- If the response to the above question is abnormal, e.g. single words or short sentences owing to difficulty breathing, call for help and continue the ABCDE evaluation:
  - A—airway.
  - B—breathing.
  - C—circulation.
  - D—disability (central nervous system [CNS]).
  - E—exposure (permitting full examination).
- Assess and manage each element in turn, using the 'look, listen, and feel' approach. When the patient has been stabilized, carry out a full assessment, including a head-to-toe examination, chart review, and medical history. Review the results of investigations.
- A clear management plan should then be made—e.g. outlining interventions or tests needed, observations required, and speciality input.

Practice tips

- If the patient's condition deteriorates or becomes unstable reassess the patient using the ABCDE approach, beginning at A, and call for help, as appropriate.
- All critically ill patients should receive oxygen.
- Study the patient's charts and medical records carefully. Attention to detail is important.

Pitfalls

- Not getting help early enough.
- Not reassessing the patient systematically, commencing at the airway, if their condition deteriorates.
- Not having a specific management plan—e.g. '↓ oxygen' is vague, whereas '↓ oxygen by 10% every 10min to keep oxygen saturation >95%' is a clear plan of management.

Recognition of airway obstruction

Background

Partial or total airway obstruction can occur at any level, from the nose and mouth to the trachea. Prompt recognition and treatment are vital to prevent death or irreversible hypoxic damage. Causes include loss of consciousness, obstruction by vomit, blood, or foreign bodies, bronchospasm, pulmonary oedema, excessive bronchial secretions, or aspiration of stomach contents. Normal airflow should be quiet. Total obstruction causes silent, laboured breathing, whereas in partial obstruction there is diminished, noisy air entry.

Equipment

- Stethoscope.

Procedure

- Use the 'look, listen, and feel' approach for patient assessment.

Look

- Movement of the chest and abdomen.
- Respiratory effort—is it abnormal or 'see-saw' in nature (movement of the chest and abdomen in opposite directions with every breath)?
- Use of the accessory muscles and intercostal recession.
- Cyanosis—remembering that this is a late sign.

Listen

- Inspiratory stridor caused by obstruction at or above the level of the main bronchi.
- Snoring—heard if the tongue or palate partially occludes the pharynx.
- Crowing or stridor associated with laryngeal spasm.
- Gurgling that occurs in the presence of semisolid material or liquid in the main airways.
- Expiratory wheeze, suggesting obstruction of the lower airways.

Feel

- Movement of air at the mouth and nose. If airway obstruction is present, open the mouth, clear secretions and foreign bodies, and open the airway (🕮 on p. 204) and administer oxygen at a high concentration.
- The patient's chest to ensure that is moving.

Practice tip

- New onset abnormal airway sounds often indicate a problem that should be dealt with immediately.

Pitfalls

- Not calling for help early enough.

Manoeuvres for opening the airway

Background

Once airway obstruction has been recognized, prompt opening of the airway and ventilation are vital to prevent hypoxia and further deterioration of the patient's condition. There are three manoeuvres that can be used to relieve obstruction of the upper airway: head tilt, chin lift, and jaw thrust. Jaw thrust is the technique of choice for patients with known or suspected cervical spine injury, in combination with manual in-line stabilization of the head and neck.

Procedure

Head tilt

- Place one hand on the patient's forehead.
- Place the fingers of your other hand under the patient's chin.
- Gently lift the chin and tilt the head backwards.

Chin lift

- Place the fingers of one hand under the patient's mandible.
- Place the thumb of the same hand on the patient's chin.
- Lift the mandible forwards.

Jaw thrust

- Identify the angle of the mandible.
- Place your fingers behind the angle of the mandible on each side.
- Displace the mandible forwards.
- Use your thumbs to open the mouth slightly, by downwards displacement of the chin.
- After any manoeuvre for opening the airway, check the airway using the 'look, listen, and feel' approach (🕮 p. 203). It might be necessary to insert an airway adjunct to maintain or augment the airway after the initial manoeuvre.
- Document the episode of care.

Practice tip

- Remove broken or displaced dentures. Leave well-fitting dentures in place because they improve the seal for ventilation.

Pitfalls

- Failing to maintain the airway after the initial manoeuvre.
- Moving the neck excessively in trauma victims.

Insertion of an oropharyngeal airway

Background

Oropharyngeal (Guedel) airways are curved plastic tubes, flanged at the oral end and flattened to fit neatly between the tongue and the hard palate. The airway sits over the tongue, preventing backwards displacement in an unconscious patient. The most common sizes are 2, 3, and 4, ranging from small to large adults. Oropharyngeal airways should only be used in deeply unconscious patients or patients who have had a cardiac arrest, because they can induce vomiting or larygospasm.

Equipment

- Oropharyngeal airway.
- Suction catheter and tubing.
- Functioning suction unit.
- Disposable gloves.

Procedure

- Explain the procedure. Although the patient is unconscious, they might still be able to hear.
- Size—choose the oropharyngeal airway with a length corresponding to the distance between the corner of the patient's mouth and the angle of the patient's jaw (Fig. 9.1).
- Open the patient's mouth and check that it is free of foreign bodies or secretions. Suction, if required.
- Insert the airway into the patient's mouth, past the teeth, with the concavity and tip facing upwards (i.e. 'upside down').
- Rotate the device 180° beyond the hard palate into the oropharynx.
- Alternatively hold the tongue down and forward with a tongue depressor and insert the airway with the tip facing downwards until it sits in the oropharynx. This method is preferred in children.
- The oropharyngeal airway sits over the tongue, with the flange between the teeth.
- After insertion, check the airway using the 'look, listen, and feel' approach.
- Document the episode of care.

Practice tip

- A fine-bore suction catheter can be used to suction through an oropharyngeal airway.

Pitfalls

- Continuing to try to insert the airway if the patient gags or coughs. If the patient cannot tolerate an airway, they do not need one.
- Causing obstruction by displacing the tongue backwards and downwards with the oropharygeal airway.
- Not maintaining the head tilt, chin lift, or jaw thrust manoeuvre if an oropharyngeal airway alone is insufficient to maintain a patent airway.

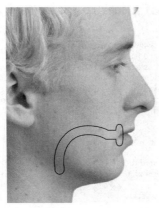

Fig. 9.1 Choose the size of the oropharyngeal airway by measuring from the patient's teeth to the angle of the mandible. Reproduced from Thomas and Monaghan (2007) *Oxford Handbook of Clinical Examination and practical skills.* With permission from Oxford University Press.

Insertion of a nasopharyngeal airway

Background
Nasopharyngeal airways are made of malleable plastic, which is bevelled at one end and flanged at the other. They are suitable for semi-conscious patients who need assistance to maintain a patent airway. They are ideal for patients with clenched jaws or trismus and are used in patients with maxillofacial injuries. They should be avoided in patients with basal skull fractures, nasal fractures, and orbital injuries. The commonest sizes used in adults are 6mm and 7mm.

Equipment
- Nasopharyngeal airway.
- Safety pin.
- Suction catheter and tubing.
- Functioning suction unit.
- Disposable gloves.
- Water-soluble lubricant.

Procedure
- Explain the procedure and gain consent.
- Insert the safety pin through the flange to prevent the airway being inhaled.
- Size the tube by measuring the distance from the nostril to the tragus of the ear.
- Lubricate the tube with water-soluble lubricant.
- Inspect the nostrils for any infection, trauma or obstruction—e.g. a polyp or deviated nasal septum. Choose the wider unobstructed side.
- Insert the bevelled end of the airway into the chosen nostril. Slide the tube posteriorly along the floor of the nose, with a slight rotating motion.
- Once *in situ*, the flange should rest against the nostril.
- Check the airway using the 'look, listen, and feel' approach (🕮 on p. 203).
- Document the episode of care.

Practice tips
- Ensure adequate lubrication of the tube.
- Be aware of the anatomy of the nasal floor when inserting the tube. Push the tube backwards, rather than upwards.
- A degree of resistance might be felt when the narrow part of the nostril is reached. Give a firm (but not forceful) push to pass the tube through.
- Do not panic if a small amount of bleeding occurs.
- Using the diameter of the patient's little finger to size the tube is no longer recommended.

Pitfalls
- Causing excessive bleeding by exerting too much force.
- Inducing vomiting or laryngospasm with a tube that is too long.
- Not maintaining the head tilt, chin lift, or jaw thrust manoeuvre if the nasopharyngeal airway alone is insufficient to maintain a patent airway.

Assessment of breathing

Background

When the airway has been assessed and managed, breathing should be assessed. Breathing problems might be caused by respiratory conditions (e.g. asthma or pneumonia), chest trauma, cardiac failure, some muscular and neurological conditions, high spinal injuries or occur 2° to abdominal distension. Metabolic acidosis (e.g. diabetic ketoacidosis) can cause tachypnoea and deep sighing breathing known as Kussmaul's respiration.

Equipment

- Stethoscope.
- Watch with a second hand.
- Pulse oximeter.

Procedure

Look

- Cyanosis.
- Rate, rhythm, and depth of breathing.
- Signs of respiratory distress—tachypnoea, use of accessory muscles, intercostal recession, and nasal flaring.
- Symmetry of chest movement—unilateral chest movement might indicate pneumothorax, pleural effusion, or pneumonia.
- ↑ jugular venous pulse.
- Scars from previous surgery or chest drains.
- Bruising in trauma.

Listen

- The patient's communications—are they responding; are they able to complete sentences; and are they orientated, agitated, or confused?
- The patient's breathing—do they have an audible wheeze?
- The chest—for breath sounds, bronchial breathing, and additional sounds, e.g. crackles or wheeze. Auscultation with a stethoscope is generally performed after palpation and percussion.

Feel

- Tracheal deviation.
- Chest expansion.
- Tenderness.
- Rib fractures (tenderness and crepitus).
- Surgical emphysema.
- Dullness or hyperresonance on percussion. 📖 on p. 292.

Check

- Oxygen saturation using a pulse oximeter. 📖 on p. 302.
- Peak flow. 📖 on p. 298.
- Arterial blood gases. 📖 on p. 258.

Practice tip

- 📖 See practice tips on p. 54 and p. 291.

Pitfalls

- Not calling for help early if there are signs of respiratory distress.
- Not applying oxygen early.
- Removing oxygen from an acutely ill patient to measure oxygen saturation or arterial blood gases.
- Not recognizing that a slowing respiratory rate could be a sign of impending respiratory arrest.
- Failing to recognize the seriousness of a low or falling peak flow rate.
- Not counting respiratory rate, or counting inaccurately.

Mouth-to-mouth ventilation

Background

In the absence of equipment, mouth-to-mouth ventilation should be commenced as soon as possible in any patient who develops inadequate or absent breathing. Expired air ventilation (rescue breathing) delivers an oxygen concentration of ~16%.

Equipment

- None.

Procedure

- Ascertain whether the patient has stopped breathing using the 'look, listen, and feel' approach. 📖 on p. 203.
- Open the patient's mouth and check that it is free of foreign bodies, vomit or copious secretions.
- Lie the patient supine and open their airway, with the neck slightly flexed and head tilted backwards.
- Pinch the nose firmly to seal it using the thumb and forefinger of one hand.
- Using the other hand, lift the patient's chin.
- Take a deep breath and seal your lips around the patient's mouth.
- Blow into the patient's mouth until their chest rises.
- Remove your mouth from the patient's and allow the chest to fall.
- Continue at a rate of 10–12 breaths/minute. If cardiac compressions are being performed, the ratio should be 2 breaths to 30 compressions.
- Reposition the patient's airway or your mouth if adequate ventilation is not taking place (i.e. the patient's chest is not rising) and re-evaluate.
- If the patient starts breathing spontaneously, place them in the recovery position.
- Document the episode of care.

Practice tips

- If you cannot get a good seal around the patient's mouth to deliver a breath, you can blow into the patient's nose and occlude their mouth instead.
- Avoid inhaling the patient's expired air because it will result in you providing air of a ↓ oxygen concentration.
- Carry a pocket resuscitation mask (📖 on p. 213) because mouth-to-mouth ventilation is aesthetically unpleasant and carries a risk of infection.

Pitfalls

- Failing to recognize inadequate ventilation.
- Not identifying obstruction by a foreign body.

Mouth-to-mask ventilation

Background
Mouth-to-mask ventilation is performed using a pocket resuscitation mask. It is aesthetically more acceptable and safer for the rescuer than mouth-to-mouth ventilation. This method can also facilitate the delivery of oxygen if it is available.

Equipment
- Pocket mask.
- Oxygen tubing and source.
- Oral airways.
- Wide-bore, rigid suction catheter.

Procedure
- Open the patient's mouth and check that it is free of foreign bodies or copious secretions.
- Suction, as required.
- Place the patient supine in the 'sniffing' position—i.e. the neck slightly flexed and head tilted backwards.
- Place the mask over the patient's mouth and nose using the thumbs of both hands.
- Lift the patient's jaw into the mask using a jaw thrust (📖 p. 204) and press the mask into the patient's face to make a tight seal.
- Blow through the valve. The chest should rise with each breath.
- Watch the chest falling between inflations.
- Reposition the patient or mask if airflow is impeded or there are any leaks between the face and the mask.
- If oxygen is available, attach it through the nipple on the mask at a flow rate of 10L/minute. The tidal volume (i.e. the amount of expired air blown into the valve) can be ↓ if supplemental oxygen is used.
- Document the episode of care.

Practice tip
- If the pocket mask does not have a nipple, supplemental oxygen can be administered by placing the oxygen tubing under the face mask.

Pitfalls
- Not achieving an airtight seal because of inadequate pressure on the mask and/or poor jaw-thrust technique.

Bag–valve–mask (BVM) ventilation

Background

Self-inflating bags connected to a face mask can be used to ventilate a patient who has stopped breathing or is breathing inadequately. The patient's expired gas is diverted to the atmosphere through a one-way valve—hence the name 'BVM'. Without supplemental oxygen, the self-inflating bag delivers an oxygen concentration of 21% (ambient air). This can be ↑ to 45% by the addition of high-flow oxygen and 85% if a reservoir bag is also attached to the self-inflating bag.

Equipment

- Self-inflating bag and reservoir.
- Oxygen tubing and source.
- Oral airways.
- Suction apparatus (wide-bore, rigid suction catheter).

Procedure

- This procedure should ideally be performed with an assistant. Although the bag can be used by one person, it requires considerable skill and this is generally not recommended.
- Open the patient's mouth and check that it is free of foreign bodies or copious secretions.
- Suction, as required.
- Place the patient supine, with the neck slightly flexed and head extended—the 'sniffing' position.
- Place the mask over the patient's mouth and nose while maintaining a jaw thrust. The mask should fit snugly against the cheeks.
- If an oxygen supply is available, attach the oxygen (at a rate of 10L/minute) to the inlet at the end of the bag.
- The assistant should squeeze the bag. The chest should rise with each breath, and airflow should be unimpeded. If not, reposition the mask and try again. In respiratory arrest and in cardiorespiratory arrest with a protected airway, perform approximately 10 ventilations a minute. In cardiorespiratory arrest with an unprotected airway give 2 ventilations after every sequence of 30 chest compressions.
- Insert an oral airway to facilitate ventilation, particularly in elderly edentulous patients.
- Document the episode of care.

Practice tips

- If a leak is noted, reposition the mask and re-check.
- If no air is entering the chest, and the position of the patient and seal of the mask are optimal, consider obstruction by a foreign body in the airway.

Pitfalls

- Putting the mask on upside down in the heat of the moment, with the nose end over the mouth.
- Not achieving an airtight seal because of inadequate pressure and/or poor jaw-thrust technique.
- Pressing down too hard on the mask or on soft tissues of the neck, causing obstruction of the airway. The latter is easy to do in children.
- Compressing the bag excessively. This causes gastric distension, which can result in regurgitation and aspiration. Gastric distension also impairs ventilation. When supplemental oxygen is used, low tidal volumes in the region of 400–600mL (6–7mL/Kg) will provide adequate oxygenation and ventilation.

Care of a patient undergoing mechanical ventilation

Background
Patients might require positive-pressure ventilation with a mechanical ventilator for a variety of reasons, including type II respiratory failure, neuromuscular weakness, neurological injury, and surgical procedures. The ventilators require oxygen, air, and electricity to work. The modes of ventilation can vary. Ventilation can be set to support a patient-initiated breath, deliver a mandatory number of breaths, deliver a set volume, or a combination of these functions.

Equipment
- Mechanical ventilator.
- Piped oxygen supply.
- Piped air supply.
- Electricity.
- Bag–valve–mask and reservoir.
- Reintubation equipment.
- Suction equipment.
- Stethoscope.

Procedure
- Explain the procedure and gain consent.

Care of the patient
- Record the patient's vital signs at least every hour or more frequently if their condition dictates.
- Observe for complications associated with ventilation—e.g. barotrauma, hypotension, or hypertension.
- Record the oxygen saturation (SpO_2) continuously and regularly check arterial blood gases.
- Observe for chest movement and listen for breath sounds.
- Perform regular tracheal suction and assist with physiotherapy to minimize the risk of ventilator-associated pneumonia (VAP).
- Monitor and assess the patient's level of sedation and analgesia—use the minimum amount possible.
- Support the ventilator tubing, for the patient's comfort and to minimize the risk of disconnection or extubation.
- Ensure the head of the bed is elevated to 45° to ↓ the incidence of VAP.
- Explain to the patient and their visitors that the patient will not be able to talk. Ensure alternative methods of communication are available (e.g. communication charts and picture boards).

Care of the ET (endotracheal) tube and the ventilator
- Secure the endotracheal tube and maintain its position with linen tape. Reposition the tube regularly to prevent lip ulceration.
- Document the position of the ET tube (in centimetres at the lips) in case the tube might slip into the right main bronchus when the patient is moved.

- Nominate one person to be responsible for supporting/securing the endotracheal tube when moving the patient, to ↓ the risk of accidental removal of the tube.
- Check the cuff pressure every 8 hours or more frequently if a leak is suspected.
- Assess the effectiveness of humidification and alter the level accordingly.
- Change the ventilator tubing and equipment every 48 hours.
- Ensure a nasogastric tube is present to minimize the risk of aspiration and prevent accumulation of gastric secretions.
- Record and document the ventilator observations, depending on the ventilation mode, to include frequency, tidal volume, minute volume, airway pressures, inspired oxygen concentration, inspiratory pressure, inspiratory time, ramp pressure support, positive end expiratory pressure (PEEP), and air entry.
- Ensure a bag–valve–mask device, Water's circuit, and portable oxygen cylinder are at the bedside in case of mechanical failure, to enable manual ventilation of the patient.
- Ensure re-intubation facilities are always available.
- Set the alarm limits within 10% of the preset values.
- Answer all alarms immediately. If you cannot quickly identify the problem and ventilation is compromised, remove the patient from the ventilator and ventilate with a Water's (resuscitation) bag. Summon help immediately.
- Following any procedure during which the ventilator circuit has had to be disconnected, reconnect the circuit and check the patient's condition.
- Document the episode of care.

Practice tip
- Reassure the patient. It is uncomfortable and frightening for an awake patient trying to breathe on a ventilator. Communication is vital to ↓ anxiety and to encourage a natural breathing pattern.

Pitfall
- Silencing an alarm and not identifying and resolving the cause of it. Once you have identified the cause it is best to then silence the alarm to prevent greater anxiety and distress to the patient, relatives and other patients in the area.

Insertion of a laryngeal mask airway (LMA)

Background

LMAs are advanced airway devices that are designed to facilitate ventilation in deeply unconscious, anaesthetized, or arrested patients. They consist of a wide-bore tube with an elliptical inflation cuff. They are more effective than bag–valve–mask (BVM) devices and relatively easy to insert. LMAs do not provide the 'gold standard' protection of the airway afforded by intubation, but pulmonary aspiration is uncommon. They are valuable in suspected cervical spine injury when it is essential that movement of the neck is minimized. Sizes 4 and 5 are suitable for most ♀ and ♂, respectively; size 3 is used for small adults.

Equipment

- LMA—reusable LMAs should have had the cuff inflated on return from sterile services, to ensure that they are correctly functioning and that no herniation of the cuff has occurred.
- Suction catheter and tubing.
- Functioning suction unit.
- Disposable gloves.
- Water-soluble lubricant.
- BVM device, with oxygen attached.
- 50mL syringe.
- Stethoscope.
- Bite block or oropharyngeal airway.
- Tape to secure the LMA.

Procedure

- Put on the gloves.
- Check the interior and exterior of the LMA and inflate the cuff to test it—sizes 3, 4, and 5 require 20, 30 and 40mL of air, respectively, to inflate the cuff.
- Deflate the cuff fully and apply lubricant to the rear/outer face of the LMA only.
- Place the patient in the supine position, with the head and neck aligned. Ideally, the neck should be slightly flexed and head extended, unless cervical spine injury is suspected.
- Pre-oxygenate the patient with a BVM device and 10L of oxygen.
- Hold the LMA like a pen, just above the cuff.
- Advance the tip of the LMA, with the upper outer surface following the palate of the mouth and using your index finger as a splint.
- Keeping the tube central, push the LMA downwards and backwards into the oropharynx.
- Stop when resistance is felt. The index finger should have disappeared into the mouth.
- Once in place, hold the LMA with the other hand before removing your finger from the patient's mouth.

- Release the LMA and inflate the cuff. The LMA will move slightly out of the mouth as the cuff finds its correct position.
- Attach the BVM/O_2 and ventilate the patient. The chest should rise.
- If the chest rises, listen to the lungs and over the stomach with a stethoscope to confirm the placement. A small leak is acceptable, but a large leak suggests misplacement. If the chest does not rise, remove the LMA and re-insert it, oxygenating the patient again before a further attempt.
- Insert a bite block or small oropharyngeal airway and tie it in place.
- Secure/tie LMA in place.
- Document the episode of care.

Practice tip

- If there is minimal air escaping at the mouth during cardiac arrest, asynchronous chest compressions and ventilations can be performed. If there are persistent leaks and hypoventilation, return to alternating compressions and ventilations at a ratio of 30:2.

Pitfalls

- Inserting the tube the wrong way round—the cuff should be in the mouth with the pipe at the top.
- Failing to be aware of hypoventilation owing to a leak around the cuff, particularly in patients with stiff lungs or increased airway resistance.
- Inducing coughing, straining, or laryngeal spasm in patients who are not deeply unconscious.
- Folding the epiglottis over the laryngeal inlet on insertion of the LMA, this can cause complete obstruction.

Assisting with endotracheal intubation

Background

Endotracheal intubation is the placement of a tube into the trachea to maintain a patent airway and enable ventilation. It is indicated in patients who are not breathing, breathing inadequately, or unable to protect their airway. It is ideally a two-person procedure.

Equipment

- Self-refilling bag–valve combination—e.g. Ambu bag, face mask, tubing, and oxygen source.
- Premedication and induction equipment—intravenous (IV) access and a laryngoscope with curved (Macintosh-type) and straight (Miller-type) blades of a size appropriate for the patient (the commonest size is 3).
- Endotracheal tubes of several different sizes. Low-pressure, high-flow cuffed balloons are preferred (commonly 7.5–8mm for ♀ and 8–8.5mm for ♂).
- Oral airways.
- Pre-cut tape.
- Introducer—Bougie or Magill's.
- Suction equipment.
- 10mL syringe to inflate the cuff.
- Water-soluble sterile lubricant.
- Monitoring equipment—pulse oximeter, blood pressure cuff and cardiac monitor.

Procedure

The assistant, health care worker (HCW) 2 will:

- Ensure that the procedure has been explained and consent gained.
- Assemble all items before intubation is attempted.
- Draw up and label premedication, induction, and paralytic agents.
- Position the patient supine, with the neck slightly flexed and head extended.
- Place a pillow under the patient's head and neck but not under the shoulders. This enables a straight line of vision from the mouth to the vocal cords. If cervical spine trauma is suspected, another HCW will need to hold the neck in a neutral position.

The person carrying out the intubation, HCW 1, will:

- Choose an appropriately sized tube for the patient.
- Inflate the balloon with 5–8ml of air from the 10-mL syringe to ensure the balloon is functional and intact.
- lubricate the end of the tube (optional).
- Pre-oxygenate the patient (with at least 85% oxygen) using the bag–valve–mask combination for 1–2min.
- For elective intubation, administer a sedative and paralyzing agent (e.g. midazolam and succinylcholine).
- Open the patient's mouth and insert the laryngoscope, checking that the mouth is free of secretions/foreign bodies and suctioning, as required.
- Indicate whether cricoid pressure is required and then insert the tube.

- If requested, the assistant should apply cricoid pressure. The cricoid cartilage is the ring felt below the thyroid cartilage (Adam's apple). If this is displaced posteriorly, it compresses and closes the oesophagus, preventing passive regurgitation of gastric contents. Pressure should be maintained until the tube is inserted through the vocal cords and cuff inflated (no longer than 30sec). The person carrying out the intubation has control and will indicate when the pressure can be released.
- Connect the bag–valve combination, and begin ventilation with oxygen-enriched air.
- Confirm that the tube is properly positioned. First, listen over the stomach with a stethoscope while ventilating the patient. If sounds of airflow are heard or distension of the stomach occurs, the tube is in the oesophagus. If the oesophagus has been intubated instead of the trachea, remove the tube and pre-oxygenate the patient before trying again.
- Listen to each side of the chest; be sure that breath sounds are equal in both sides of the thorax. If not, reposition the tube. When breath sounds are equal on both sides and the thorax rises equally on both sides with each inspiration, note the position of the tube (mark the tube at the patient's mouth) and inflate the cuff with the 10mL syringe until there is no air leak around the tube when positive pressure is applied.
- Secure the tube with tape.
- Obtain a chest X-ray film immediately to check the placement of the tube and also obtain measurements of arterial blood gases to assess the adequacy of ventilation.
- Document the episode of care.

Practice tips

- To estimate the size of the laryngoscope blade required, hold the blade next to the patient's face—the blade should reach between the lips and the larynx.
- Intubation should take no longer than 30sec.
- In patients with suspected cervical spine injury, counter-pressure should be applied to the back of the neck during application of cricoid pressure to prevent movement of the cervical spine.

Pitfalls

- Maintaining cricoid pressure while the patient is actively vomiting. This might result in damage to or perforation of the oesophagus.
- Applying cricoid pressure incorrectly can make intubation more difficult.
- Releasing cricoid pressure before being requested to by the person carrying out the intubation.

Extubation

Background

Extubation refers to the removal of an endotracheal tube from the airway. Patients are ready for extubation when they no longer need ventilatory support and can protect their airway. It is a potentially dangerous procedure, with a risk of aspiration, laryngospasm, hypoventilation, or a cardiac response (e.g. arrhythmia). The patient should receive nil by mouth for 3–4 hours before a planned extubation. The procedure should ideally be performed with an assistant. Appropriately trained personnel, who can treat complications or re-intubate if required, should be on standby.

Equipment

- Wide-bore, rigid suction tube.
- Sterile, multi-eyed suction catheter—of an appropriate size for the internal diameter of the endotracheal tube (sizes 8, 10, 12, and 14FG).
- Functional suction unit—15–20kPa, 100–150mmHg, and 150–200cmH$_2$O.
- 10mL syringe.
- Disposable sterile PVC (latex-free) glove.
- Disposable gloves and apron for the assistant.
- Protective eyewear.
- Oxygen therapy and humidifier.
- Oxygen supply.
- Bag–valve–mask device.
- Monitoring equipment—pulse oximeter blood pressure cuff, and cardiac monitor.

Procedure

- Explain the procedure and gain consent.
- Wash your hands and prepare the trolley and oxygen therapy.
- Position the patient supine with the neck slightly extended.
- Aspirate nasogastric tube, if present.
- Suction to remove any excess secretions.
- Assess the need for pre-oxygenation before the procedure.
- Remove the air from the cuff until the pilot balloon indicates that the cuff is deflated (this should be carried out by the assistant).
- Cut the ties securing the endotracheal tube.
- Turn on the suction apparatus and set the suction pressure—a maximum of 20kPa, 150mmHg, and 200cmH$_2$O.
- Attach the correct size of sterile catheter to the suction apparatus, ensuring that the catheter remains in the sterile packaging.
- Put the sterile PVC glove on your dominant hand.
- Remove the packaging with your non-dominant hand while holding the exposed catheter with your dominant hand.
- Remove any caps on the catheter mount/T-piece with your non-dominant hand.
- Insert the suction catheter gently and slowly, without suction pressure until resistance is felt at the carina.

- Withdraw the catheter 1–3cm when this resistance is felt.
- Withdraw both the endotracheal tube and the suction catheter slowly and steadily, while applying continuous suctioning.
- When the tube is removed, release the suction.
- Discard the endotracheal tube and suction catheter in clinical waste.
- Re-commence oxygen therapy.
- Observe the patient for signs of respiratory distress and compare pre-extubation and post-extubation observations.
- Dispose of the equipment in clinical waste.
- Wash your hands.
- Document the episode of care.

Practice tip

- Prepare the equipment before use, particularly oxygen therapy.

Pitfalls

- Not suctioning both orally and through the endotracheal tube.
- Forgetting to stop the nasogastric feed before removal, ↑ the risk of aspiration.

Assisting with needle cricothyroidotomy

Background

Needle cricothyroidotomy is performed as an emergency procedure, to provide a temporary airway if there is an obstruction at or above the level of the larynx such that intubation is impossible. It involves insertion of a needle or cannula into the airway through the cricothyroid membrane, which lies between the thyroid and cricoid cartilages. The technique described uses a simple over-the-needle cannula. Commercial needle cricothroidotomy kits are available. A needle cricothyroidotomy will oxygenate the patient. It is time-limited to ~45min because it does not allow sufficient expiration of carbon dioxide, resulting in lethal hypercapnia.

Equipment

- Dressing pack.
- Size 12 or 14 gauge over-the-needle cannula.
- 5mL syringe.
- Gauze swabs.
- 2% chlorhexidine in 70% isopropyl alcohol.
- Disposable scalpel blade, size 11 (optional).
- Sterile gloves.
- Oxygen supply.
- Oxygen tubing and a Y-shaped connector.

Procedure

- If the patient is conscious, ensure that the procedure has been explained and consent obtained. Continue to reassure the patient throughout.
- Place the patient in a supine position.

The health care worker (HCW) carrying out the cricothyroidotomy (HCW 1) will then:

- Attach a 5mL syringe to a 12 or 14 gauge over-the-needle cannula.
- Clean the neck with antiseptic solution (2% aqueous chlorhexidine solution).
- Identify the cricothyroid membrane and puncture the skin in the midline with the needle attached to the syringe. Then, carefully insert the needle through the lower half of the cricothyroid membrane. Aspiration of air signifies entry into the trachea.
- Remove the syringe and withdraw the needle while advancing the catheter downwards into position, being careful not to perforate the posterior wall of the trachea.

You should:

- help to keep the patient as still as possible during the procedure. A conscious patient is likely to be agitated and moving about.
- Secure the cannula in the neck with tape as soon as it is in position.

HCW 1 will:
- Attach the oxygen tubing to the cannula by use of a Y-connector.
- Place a thumb on the patent part of the Y-connector to allow oxygen to flow for 1 second. Then remove the thumb for 4sec to allow expiration thorough the upper airway.

You should:
- Ensure preparations are underway for insertion of a more secure airway (cricothroidotomy or tracheostomy) as a matter of urgency.

Practice tip
- If a Y-connector is unavailable, fold the oxygen tubing over and cut a hole in it. This can then be occluded and uncovered in the 1:4 ratio described above.

Pitfalls
- Failing to secure the cannula when it is inserted.
- Not having the equipment readily available when required.
- Failing to convert to a definitive airway as soon as possible.

Assisting with insertion of a percutaneous tracheostomy

Background

A tracheostomy is a surgical opening in the anterior wall of the trachea to facilitate ventilation. It might be performed as an emergency or elective procedure. The commonest indication is long-term ventilation. In a controlled setting, percutaneous tracheostomy can be performed at the bedside by a trained clinician with the assistance of another health care worker (HCW).

Equipment

- Dressing pack/intravenous cut-down set.
- Percutaneous introducer set.
- Tracheostomy tube—size requested by person performing the procedure and one size smaller.
- Gauze swabs.
- 2% chlorhexidine in 70% isopropyl alcohol.
- One sterile gown.
- Three sterile towels.
- One suture and needle (optional).
- Sterile gloves, assorted sizes.
- Tracheal dilators.
- Water-soluble sterile lubricant.
- A selection of needles.
- Two 20mL ampoules of 0.9% saline solution.
- A selection of syringes.
- Tracheostomy tapes/ties.
- Tracheostomy dressing.
- 1% lidocaine/adrenaline solution.
- Re-intubation equipment.
- Monitoring equipment—pulse oximeter, blood pressure cuff, and cardiac monitor.
- Bag–valve–mask device and oxygen supply.
- Bronchoscopy trolley and equipment (optional, although recommended).

Procedure

- Ensure that the procedure has been explained. Although the patient is unconscious, they might still be able to hear.
- The patient will already be intubated and ventilated. ↑ the inspired oxygen concentration to 100% for at least 5min before the procedure.
- Ensure the patient is adequately anaesthetized.
- Ensure that all equipment and monitoring devices are working, including electrocardiogram (ECG), blood pressure, SpO_2, and end tidal CO_2 monitoring.
- Place the patient in a supine position, with the neck extended by placing a sandbag/rolled-up pillow under the shoulders.

The health care worker carrying out the procedure (HCW 1) will then perform the following actions:

- Clean and drape the area around the intended tracheostomy site.
- Deflate the cuff of the existing endotracheal tube and withdraw the tube under direct vision of the bronchoscope until the cuff is just under the vocal cords.
- Secure the endotracheal tube to prevent dislodgement and reinflate the cuff.
- Make an incision in the trachea between the second and the third cartilaginous rings and insert the tube, using either a dilatation or the Seldinger technique.
- Inflate the cuff of the tracheostomy tube and connect the ventilator breathing circuit.
- Secure the tube using tracheotomy ties.
- Ventilation is verified by the 'look, listen, and feel' approach.

You should:

- Place a tracheostomy dressing around the tube.
- Suction through the tracheostomy to remove blood and secretions.
- Document the episode of care.
- A chest X-ray is obtained to check the tube position and exclude a pneumothorax.

Pitfalls

- Failing to secure the tracheal tube during the procedure, resulting in accidental extubation.
- Failing to monitor the patient closely and missing hypoxia and hypoventilation caused by an air leak after the trachea is opened.

Measurement of cuff pressure

Background

The tracheal cuff on an artificial airway, e.g. tracheostomy tube or endotracheal tube (ETT) provides a seal for positive-pressure ventilation and might prevent aspiration. The cuff pressure should be checked and documented at least every 8 hours to prevent tracheal damage. Most gauges have colour-coded zones, with green an acceptable pressure (20–25cmH$_2$0) and red unacceptable.

Equipment

- Cuff pressure gauge.
- Manometer tubing.
- Gloves.
- Suction.

Procedure

- Explain the procedure and gain consent.
- Wash your hands and put on the gloves.
- Attach the pressure manometer tubing between the port on the cuff pressure gauge and the ETT, tracheostomy external cuff, or pilot balloon.
- Record the pressure displayed on the gauge. The reading should be taken at the end of expiration.
- If the cuff pressure is >25cmH$_2$O, suction the patient orally before removing the air from the cuff, to prevent oral secretions from entering the lungs.
- Do not add more air if a leak is suspected, because over-inflation might cause tracheal damage. Contact the senior clinical staff or outreach team immediately, according to your local policy. Experienced, competent practitioners might deal with a leakage by removing all the air from the cuff following oral suctioning. The cuff is then inflated using a syringe or by squeezing the bulb of the manometer to the minimal occlusion volume needed.
- Re-check the cuff pressure with the pressure gauge.
- Document the episode of care.

Practice tip

- It is easier to manipulate the amount of air in the cuff using a syringe than with the bulb of the manometer.

Pitfall

- Accidentally depressing the automatic deflate button which is on the side of some of the gauges which could potentially lead to aspiration.

Suction through a tracheostomy

Background

One of the commonest problems associated with a tracheostomy tube is blockage owing to the accumulation of secretions. Suctioning is essential to maintain the artificial airway. The frequency of suction will depend on an individual patient's needs. Indications include excess secretions, abnormal breath sounds, or breathing difficulties. The health care worker (HCW) should be aware of the type of tracheostomy tube *in situ* and any accompanying inner cannulae. The size of the suction catheter is calculated using the following formula:

(Size of the tracheostomy tube − 2) × 2

Example

For a size 8 tracheostomy tube:
(8 − 2) × 2 = a size 12 suction catheter is required.

Equipment

- Functional suction unit—15–20kPa, 100–150mmHg, 150–200cmH$_2$O.
- Sterile, multi-eyed suction catheters—sizes 8, 10, 12, and 14FG, according to the internal diameter of the tracheotomy tube *in situ*.
- Wide-bore, rigid suction tube.
- Sterile gloves.
- Disposable apron.
- Jug or bowl of water.
- Protective eyewear.
- Bag–valve–mask device.
- Oxygen supply and a humidifier.

Procedure

- Explain the procedure and gain consent.
- Pre-oxygenate the patient, if required.
- Clean your hands. Put on clean disposable gloves and an apron.
- Check the inner cannula, if applicable. If it is fenestrated, replace it with a non-fenestrated/plain inner cannula.
- Turn on the suction apparatus and set the suction pressure to a maximum of 20kPa, 150mmHg, 200cmH$_2$O.
- Attach the correct size of sterile catheter to the suction apparatus, ensuring the catheter remains in the sterile packaging.
- Put a sterile glove on your dominant hand.
- Hold the exposed catheter in your dominant hand while removing the packaging with your other hand.
- Remove any caps on the catheter mount/T-piece with your non-dominant hand.
- Insert the suction catheter through the tracheostomy tube slowly and gently, without suction pressure until resistance is felt at the carina.

- When resistance is felt, withdraw the catheter 1–3cm and then apply continuous suctioning while withdrawing the catheter slowly and steadily for a maximum duration of 10–15sec.
- Release the suction and wrap the catheter in your dominant hand.
- Invert the glove and discard the catheter and glove in clinical waste.
- Assess the patient's requirements for further suctioning. If it is required, a pair of clean gloves and a new sterile catheter will be needed. The process is then repeated following the same steps above.
- Evaluate the colour, consistency, and amount of secretions removed.
- Document the episode of care.

Practice tips

- If you put the suction tubing with the suction catheter attached but still in its packaging under your armpit, it is easier to hold it and remove the packaging.
- Suction catheters that are specifically designed for tracheostomies are available, although not commonly used. These are shorter in length than the standard types and will minimize damage to the mucosa/carina caused by inserting the suction catheter too far.

Pitfall

- Spending excess time performing suction, leading to hypoxia and bradycardia.

Tracheostomy care

Background

Meticulous routine care of a tracheotomy tube and site helps to prevent complications. Humidification is usually necessary to avoid dry secretions, which can cause retention of sputum and blockage of the tube. Care of an inner tube, if present, prevents occlusion of the airway. Assessment and cleaning of the stoma site ↓ the risk of skin breakdown.

Equipment

- Working suction equipment.
- Suction catheters of an appropriate size.
- Disposable gloves (not powdered).
- Tracheostomy tubes (one tube the same size as the tube *in situ* and another tube one size smaller).
- Tracheal dilators.
- Scissors.
- Ambu bag, reservoir, and face mask.
- Spare inner cannula (if applicable).

Procedure

- Explain the procedure and gain consent.
- Check humidification is adequate, as follows:
  - Does the bottle of water need changing for a cold-water humidifier?
  - Is the temperature correct on the heated circuit?
  - Is the heat–moisture exchanger (HME); e.g. Swedish nose or Thermovent still patent?
  - Does the patient require a nebulizer, in addition to humidification?
- Check the inner cannula (if present) every 4 hours or more if copious or very dry secretions are present.
  - Unlock the inner cannula, withdraw it slowly, and inspect the tube. If the patient is ventilated or requires positive end expiratory pressure (PEEP) or high concentrations of oxygen, they might require pre-oxygenation before doing this.
- If cleaning the inner tube is required, you will need to:
  - Remove the inner tube and replace it with a spare inner cannula.
  - Rinse the tube with sterile or warm tap water to remove any particles.
  - Clean the tube with specifically designed swabs.
  - When clean, rinse the tube through with sterile water and replace it.
- Check the stoma site—cleaning of the stoma site should take place at least once daily or more frequently if required (📖 on p. 234).
- Suction, as required (📖 on p. 230).
- Check the cuff pressure (📖 on p. 228).
- Document the episode of care.

Practice tip
- Tracheostomy dressings might not be required long term. They are used to absorb drainage from the tracheostomy site and ↓ irritation.

Pitfalls
- Using HMEs (e.g. Swedish nose) in patients with excess secretions. They can become blocked by secretions and cause airway occlusion.
- Some manufacturers have temporary inner cannulae, which are only to be used while the standard inner cannula is being cleaned.

Changing a tracheostomy dressing

Background

Secretions from around a tracheostomy tube can cause irritation and skin breakdown. Cleaning and changing dressings will prevent this. This should be done at least once daily if secretions are present and more frequently if required. The procedure requires the involvement of two health care workers (HCWs) because one HCW needs to hold the tube throughout. Tracheostomy dressings might not be required long term.

Equipment

- Apron and gloves.
- Sterile dressing pack.
- Pre-cut/keyhole dressing.
- Tracheostomy dressing.
- Sterile gauze.
- Sterile 0.9% saline solution.
- Tracheostomy ties.

Procedure

- Explain the procedure and gain consent.
- Wash your hands, prepare the equipment, and put on the gloves and apron.
- Position the patient supine with the neck slightly extended.
- Suction the patient, if required.
- The other HCW holds the tracheostomy tube securely on either side of the flange throughout the procedure.
- Cut the old/soiled tapes.
- Remove the old stoma dressing and discard it in clinical waste.
- Clean your hands again and put on clean gloves.
- Assess the stoma site and take a wound swab if required.
- Clean around the stoma using 0.9% sodium chloride solution and dry the area thoroughly with sterile gauze.
- Apply the keyhole dressing.
- Fasten the tube with ties, adjusting them to fit the patient's neck but allowing enough slack to slide two fingers under the tapes.
- Dispose of the equipment in clinical waste.
- Both HCWs wash and dry their hands.
- Document the episode of care.

Practice tip

- Minimal movement of the tube throughout the procedure will ↓ the probability of the patient coughing, making it easier to carry out the procedure.

Pitfall

- Cutting the external balloon of a cuffed tracheostomy tube. Seek senior help if this occurs.

Changing a tracheostomy tube

Background

Tracheostomy tubes are usually changed once every 7–14 days to prevent infection and blockage of the tube by secretions. Tubes should not be changed unnecessarily. Manufacturers issue guidelines for the frequency of change required for specific tubes. Newly formed tracheostomies need sufficient time to enable a tract to form. The first change is ideally performed by an appropriately trained senior clinician. If the change was not problematic, subsequent changes can be performed by a health care worker (HCW) deemed competent in the procedure. The patient should receive nil by mouth for 3–4 hours before the procedure. Personnel competent in emergency intubation and appropriate equipment should be close by while the tracheostomy tube is changed.

Equipment

- Tracheostomy tubes (one tube the same size as the tube *in situ* and one tube one size smaller).
- Apron and gloves.
- Working suction equipment.
- Sterile dressing pack.
- Sterile gloves.
- 10mL syringe.
- 0.9% sodium chloride solution.
- Water-soluble sterile lubricant.
- Pre-cut/keyhole tracheostomy dressing.
- Sterile gauze.
- Tracheostomy ties.
- Cuff pressure gauge.
- Monitoring equipment—pulse oximeter and blood pressure cuff.
- Bag–valve–mask device and oxygen supply.
- Tracheal dilators.
- Re-intubation equipment.

Procedure

- Explain the procedure and gain consent.
- Ideally, this procedure should be performed by two HCWs.
- Wash your hands and prepare the trolley.
- Position the patient supine with the neck slightly extended.
- Put on the gloves and apron.
- Aspirate through the nasogastric tube, if present.
- Suction the patient to remove secretions, if required.
- Check the new tracheostomy tube by inflating the cuff with air and observing for any leaks. The pilot balloon should indicate that the cuff is inflated. Remove all the air.
- Lubricate the tube and place it on a sterile surface.
- Pre-oxygenate the patient before the procedure if they are receiving oxygen therapy.
- Ask the patient to breathe out. Expiration should prevent them coughing, which can cause the tracheostomy to close over.

- As the patient exhales, cut the ties and remove the old tube in an upwards and outwards motion.
- Insert the new tracheostomy tube with the obturator in place while the patient is still exhaling.
- Remove the obturator immediately and insert the inner cannula, if applicable.
- Re-commence oxygen therapy.
- Inflate the cuff using a syringe.
- Check the cuff pressure with a pressure gauge (📖 on p. 228).
- Observe the patient for signs of respiratory distress and compare pre-insertion and post-insertion observations.
- Clean the stoma site, if required.
- Apply a keyhole dressing.
- Fasten the tube with ties, adjusting them to fit the patient's neck but allowing enough slack to slide two fingers under the tapes.
- Dispose of the equipment in clinical waste.
- Both HCWs wash their hands.
- Document the episode of care.

Practice tips
- Consider whether the patient is ready for decannulation/removal of the tracheostomy tube instead.
- If the tube change fails and the patient becomes distressed or cyanosed, call for senior medical help immediately. Use a tracheal dilator to attempt to insert a smaller tube. If this fails, administer oxygen through the stoma. Alternatively, cover the stoma site with a dressing, open the patient's airway, and administer oxygen by use of a face mask until help arrives.

Pitfall
- Not having all the equipment available before commencing the procedure.

Tracheostomy care in an emergency

Background

In the event of a cardiac or respiratory arrest, it is essential to secure the airway. The reason for the tracheostomy and type of tube in place will determine the method used if a patient with a tracheostomy has a respiratory or cardiac arrest. If the patient has had part of their trachea removed, resuscitation must occur through the stoma site.

Equipment

- Ambu bag and reservoir.
- Face mask.
- Suction equipment.
- Oxygen.
- Resuscitation trolley.

Procedure

- If the patient is unresponsive, follow standard advanced life support (ALS) guidelines (📖 on p. 384, 385).
- If the patient is not breathing, check that the tracheotomy cuff is inflated and manually ventilate the patient by use of a bag–valve–mask device and catheter mount attached to the tracheostomy tube using 10L of oxygen.
- If you are unable to inflate the lungs, suction the tracheostomy tube because it might be blocked.
- If you are still unable to ventilate the patient, check the patency of the inner tube, if applicable.
- Remove the inner cannula tube and replace it. If it is fenestrated, change it to a plain inner cannula (one without a hole) or seal the nose and mouth to prevent air escaping.
- If the tube is uncuffed, manually ventilate the patient using the Ambu bag. Occlude the patient's nose and mouth in these circumstances to prevent excessive loss of air.
- A small, soft face mask can also be placed over the stoma and ventilation applied in this way.
- If ventilation is still inadequate and the patient has not had part of their trachea removed, consider removing the tracheostomy tube, occluding the stoma with a dressing/gauze, and performing manual ventilation by use of a face mask until help arrives.
- If you are still unable to maintain a patent airway, continue with basic life support.

Practice tip

- Call for help early.

Pitfall

- Not knowing the type of tracheotomy tube or indications for its insertion.

Assessment of the circulation

Background
Assessment of the circulation in a critically ill patient takes place after the airway and breathing have been managed. Cardiovascular compromise might be owing to 1° cardiac problems or the result of hypovolaemia, sepsis, or, less commonly, head or spinal injury.

Equipment
- None.

Procedure
Look
- Skin colour—is the patient cyanosed or pale? Is the patient sweating? In sepsis, the patient might appear red or pink and flushed.
- Obvious signs of haemorrhage—check wound drains, if present.
- ↑ jugular venous pulse.
- Obvious pulsations in the chest or abdomen.
- The capillary refill time should be <2sec.

Listen
- With a stethoscope to the heart and lungs for added heart sounds, murmurs and evidence of fluid in the lungs (crackles or cardiac wheeze).
- Blood pressure might be measured manually with auscultation, but more commonly it is measured electronically.

Feel
- Pulses (peripheral and central) for rate, regularity, volume, and character.
- Peripheral limb temperature compared with the central temperature. Peripheral cooling and shutdown are usually present in hypovolaemic and cardiogenic shock. Warm peripheries might indicate sepsis as a cause of shock.

Insert
- Consider insertion of a urinary catheter to measure urinary output.
- Consider insertion of a central line to measure central venous pressure.

Practice tips
- Airway Breathing Circulation and Disability (ABC and D) are linked inextricably and a problem with the circulation might manifest as airway compromise, ↑ respiratory rate, or an altered level of consciousness.
- A narrow pulse pressure may be an early sign of hypovolaemic shock (amongst other causes).
- A low diastolic pressure suggests vasodilatation, as seen in sepsis.

Pitfalls
- Failing to call for appropriate help early.
- Not being aware that hypotension is a late sign in shock and ignoring earlier signs, e.g. tachycardia, tachypnoea, and a narrow pulse pressure.

Assisting with insertion of a central line

Background

A central venous catheter (CVC) is a hollow radio-opaque cannula that is inserted into the subclavian, internal jugular, femoral, or brachial vein. Central lines have several indications, including monitoring of central venous pressure (CVP), access for drugs and fluids that are irritants to peripheral veins (e.g. inotropes, cytotoxic drugs, and parenteral nutrition), and fluid administration, particularly if peripheral access is difficult.

Equipment

- Sterile CVP/intravenous (IV) cut-down set.
- CVC set.
- Gauze swabs.
- 2% chlorhexidine in 70% isopropyl alcohol.
- One sterile gown and mask.
- Three sterile towels.
- One non-dissolvable suture and needle.
- Sterile gloves, assorted sizes.
- A selection of needles.
- Two 20mL ampoules of 0.9% saline solution.
- A selection of syringes.
- 1% or 2% lidocaine solution.
- Two sterile semi-occlusive dressings.
- Equipment for reading CVP, if required.
- Monitoring equipment—pulse oximeter, blood pressure cuff, and cardiac monitor.
- Ultrasound machine (optional, although recommended).

Procedure

- Ensure that the procedure has been explained and consent gained. Re-assure the patient and answer any further questions.
- Obtain baseline observations before the procedure.
- Prepare the equipment.
- Wash your hands and open all equipment onto the sterile field.
- Assist the health care worker (HCW) carrying out the procedure to put on a sterile gown.
- Position the patient supine, with the head tilted downwards (if tolerated)—reverse Trendelenburg position.
- Ensure all standard monitoring equipment is working—e.g. cardiac, blood pressure and oxygen saturation monitoring.

The HCW carrying out the procedure (HCW 1) will then perform the following actions:

- Clean and drape the area around the intended insertion site and administer local anaesthetic into the surrounding skin.
- Prime the central line and ensure all ports are capped off.
- Insert the line using an ultrasound-guided technique.
- Suture the cannula to the skin.

Following insertion and suturing of the line, you (the assistant) will perform the following actions:

- Apply a sterile, transparent, non-occlusive dressing to the line using a sandwich technique.
- Discard any waste in the clinical waste disposal and ensure that all sharps have been disposed of in the sharps bin by HCW 1.
- Put instruments aside for return to sterile services.
- Reposition the patient.
- Record post-insertion observations.
- Label the line with the date and time of insertion.
- Document the episode of care.
- A chest X-ray should be obtained after the procedure to check the position of the CVC line.
- Ensure that it is documented in the notes that the line can be used before infusion of fluid or drugs.

Practice tip

- Use a checklist to ensure all the equipment is ready before the procedure commences. This will speed up the process.

Pitfalls

- Reassure the patient throughout the procedure. They usually cannot see what is going on and can become anxious.
- Not maintaining strict asepsis during the procedure, leading to catheter-related bloodstream infection (CRBI), which is potentially fatal.

Care of a central line

Background
Good care of a central line minimizes the possibility of inadvertent displacement, air embolism, and line-associated infection.

Equipment
- Sterile dressing pack.
- Gauze swabs.
- 2% chlorhexidine in 70% isopropyl alcohol.
- Sterile gloves, assorted sizes.
- Disposable gloves.
- Two sterile semi-occlusive dressings.
- Microbiology swab.
- 10–20mL 0.9% saline solution.
- 10 and 20mL syringes.

Procedure
- Review the necessity for the central line daily. Routine changes of line are not recommended. If the line is no longer required, it should be removed promptly.
- Avoid access hubs and frequent connection and disconnection.

Cleaning the insertion site
- If the insertion site requires cleaning, e.g. after a dressing displacement, explain the procedure and gain consent.
- Prepare the equipment.
- Wash your hands and open the dressing pack.
- Put on the disposable gloves and remove the dressing from the insertion site.
- If the site is red or oozing fluid, send a swab for microscopy, culture, and sensitivity.
- Remove the gloves and discard.
- Wash your hands.
- Put on sterile gloves.
- Clean the insertion site and surrounding skin with antiseptic solution (2% chlorhexidine in 70% isopropyl alcohol) using a circular motion, starting nearest the insertion site and working outwards.
- Allow the area to dry before applying a dressing.
- Apply a sterile, transparent, non-occlusive dressing to the line using a sandwich technique.
- Discard waste in clinical waste.
- Document the episode of care.
- Clearly label all infusions with the date and time next to the port of the central line and on the drug or infusion fluid.
- If the central line is not in constant use, it might require flushing to maintain patency.

Flushing a central line
- Prepare the equipment.
- Wash your hands and put on gloves.
- Clean the needleless injection cap with antiseptic solution and allow the area to dry.
- Attach a 5mL syringe and aspirate 2–3mL. Observe for withdrawal of blood.
- Clamp the line before removal of this syringe to prevent air embolism.
- Attach a 10mL syringe filled with 0.9% saline to the injection cap and unclamp the line when this syringe is engaged.
- Slowly inject up to 10mL of 0.9% saline solution into the port.
- Repeat for any further ports.
- Dispose of equipment and wash your hands.
- Document the episode of care.

Practice tips
- Try to ensure there are no folds or creases in the dressing because this will minimize the need to re-dress the site.
- Ask the patient to tilt their head to one side, if possible, when applying the dressing because this will stop the dressing pulling on the skin.

Pitfalls
- Not inspecting the line site daily.
- Not removing the line if signs of phlebitis or infection are noted.

Measurement of central venous pressure

Background

Central venous pressure (CVP) is equivalent to right atrial pressure. It is used as a guide for fluid management and determined by blood volume, vascular tone, and cardiac function. A normal CVP ranges from $7cmH_2O$ to $14cmH_2O/5mmHg$ to 10mmHg when recorded midaxilla.

Equipment

- Manometer/tape measure.
- Drip stand.
- Spirit level.
- CVP monitoring infusion set.
- Intravenous crystalloid—e.g. 0.9% sodium chloride and 5% glucose solutions.

Procedure

- Explain the procedure and gain consent.
- Prepare the equipment.
- Connect the infusion fluid to the CVP monitoring set.
- Prime the line, ensuring that the three-way tap is turned off to the manometer initially.
- Prime the manometer slowly, ensuring that the fluid does not reach the air vent.
- Connect the primed line to the distal lumen of the central venous catheter (if using a multilumen catheter).
- Stop any other infusions.
- Position the patient supine, if tolerated. If not tolerated, the head of the bed could be raised up to 45°. The reading should not be taken with the patient on their side.
- Place the manometer so that the zero ('0') is level with the right atrium. Use a spirit level to ensure accuracy. Two reference points can be used, as follows:
  - The fourth intercostal space midaxilla—the phlebostatic axis.
  - The sternal angle can be used if the patient is supine. These readings will be 5cm lower than those from the midaxilla.
- Mark the patient (with their agreement) and document the zero reference point on a chart.
- Check the patency of the line. Flush it, if required.
- Switch the three-way tap at the base of the manometer off to the patient and on to the manometer and infusion fluid.
- Slowly fill the manometer, ensuring the fluid does not reach the air-vent cap.
- Turn the three-way tap off to the infusion fluid and on to the patient and the manometer.
- The column of water should ↓ steadily. When the fluid level ceases to ↓, it should fluctuate in synchrony with the patient's respiration.
- Record the end expiratory reading.

- Turn the three-way tap off to the manometer and readjust the infusion rate.
- Re-commence other infusion lines and pumps, as appropriate.
- Reposition the patient.
- Alert senior clinical staff if the reading is outside the expected limits.
- Document the episode of care.

Practice tips

- Trends in CVP readings are more significant than single readings.
- To convert cmH_2O to mmHg, divide cmH_2O by 1.36.

Pitfalls

- Allowing the filter at the top of the tubing to become wet. This can allow airborne organisms to enter the system and prevent accurate CVP readings.
- Obtaining inaccurate readings if the patient is not positioned in the same place for consecutive readings or other infusions are running at the same time.
- Allowing bubbles into the system, which can affect readings.

Removal of a central line

Background
If a central venous catheter is no longer required, it should be removed promptly to minimize the risk of complications, particularly sepsis and thrombosis.

Equipment
- Sterile dressing pack.
- Sterile drape/dressing towel.
- Sterile gloves.
- Disposable gloves.
- A selection of syringes.
- Stitch cutter.
- Sterile forceps.
- 2% chlorhexidine in 70% isopropyl alcohol.
- Sterile gauze swabs.
- Sterile adhesive plaster (waterproof).
- Sterile scissors.
- Sterile specimen container.
- Sharps box.

Procedure
- Explain the procedure and gain consent.
- Obtain baseline observations before the procedure.
- Prepare the equipment.
- Wash and dry your hands and open the dressing pack.
- Switch off all infusions and clamp lines.
- Position the patient supine, with the head tilted downwards (if tolerated)—reverse Trendelenburg position.
- Put on disposable gloves and remove the dressing.
- Remove the gloves and discard.
- Wash your hands.
- Put on sterile gloves and place a drape around the insertion site.
- Clean the insertion site and surrounding skin with antiseptic solution (2% chlorhexidine in 70% isopropyl alcohol) using a circular motion, working outwards from the insertion site.
- Remove the suture using the stitch cutter and forceps.
- Place a pad of gauze swabs over the insertion site and ask the patient to take a deep breath in and hold it. If the patient is receiving positive-pressure ventilation, synchronize the removal of the catheter with the end of the expiratory phase.
- Pull the catheter out while applying pressure with the gauze swabs.
- Place the catheter on the sterile field and ask the patient to breathe normally.
- Apply pressure to the puncture site until the bleeding stops (usually ~5min).
- Cover the site with an occlusive dressing.
- Reposition the patient.

- If microscopy, culture, and sensitivity (MC&S) are required, cut off the catheter tip using the sterile scissors and place it in a sterile specimen pot.
- The puncture site should remain covered for at least 24 hours to prevent an air embolism.
- If an air embolism is suspected, call for help, administer 100% oxygen, and position the patient on their left side, with the bed or trolley tilted head down—signs and symptoms of an air embolism include shortness of breath, anxiety, hypotension, chest pain, and collapse.
- Document the episode of care. This should include the time, date and the type and the condition of the catheter removed. The condition of the patient's skin around the insertion site should also be recorded.

Practice tip

- If the patient cannot tolerate the reverse Trendelenburg position or they are receiving an epidural infusion, a valsalva manoeuvre can be carried out when removing the line.

Pitfalls

- Taking an excessive amount of time to remove the catheter and making the patient hold their breath for too long.
- Allowing the catheter to migrate out accidentally when the holding suture is removed.

Assisting with venous cut-down

Background

Venous cut-down is used if peripheral venous cannulation is not possible. The vein is exposed surgically and a cannula is inserted into the vein under direct vision. It is potentially life-saving in patients who are in shock. The commonest veins used are the basilic vein in the antecubital fossa and the great saphenous vein at the ankle. The following describes the procedure on the basilic vein.

Equipment

- Sterile intravenous (IV) cut-down pack.
- A size 11 blade.
- Sterile drape/dressing towel.
- Sterile gloves.
- 2% chlorhexidine in 70% isopropyl alcohol.
- Sterile gauze swabs.
- Sharps box.
- 2mL and 5mL syringes.
- 1% or 2% lidocaine solution.
- 4.0 silk ties.
- 4.0 silk or nylon sutures on a cutting needle for skin closure.
- A selection of needles.
- IV cannula.
- Tourniquet.
- IV infusion fluid connected to an administration set and primed.
- Sterile semi-occlusive dressing.

Procedure

- Ensure that the procedure has been explained and consent gained.
- Prepare the equipment.
- Wash and dry your hands and open the dressing pack.
- Place the patient in the supine position.
- You might need to hold the patient's arm during the procedure.
- Apply a tourniquet around the patient's upper arm.

The person carrying out the procedure health care worker (HCW) 1 will:

- Wash their hands and put on sterile gloves.
- Clean and drape the area around the intended insertion site.
- Administer local anaesthetic into the surrounding skin.
- Make a 2–3cm transverse incision over the vein.
- Bluntly dissect the vein out.
- Place two ligatures (sutures) around the vein. The distal ligature is then used to tie off the vein distally, but the ends are not cut.
- Hold the ends of both ligatures with the artery forceps to maintain traction. HCW 2 might be asked to assist at this point.
- Make a V-shaped incision in the vein and insert the cannula into it. The tourniquet is then released and blood should be seen flowing into the catheter.
- Tie the proximal ligature over the cannulated vein to secure it.
- Connect the cannula to the giving set and commence the infusion.

- Check for any bleeding in the wound.
- Close the skin with sutures and apply a dressing.
- Discard any waste in clinical waste disposal.
- Wash their hands.
- Document the episode of care.

Practice tips

- Maintaining traction on the vein during the procedure makes it easier to insert the cannula.
- Try to distract the patient from looking at the procedure, because this tends to cause excessive movement and makes holding and cannulating the vein difficult. It may also be distressing for the patient.

Pitfalls

- Not securing the cannula adequately can result in it slipping out.
- Poor asepsis particularly in emergencies resulting in infection.

Insertion of an intraosseous needle

Background

The intraosseus route is used for vascular access if other routes have failed. It is a temporary measure to buy time and most commonly used in babies, infants, and children. The anterior aspect of the upper tibia is the most commonly used approach, as described below. Contraindications include local fractures or infection. Other sites include the lateral femoral condyle, iliac crest, and sternum. The marrow cavity can be used for the administration of fluids and drugs because it is in continuity with the venous circulation.

Equipment

- Sterile dressing pack.
- Sterile gloves.
- 2% chlorhexidine in 70% isopropyl alcohol.
- Sterile gauze swabs.
- Sharps box.
- 2mL and 5mL syringes.
- 1% or 2% lidocaine solution.
- Intraosseous or bone-marrow needle.
- 50mL syringe.
- Tape.

Procedure

- Explain the procedure and gain consent.
- Prepare the equipment.
- Wash your hands.
- Flex the knee and support with a rolled-up blanket or sandbag.
- Clean the skin.
- Inject a small amount of local anaesthetic into the skin and continue infiltration down to the periosteum.
- Insert the intraosseus needle at 90° to the skin (perpendicular).
- Advance the needle until a 'give' is felt; this occurs when the needle penetrates the cortex of the bone.
- Remove the trochar. Confirm the correct position by aspirating blood using the 5mL syringe.
- Secure the needle in place with sterile gauze and strapping.
- Give boluses of fluid (the infusion volume depends on the clinical situation) using the 50mL syringe to push the fluid in gently.
- Discard any waste in the clinical waste disposal.
- Decontaminate your hands.
- Document the episode of care.

Practice tips

- Ensure the needle is at 90° and apply firm pressure because it is easy for the needle to slip off the surface of the bone.
- Fluids might be infused under gentle pressure using a pressure bag set at 100mmHg. The infusion is best limited to a few hours until intravenous access is achieved.

- Blood can be taken from the intraosseus needle for most routine blood tests.
- Drugs can be given provided they are gently syringed in.

Pitfalls

- Not securing the needle well can cause inadvertent displacement.
- Not observing strict asepsis, with the consequent risk of osteomyelitis.

Insertion of an arterial line

Background

Arterial lines provide easy access to an artery in critically ill patients who require frequent analysis of blood gases and other blood tests. They enable continuous direct measurement of arterial blood pressure. Caution is advised in patients with peripheral vascular disease and haemorrhagic disorders. Cannulation is relatively contraindicated in areas of infection, sites of previous vascular surgery, through synthetic vascular grafting, or if there is no collateral blood supply to the site of the arterial line.

Equipment

- 500mL pressure-infuser cuff/pressure bag.
- 1500mL bag of 0.9% saline solution ± 500U of heparin.
- 22 gauge, or similar, arterial cannula.
- Guide wire—optional.
- Sterile dressing pack.
- Sterile gloves.
- 2% chlorhexidine in 70% isopropyl alcohol.
- Local anaesthetic—injection of 1% lidocaine solution.
- 2, 5, and 10mL syringes.
- Semi-occlusive dressing.
- Arterial line label.
- Pressure monitoring system, transducer set, cable, and monitor if invasive blood pressure readings are required (📖 on p. 256).

Procedure

- Explain the procedure and gain consent.
- Choose the insertion site. The most common site is the radial artery, followed by the brachial, femoral, or dorsalis pedis.
- If the radial artery is chosen, assess for collateral circulation using Allen's test. Ask the patient to clench their fist as you compress their radial and ulnar arteries. When the hand is white, release the pressure on the ulnar artery and watch for the colour to return to the patient's hand. If it doesn't, the radial artery on that side should not be used because the test demonstrates inadequate collateral circulation and the potential for an ischaemic hand if the artery became occluded.
- Prepare a sterile field and administer local anaesthetic. Allow time for it to work before proceeding.
- Rest the patient's forearm on a pillow, palm upwards, allowing the wrist to dorsiflex over it.
- Attach a syringe to the arterial catheter.
- Palpate for the artery.
- Insert the catheter into the artery at ~30° to the skin.
- When a flashback of bright red blood is seen, remove the introducer and pull the catheter back a little so that the tip of it is at the puncture site in the artery. Do this with extreme caution as there is a risk of coming out of the artery if you withdraw too much.
- Feed the guidewire through the catheter and along the lumen of the artery. Be careful not to feed all of the wire in and never let go of it.

- Slide the catheter into place, holding the wire at all times.
- Remove the wire.
- Occlude the end of the catheter with your gloved hand until it is attached to the transducer line.
- Suture the line in place.
- Use a sterile, occlusive dressing to cover the entry site and secure the line.
- Ensure the insertion site is clearly visible.
- Label the line.
- Dispose of sharps in the sharps box and waste in clinical waste disposal.
- Document the episode of care.

Practice tips

- Locate the position of maximal pulsation in the artery before attempting to insert the cannula.
- Ensure the transducer set is primed for use before insertion of the line.
- An arterial catheter with a valve to stop blood flow is preferable because it facilitates changing transducer sets or dressings.

Pitfalls

- Poor asepsis, leading to infection around the catheter insertion site.
- Disconnection of the catheter from the tubing, which might result in bleeding.

Care of an arterial line

Background

An arterial line is a percutaneous cannula placed within an artery, which is used for continuous blood pressure monitoring and arterial blood sampling. It is kept patent by a continuous intravenous infusion (usually 0.9% saline solution) by use of a pressurized flushing device.

Equipment

- 500mL pressure-infuser cuff/pressure bag.
- 1 × 500mL bag of 0.9% saline solution ± 500U of heparin.
- Sterile dressing pack and gloves.
- 2% chlorhexidine in 70% isopropyl alcohol.
- Semi-occlusive dressing.
- Arterial line label.
- Pressure monitoring system, transducer set, cable, and monitor if invasive blood pressure readings are required (📕 on p. 256).

Procedure

Care of the line

- Review the necessity for an arterial line daily. If it is no longer required, it should be removed promptly.
- Ensure that the line is clearly labelled with the date and time of insertion, usually in red. No infusions of fluid or drugs should be given into the line, apart from that keeping it patent.
- Ensure a needleless hub is *in situ* for removal of arterial blood.
- Check the flush bag every 2 hours to ensure that the pressure is maintained at 300mmHg and there is still fluid in the bag. Replace the fluid, if necessary.
- Avoid frequent connection or disconnection.

Care of the patient

- Observe the limb distal to the cannula for numbness or signs of ischaemia, e.g. pallor or coldness. If present, inform senior clinical staff immediately and remove the cannula.

Cleaning the insertion site

- If the insertion site requires cleaning, e.g. following displacement of a dressing, explain the procedure and gain consent.
- Prepare the equipment
- Wash your dry your hands and open the dressing pack.
- Put on disposable gloves and remove the dressing.
- If the site is red or oozing fluid, send a swab for microscopy, culture, and sensitivity.
- Remove the gloves and discard.
- Wash your hands.
- Put on sterile gloves.

- Clean the insertion site and surrounding skin with antiseptic solution (2% chlorhexidine in 70% isopropyl alcohol) using a circular motion, starting nearest the insertion site and working outwards.
- Allow the area to dry before applying a dressing.
- Apply a sterile, transparent, non-occlusive dressing.
- Discard waste in clinical waste.
- Document the episode of care.

Changing the transducer
- Change the transducer set according to the manufacturer's guidelines.
- Clearly label and date the line following this procedure.
- Document the episode of care.

Practice tip
- If the arterial catheter does not have a valve to stop blood flow, an assistant should ideally secure the line and occlude the blood flow while the transducer is being changed.

Pitfalls
- Not securing the line adequately, leading to disconnection.
- Poor labelling of the arterial line, leading to inadvertent administration of fluids or drugs into it.

Invasive measurement of blood pressure by an arterial line

Background

Arterial blood pressure can be continuously and accurately measured by an indwelling arterial line. This is valuable in patients at risk of sudden haemodynamic changes, including those on drugs that have a direct effect on mean arterial pressure (MAP), e.g. inotropes.

Equipment

- Indwelling arterial catheter.
- Disposable transducer set.
- Transducer cable.
- 500mL 0.9% saline solution/heparinized saline.
- Pressure bag.
- Monitor.

Procedure

- Explain the procedure and gain consent.
- Prime the transducer set with saline/heparinized saline (1U/mL) to remove all air bubbles.
- Place the saline/heparinized saline bag inside the pressure bag.
- Pump the pressure bag up to 300mmHg to prevent backflow of blood and ensure a continuous flow of fluid at 3mL/hour.
- Attach the primed transducer set to the indwelling arterial catheter. Ensure all hubs/stopcocks are secure.
- Two types of 'zeroing' are needed to obtain accurate pressure readings:
  - Zero the transducer—place the transducer in the midaxilla at the level of the right atrium (fourth intercostal space, known as the 'phlebostatic axis'). Use a spirit level to ensure accuracy.
  - Zero the monitor to negate the effects of atmospheric pressure. Once correctly positioned, turn the three-way tap nearest to the arterial catheter off to the patient and on to air and the transducer. The transducer and monitor should then be calibrated by pressing 'zero'/'calibrate' on the monitor. The monitor will then display a straight waveform and a zero reading. Turn the three-way tap off to air and on to the patient to enable monitoring to begin. Adjust the scaling on the monitor, as appropriate.
- Set the alarm limits within predefined limits or 10% of the patient's normal values.
- Observe the waveform—a normal arterial waveform has three parts, as follows:
  - A systolic peak.
  - A diacrotic notch.
  - End diastole.
- Check the flush bag every 2 hours to ensure that the pressure is maintained and there is still fluid in the bag.
- Monitor the circulation in the extremity every 2–4 hours.
- Calibrate and zero the system at least every 8 hours and after repositioning the patient.

- Label the line clearly, usually in red. Ensure that no infusions are given through the line.

Practice tip
- Check the blood pressure with a manual cuff every 8 hours to compare readings. A variation of <20mmHg is acceptable.

Pitfalls
- Not checking a clear waveform is displayed before recording the readings.
- Inaccurate readings owing to kinking of the arterial catheter or partial obstruction by a clot.
- A damped trace owing to air bubbles.
- Not re-zeroing the system every 8 hours or after moving the patient.

Arterial blood gas sampling by an arterial line

Background

Analysis of arterial blood gases (ABG) is used to evaluate the adequacy of ventilation, acid–base status, oxygenation, and the oxygen-carrying capacity of blood. Arterial blood can be drawn from an indwelling arterial cannula sited in a peripheral artery (radial, brachial, femoral, or dorsalis pedis), avoiding the need for repeated arterial stabs.

Equipment

- 2mL pre-heparinized syringe.
- 5mL syringe.
- Sterile protective bung/blind hub.
- Protective gloves.
- Isopropyl alcohol-impregnated swab.
- Cardboard procedure tray.
- Sterile gauze.
- If other blood samples are required, appropriate blood bottles and forms.
- Sharps bin.

Procedure

- Explain the procedure and gain consent.
- Locate the arterial line and the three-way tap nearest to the arterial cannula.
- Ensure the three-way tap is turned off to the sample port.
- Remove the sterile bung/blind hub from this three-way tap and wipe the sample port with an alcoholic pre-injection swab.
- Attach a sterile 5mL syringe to the sample port on the three-way tap. If an arterial 'bionector' is in place, wipe down the port and insert a 5mL syringe.
- Open the three-way tap so that it is on to the sample port and the arterial catheter.
- Aspirate 2.5mL of blood from the 15cm dead space between the sample port and the cannula. If the line is >15cm, you might need to aspirate a larger amount.
- Turn the three-way tap 45° to the half-closed position and remove the blood-filled syringe. Discard it into the sharps bin.
- Attach the pre-heparinized syringe to the sample port, open the three-way tap to the patient, and gently aspirate an ABG sample (~1.5mL of blood). Many pre-heparinized syringes self-fill and ∴ will not require any active aspiration.
- Close the three-way tap and remove the syringe containing the ABG sample.
- Evacuate any air bubbles immediately by gently pushing the plunger into the syringe barrel.
- Seal the ABG syringe with the impermeable cap/bung supplied.
- Gently invert the sample to ensure mixing of the heparin. Do not shake it.

- Turn the three-way tap off to the arterial catheter and on to the transducer and sampling port. Flush the line gently (using the flushing device on the transducer) into a syringe until all the blood is cleared from the three-way tap.
- Close the three-way tap to the sample port, clean it with an alcoholic pre-injection swab, and apply a new sterile protective bung/blind hub.
- Activate the flush device until the arterial line is clear of blood. Check the pressure-infuser cuff is still inflated to 300mmHg to ensure the flushing device works.
- Take a sample for analysis immediately. If there is an unavoidable delay before analysis, the sample should be stored in ice.
- Insert the syringe into a blood gas analyser and follow the manufacturer's guidelines for use of the analyser.
- Insert the patient's details, in addition to the temperature and oxygen percentage, to ensure correct measurements.
- Discard the syringe into a sharps bin and waste into clinical waste disposal.
- Document the episode of care.

Practice tip
- Ensure the sample is sealed with an impermeable bung before transport, to prevent mixing with atmospheric gases.

Pitfalls
- Failing to remove air bubbles before transport of the sample.
- Not entering the patient's details when analysing the results.

Analysing arterial blood gases 1

Background

ABG analysis can be performed quickly and is one of the first tests performed in a critically ill patient. It can give useful information about oxygenation, ventilation, perfusion and acid-base status and can aid diagnosis. The results (see Box 9.1 for the normal reference range) should be analysed in a systematic fashion and correlated with the patient's clinical condition.

- **Oxygenation** Hypoxaemia—a PaO_2 < 8.0kPa can result from ventilation–perfusion (V/Q) mismatch, e.g. pulmonary embolism or from hypoventilation e.g. chronic obstructive pulmonary disease (COPD). It is important to know the fraction of inspired oxygen (fio_2) when the A36 sample was taken.

- **Ventilation** The $PaCO_2$ tells us about the ventilatory status of the patient. A low $PaCO_2$ means that the patient is hyperventilating (over-breathing and blowing CO_2 off) and a high $PaCO_2$ signifies hypoventilation. An abnormal $PaCO_2$ may be due to a primary ventilatory problem or compensation for a primary metabolic disturbance (see below).

- **Acid-base balance** The pH is a measure of the hydrogen ion concentration. Enzymes within cells require a stable pH between 7.35 and 7.45 to function normally. In normal acid-base balance there is a normal pH and normal values of $PaCO_2$ and HCO_3^-. The body regulates acid-base balance through the three mechanisms of buffer systems, respiratory regulation and renal regulation. Acid base imbalances may be considered as either *respiratory* involving CO_2 elimination or *metabolic* involving the kidneys and linked to HCO_3^- values. When there is an abnormal pH, the primary acid-base balance is always obvious by looking at the HCO_3^- and $PaCO_2$ values. In an acidosis (pH<7.35) if the HCO_3^- is ↓ the primary disturbance is *metabolic*, but if the $PaCO_2$ is ↑ the primary disturbance is *respiratory*. In an alkalosis (pH>7.45) if the HCO_3^- is ↑ the primary disturbance is metabolic but if the $PaCO_2$ is ↓ the primary disturbance is respiratory. *Mixed acid base disorders* can occur, i.e. two or more primary acid-base abnormalities can coexist, e.g. if in an acidosis the HCO_3^- is ↓ **and** the $PaCO_2$ is ↑ there is **both** a primary metabolic and a primary respiratory component to the acidosis.

- **Compensation** Compensation describes the physiological response to the primary disturbance. In a primary *respiratory* disturbance metabolic changes compensate (through renal control of H+ and HCO_3^- ion excretion). In *metabolic* derangements respiratory changes compensate (through control of CO_2 excretion from the lungs). Over-compensation does not occur.

📖 See Table 9.1, p. 263, for a summary of the changes that occur in the various acid base disorders.

Equipment

- Blood gas sample (📖 on p. 258).
- Blood gas analyser.

Procedure

- Ensure that you have the correct printout for your patient.
- Assess the oxygenation. Note the FiO_2 that the patient was breathing at the time the sample was taken. Is the patient hypoxaemic (PaO_2 <8.0kPa)? Calculate the alveolar arterial gradient.
- Look at the pH. If it is low (<7.35) there is acidaemia and if it is high (>7.45) alkalaemia.
- Look at the $PaCO_2$ to determine the *respiratory component*.
  >6.0kPa: respiratory acidosis (or respiratory compensation for a metabolic alkalosis).
  <4.7kPa: respiratory alkalosis (or respiratory compensation for a metabolic acidosis).
- Look at the HCO_3^- to determine the *metabolic component*. <22mmol/L: metabolic acidosis (or metabolic compensation for a respiratory alkalosis).
  >26mmol/L: metabolic alkalosis (or metabolic compensation for a respiratory acidosis).
- The *base excess (or deficit)* value can be ignored. It mirrors the HCO_3^- and its value makes no difference to the interpretation of the clinical condition.
- Assimilate the information obtained. Decide whether the primary abnormality is respiratory, metabolic or mixed and whether there is any compensation.
- Measure the anion gap if metabolic acidosis is present (📖 see p. 262).
- Ask yourself is the data consistent and does the analysis fit with the clinical picture.
- Document the result and your interpretation of it, making sure to document the FiO_2.

Practice tips

- A normal pH does not exclude an acid-base disturbance. It may be the result of virtually complete compensation.
- A compensated picture on ABG analysis suggests chronic disease.
- If the PaO_2 is very low consider venous contamination either through an intrapulmonary shunt or poor technique when taking the sample.

Pitfalls

- Failing to detect relative hypoxaemia in patients on supplemental oxygen. The alveolar-arterial (A-a) gradient can be more sensitive than PaO_2 alone in detecting a problem with gas exchange. (see appendix Y).

Box 9.1 Normal reference ranges for ABG values

- pH—7.35–7.45
- PaCO2 (partial pressure of carbon dioxide): 4.4–6.0kPa.
- PaO2 (partial pressure of oxygen): 10.5–13.5kPa.
- HCO3(bicarbonate): 22.0–26.0mmol/L.
- Base excess (BE): −2 to +2

Reproduced from Wyatt *et al.*, (2006) Oxford Handbook of Emergency Medicine, 3rd edn. With permission from Oxford University Press.

Analysing arterial blood gases 2 (the anion gap in metabolic acidosis)

Background

Metabolic acidosis is associated with either a normal or an increased anion gap. The anion gap is an 'artifical' calculated measure that reflects the serum concentrations of negatively charged molecules (anions) not routinely measured (e.g. plasma proteins, sulphates and organic acids). The anion gap varies when there are changes in the concentration of the serum components contributing to acid base balance. The normal range is 10–16mmol/L. The calculation of the anion gap in metabolic acidosis is useful clinically to help distinguish causes of metabolic acidosis.

Procedure

- Calculate the anion gap with the equation

  $(Na^+ + K^+) - (Cl^- + HCO_3^-)$.

- If the anion gap > 16 mmol/L consider the causes of increased anion gap which can be classified as follows

Excess acid through the body's own production

Lactic acidosis
- anaerobic metabolism in states of hypoperfusion
- excessive exercise
- reduced lactate metabolism in liver failure
- metformin

Ketoacidosis
- insulin deficiency—diabetic ketoacidosis(DKA)
- starvation

Excess acid through ingestion (poisoning)
- Saliciylates, methanol/ethylene glycol, biguanides, tricylcics

Excess acid through inability to excrete it
- Renal failure
- If the anion gap is normal consider the following causes:
  - chronic diarrhoea or ileostomy (loss of HCO_3^-)
  - renal tubular damage
  - pancreatic fistulae
  - acetazolamide thrapy
- Correlate your findings with the clinical picture to make a diagnosis.

Practice tips

To help differentiate between lactic acidosis and ketoacidosis calculate the ratio of the decrease in plasma HCO_3^- to the increase in the anion gap. In lactic acidosis the ratio is around 1.6 to 1.0. In ketoacidosis it is closer to 1.0 because of the loss of ketoacids in the urine.

Pitfall
- Failing to calculate the anion gap in a metabolic acidosis.

Table 9.1 Summary of changes in acid–base disorders

Acid-base disorder	pH	PaCO$_2$	HCO$_3^-$	Examples of causes
Respiratory acidosis	↓	↑		Type 2 respiratory failure
				Opiate poisoning
Metabolic acidosis	↓		↓	Diabetic ketoacidosis
				Salicylate poisoning
Respiratory alkalosis	↑	↓		Hyperventilation (e.g. hysterical or excess minute volume in artificial ventilation)
Metabolic alkalosis	↑		↑	Vomiting
				Diuretic therapy
				Excess antacids
Respiratory acidosis with renal compensation	↓ *	↑	↑	
Metabolic acidosis with respiratory compensation	↓ *	↓	↓	
Respiratory alkalosis with renal compensation	↑ *	↓	↓	
Metabolic alkalosis with respiratory compensation	↑ *	↑	↑	
Mixed metabolic and respiratory acidosis	↓	↑	↓	
Mixed metabolic and respiratory alkalosis	↑	↓	↑	

* If the compensation is virtually complete the pH may be in the normal range—over-compensation does not occur.

Assessment of disability/exposure (D/E)

Background

When the airway, breathing, and circulation have been stabilized, the patient's level of disability (D) or consciousness and neurological status should be assessed. Assessment of D should also include an evaluation of pain.

Equipment

- Pen torch.
- Blood glucose meter.

Procedure

Look for
- Signs of altered consciousness—drowsiness, agitation, lethargy, or inability to talk.
- Weakness of limbs or face.
- Pupil size and response to light and accomodation.

Listen for
- Appropriate responses to questioning.
- Noisy breathing (airway obstruction) or altered breathing patterns.

Feel for
- Weakness—test the power of the patient's limbs.
- Flaccidity or spasticity.
- Skin temperature.

Assess
- The Glasgow Coma Scale score (GCS) (📖 on p. 582) or AVPU which is a simplified assessment of the level of consciousness—is the patient alert (A), responding to voice (V), pain (P), or unresponsive (U)?
- Pain levels.
- Blood glucose.

When the airway, breathing, circulation and disability (A, B, C, and D) have been assessed, the patient should have a full systematic examination. All areas of the body should be exposed (E) sequentially, while maintaining the patient's dignity and keeping them warm. Look for rashes, sites of infection, wounds, haemorrhage, abdominal distension, and calf swelling.

Practice tips

- Patients feigning unconsciousness will usually not let their arm fall onto their head/face if it is lifted up and dropped towards their face. They will move the arm to the side.
- In trauma victims with a ↓ GCS, who are at risk of spinal injury, it is not a good idea to check the pain response over the sternum or with fingernail pressure. The jaw thrust is a better manoeuvre to test response to pain in such patients. It has the added bonus of also opening the airway. Supraorbital pressure can also be used.

Pitfalls
- Not re-checking the GCS. The GCS can deteriorate and should be re-assessed regularly in patients with potential brain injury or other reasons for altered consciousness.
- Not assessing the GCS accurately by being too gentle.
- Causing bruising by excessive pressure on the sternum when checking the patient's response to pain.

Assisting with insertion of an epidural catheter

Background

An epidural catheter is inserted into the epidural space to enable administration of opioids and/or local anaesthetics by bolus or infusion. Epidural catheters can be inserted into the thoracic, lumbar, or sacral regions of the vertebral column, depending on the site of analgesia required. They are used for pain relief during labour and surgery, particularly abdominal and thoracic procedures. They are also used in the treatment of acute back pain and for analgesia in terminal illness.

Equipment

- Sterile epidural/dressing pack.
- Epidural kit.
- Gauze swabs.
- 2% chlorhexidine in 70% isopropyl alcohol.
- One sterile gown and mask.
- Sterile towel.
- Sterile gloves, assorted sizes.
- Touhey needle.
- Two 20mL ampoules of 0.9% saline solution.
- A selection of syringes.
- 1% or 2% lidocaine solution.
- Sterile semi-occlusive dressing.
- Tape, e.g. Mefix®.
- Monitoring equipment—pulse oximeter, blood pressure cuff, and cardiac monitor.

Procedure

- Ensure that the procedure has been explained and consent gained. Reassure the patient and answer any further questions.
- Obtain baseline observations before the procedure.
- Prepare the equipment.
- Ensure all standard monitoring equipment is working—including cardiac, blood pressure and oxygen saturation monitoring.
- Ensure that a patent peripheral intravenous cannula is *in situ*.
- Position the patient on their side, with their back arched to separate the vertebrae.
- Help the health care worker (HCW) carrying out the procedure (HCW 1) to put on a sterile gown. They will also wear a mask, hat, and gloves.

HCW 1 will then perform the following actions:

- Clean and drape the area around the intended insertion site.
- Administer local anaesthetic into the surrounding skin.
- Insert a Touhey needle, with a syringe attached, into the epidural space.
- Move the syringe from the Touhey needle and thread the epidural catheter through the needle into the epidural space.
- Remove the needle when the catheter is in position.

- Aspirate the catheter to ensure that there is no blood or cerebrospinal fluid (CSF) suggesting the catheter is in a blood vessel or the spinal canal.
- Attach the antibacterial filter and then administer a test dose. Severe pain indicates intrathecal administration.

When the catheter is correctly positioned the assistant (HCW 2) should perform the following actions:
- Cover the insertion site with a sterile, transparent, non-occlusive dressing.
- Secure the line up the patient's back, to the shoulder, with tape.
- Connect the epidural administration set.
- Discard any sharps in the sharps bin and waste in clinical waste disposal.
- Reposition the patient.
- Record post-insertion observations.
- Label the line with the date and time of insertion.
- Document the episode of care.

Practice tip

- Ensure that a test dose is administered by the person who has sited the epidural and that they document the procedure before leaving the area.

Pitfall

- Forgetting to insert an intravenous cannula before insertion of the epidural.

Care of an epidural catheter

Background

Epidural analgesia offers unique benefits in the relief of acute, chronic, and postoperative pain. It offers patients the potential of a virtually pain-free post-surgical recovery. Local anaesthetic and opioid drugs are given as a continuous infusion (from a syringe or pre-filled bags) through a fine catheter inserted through the back into the epidural space.

Equipment

- Valid prescription chart.
- Epidural infusion device.
- Epidural medication.
- Monitoring equipment—pulse oximeter, blood pressure cuff, and cardiac monitor.
- Disposable gloves.
- Ice cube.

Procedure

- Ensure there is a signed and valid prescription chart before commencing administration of any epidural drug.
- Before commencing an epidural infusion, check the operation sheet to ensure that a test dose has been given and the level of block is recorded.

Care of the epidural catheter and line

- Document distance marks in centimetres on the epidural catheter visible at the skin surface. The markings on the catheter will indicate the amount of catheter inserted and the initial check should be used as a baseline measurement.
- Check all connections along the epidural catheter, filter, and giving set are intact to ↓ the risk of disconnection.
- Check for fresh blood in the epidural line.
- Ensure the epidural line is clearly labelled.
- Check that the epidural catheter line and filter are secured to the patient (i.e. taped upwards to the shoulder). This is to prevent stress on the line and inadvertent disconnection or dislodgement.
- Ensure that the epidural pump is working and, if possible, connected to the mains electricity supply.

Care of the patient

- Assess and record the respiratory rate and depth, observing for signs of respiratory depression.
- Monitor the blood pressure, according to instructions on the epidural observation chart or more frequently if appropriate.
- Observe the pulse rate, according to the instructions on the epidural chart. A high level of block can cause bradycardia. Bleeding and pain might cause tachycardia.

- Monitor the patient's temperature every 4 hours. Pyrexia might indicate infection.
- Assess the sedation score—the level of sedation will ↑ before the respiratory rate ↓ and is a better indicator of opioid overdose.
- Assess the pain score at rest and on movement. Titrate the epidural to allow for deep breathing, coughing, and mobilization.
- Assess the patient's leg strength, using the motor score, before getting the patient out of bed. Severe weakness is abnormal; an ↑ motor score might be an early sign of neurological deficit caused by intrathecal infusion, spinal haematoma, or spinal cord infarction.
- Assess the level of the block every 4 hours or more frequently if the patient is complaining of pain or difficulty in breathing.
- The level of the block is assessed by applying ice in a clean glove to the patient's skin, moving from the lower limbs upwards noting where their response to the cold stimulus alters.
- A mark should be made on the body to indicate the height of the block on both sides, using a marker pen. If the level of block rises above T4 (the level of the nipples), test for tingling/numbness in the little fingers. If this occurs, stop the pump and inform the senior clinical staff immediately.
- Observe and record the urine output. Patients who are not catheterized could lose bladder sensation and develop urinary retention. An accurate fluid balance must be maintained.
- Observe for nausea and vomiting. If the patient complains of nausea or vomits, treat them with anti-emetics and assess their response to them.
- Observe for, and document, any signs of pruritus. If there are no signs of a serious anaphylactic reaction, administer medication as prescribed to alleviate symptoms. If pruritus does not resolve, request a review. It might be necessary to prescribe an opioid-free epidural infusion.
- Check the patency of the intravenous cannula daily by flushing with 5mL of 0.9% saline solution. All patients must have a patent intravenous cannula throughout the duration of the epidural and for 8 hours afterwards.
- Stop the infusion and inform the senior clinical staff if the patient complains of ↑ back pain or tenderness. This might indicate an epidural haematoma and an urgent scan might be required.
- Check pressure areas at least daily. Patients on an epidural infusion should be classified as at high risk of the development of pressure sores owing to their ↓ sensation.

Practice tip
- Observe the patient for tingling in the little fingers or around the mouth. The infusion might need to be switched off if this occurs. It might be a sign of either the toxic effects of bupivacaine or a high level of block.

Pitfall
- Changing the dressing around the site routinely. This ↑ the risk of introducing infection and accidentally dislodging the epidural.

Assisting with insertion of an intrathecal catheter

Background

An intrathecal catheter sits in the intrathecal space around the spinal cord (between the pia and arachnoid mater). It is connected to a drug-delivery system. Analgesic or local anaesthetic agents can be delivered by bolus or infusion directly into the cerebrospinal fluid (CSF). Much smaller doses are required than those administered by oral or intravenous routes, leading to fewer adverse effects. The intrathecal catheter can be attached to an infusion pump placed abdominally in a subcutaneous pouch. The catheter is tunnelled under the skin and attached to the pump. Insertion of an intrathecal catheter should ideally be carried out in theatre. The indications are outlined in 📖 272.

Equipment

- Epidural kit.
- Sterile dressing pack.
- Gauze swabs.
- 2% chlorhexidine in 70% isopropyl alcohol.
- One sterile gown and mask.
- Sterile towel.
- Sterile gloves.
- Touhey needle.
- Two 20mL ampoules of 0.9% saline solution.
- A selection of syringes.
- 1% or 2% lidocaine solution.
- Sterile semi-occlusive dressing.
- Tape, e.g. Mefix®.
- Monitoring equipment—pulse oximeter, blood pressure cuff, and cardiac monitor.

Procedure

- Ensure that the procedure has been explained and consent gained. Re-assure the patient and answer any further questions.
- Ensure all monitoring equipment is working
- Ensure that a peripheral intravenous cannula is present before the procedure is commenced.
- Obtain baseline observations before the procedure.
- Position the patient on their side, with their back arched to separate the vertebrae.
- Prepare the equipment.
- Wash your hands and open all the equipment onto the sterile field.
- Help the health care worker (HCW) person carrying out the procedure (HCW 1) to put on their sterile gown. They should also wear a mask, hat, and sterile gloves.

HCW 1 will then perform the following actions:

- Clean and drape the area around the intended insertion site.
- Administer local anaesthetic into the surrounding skin.

- Insert a Touhey needle attached to a syringe into the intrathecal space.
- Remove the syringe from the Touhey needle and thread the epidural catheter through the needle into the intrathecal space.
- Tunnel the catheter under the skin.
- Remove the needle when the catheter is in position.
- Aspirate the catheter to ensure there is no blood or CSF suggesting that the catheter is in a blood vessel or the spinal canal.
- Attach the antibacterial filter.
- Administer a test dose to ensure the catheter is correctly positioned.

When the catheter is correctly positioned, the assistant (HCW 2) should perform the following actions:
- Cover the insertion site with a sterile, transparent, non-occlusive dressing.
- Secure the line up the patient's back, to the shoulder, with tape.
- Connect the intrathecal administration set.
- Discard any sharps in the sharps bin and waste in clinical waste disposal.
- Reposition the patient.
- Record post-insertion observations.
- Label the line with the date and time of insertion.
- Document the episode of care.

Practice tips
- Ensure that a test dose is administered by the person who has sited the intrathecal catheter and that they document the procedure before leaving the area.
- All drugs given through the spinal route should be preservative-free.

Pitfall
- Not ensuring an intravenous cannula has been inserted before intrathecal insertion.

Care of an intrathecal catheter

Background

An intrathecal catheter is a fine, plastic tube inserted between the vertebrae into the intrathecal space around the spinal cord. It is attached to an administration set and used to deliver analgesic and local anaesthetic drugs into the cerebrospinal fluid and around the spinal nerves. Intrathecal analgesia is used for postoperative (e.g. major abdominal surgery), traumatic, back, and chronic pain and as an alternative to general anaesthesia in patients with respiratory, cardiovascular, or severe metabolic disease. It should not be used if there is local infection at the site of intrathecal insertion, the patient has a significant clotting defect, is receiving full anticoagulation therapy, or has a known drug allergy, or in uncooperative patients.

Equipment

- A valid prescription chart.
- Intrathecal infusion device.
- Intrathecal medication.
- Monitoring equipment— cardiac monitor, blood pressure cuff, and pulse oximeter,
- Disposable gloves.
- Ice cube.
- Skin marker.

Procedure

- Before commencing an intrathecal infusion, check the operation sheet to ensure a test dose has been given and the level of block is recorded.
- Ensure there is a signed, valid prescription chart before commencing administration of any intrathecal drug.

Care of the intrathecal catheter and line

- Ensure that the intrathecal pump is working and, if possible, connected to the mains electricity supply.
- Ensure that the intrathecal line is clearly labelled.
- Ascertain and document distance marks in centimetres on the epidural catheter visible at the skin surface, which indicates the amount of catheter inserted. The initial check should be used as a baseline measurement.
- Check that all connections along the catheter, filter, and giving set are intact to ↓ the risk of disconnection.
- Ensure the catheter line and filter are secured to the patient (i.e. taped upwards to the shoulder). This prevents stress on the line and inadvertent disconnection or dislodgement.
- Check for blood in the line. If this occurs, stop the infusion and inform the senior clinical staff.

Care of the patient
- Assess and record the respiratory rate and depth. Observe for signs of respiratory depression.
- Monitor the pulse and blood pressure with the frequency recommended on the intrathecal/spinal observation chart. A high level of block can cause bradycardia. Bleeding or pain might cause tachycardia.
- Monitor the patient's temperature every 4 hours. Pyrexia might indicate catheter-related infection.
- Assess the sedation score. The level of consciousness will ↓ before the respiratory rate ↓ and is a better indicator of opioid overdose.
- Assess the pain score at rest and on movement. Titrate the intrathecal infusion to allow for deep breathing, coughing, and mobilization.
- Assess and record the level of the block every 4 hours on both sides of the body.
- The level of the block is assessed by applying ice in a clean glove to the patient's skin, moving from the lower limbs upwards noting where their response to the cold stimulus alters.
- A mark should be made on the patient's body to indicate the height of the block on both sides, using a marker pen. If the block rises above the level of the 4th thoracic vertebra—T4, the level of the nipples—test for tingling/numbness in the little fingers. If this occurs, stop the pump and inform the senior clinical staff immediately.
- Assess the patient's leg strength, using a motor score, before getting the patient out of bed. Severe weakness is abnormal. An ↑ motor score could be an early sign of a neurological deficit caused by intrathecal infusion, spinal haematoma, or spinal cord infarction.
- Measure and record the urine output. Observe for signs of bladder distension, discomfort, or urgency. If retention of urine occurs, urinary catheterization must be considered.
- Observe for nausea and vomiting. If they occur, look for causes other than adverse effects of intrathecal medication. Treat symptomatically with anti-emetics.
- Observe for, and document, signs of pruritus. If there are no signs of a serious anaphylactic reaction, administer medication as prescribed to alleviate symptoms. If pruritus persists, request a medical review.
- Check pressure areas at least daily. Patients are at high risk of the development of pressures owing to ↓ sensation.

Practice tip
- Do not change the dressing around the insertion site routinely because this ↑ the risk of infection.

Pitfall
- Failing to label the intrathecal line clearly, leading to inadvertent insertion of fluids or drugs intended for other routes.

Care of an external ventricular drain (EVD)

Background

EVDs are inserted for emergency treatment of a malfunctioning internal shunt and/or hydrocephalus, to monitor and control intraventricular pressure and cerebrospinal fluid (CSF) output, or to divert infected CSF in ventriculitis, which can occur with an infected shunt. They are usually inserted over the non-dominant hemisphere, 1cm anterior to the coronal suture, and 2–3cm from the midline.

Equipment

- EVD system.
- Spirit level.
- Pen torch.

Procedure

- Explain any procedures and gain consent, if appropriate.

Care of the drain

- Maintain the drain at the prescribed height, usually 10–15cm above the ventricular level (13cm is ~equivalent to 10mmHg).
- Ensure the zero ('0') is level with the midline of the head, just above the external auditory meatus or bridge of the nose, when the patient is lying on their side. This point corresponds to the foramen of Munro, (the foramen between the lateral ventricles and the third ventricle). Use a spirit level for accuracy and adjust the height of the drain, if necessary.
- The entry site of the EVD into the skull should be dressed with a sterile, occlusive dressing. Observe the dressing for any signs of leakage. It should be changed if it becomes soiled or loose, using a strict aseptic technique.
- Inform the senior clinical staff immediately if the catheter becomes displaced.
- Ensure that the drain is secured to the bed to avoid it dropping, which could lead to excessive drainage and the potential for a subdural or subarachnoid haemorrhage.
- The EVD should be closed off if the patient requires repositioning and reopened once the zero point has been re-established.
- Record the CSF volume every hour and note the colour of the drainage fluid. Alert the senior clinical staff if there are any changes in the drainage pattern or colour of the CSF, e.g. if it becomes cloudy or bloodstained.
- Use a strict aseptic technique when changing the drainage bag.
- Maintain a closed system. The system should only be changed or flushed by a neurosurgeon.

Care of the patient
- Monitor the patient's temperature at least every 4 hours.
- Monitor the patient's level of consciousness using the Glasgow Coma Scale at least every 4 hours or more frequently if there are any changes in the patient's neurological status.
- Document the episode of care.

Practice tips
- If the reason for insertion has resolved or is resolving, the CSF might not drain all the time.
- Use a spirit level to ensure the zero reference point is measured accurately from the midline of the head, just above the ears.

Pitfall
- Lying the drain flat. This will cause the air filter to become wet and stop the EVD from functioning.

Care of an intracranial pressure (ICP) bolt

Background

An ICP bolt enables continuous measurement of the ICP in patients with severe head injuries and post neurosurgery. It enables early intervention in patients with an ↑ ICP. Normal ICP is 0–15mmHg and an ICP >20mmHg usually requires treatment. ICP can be monitored in three main ways:

- By a tube in the lateral ventricles—an intraventricular catheter.
- By a sensor in the epidural space—an epidural sensor.
- Most commonly, by a screw or bolt in the subarachnoid space— a subarachnoid bolt.

For insertion, all require a burr hole to be drilled through the skull.

Equipment

- ICP bolt.
- ICP monitoring system.
- Pen torch.

Procedure

- Ensure you are familiar with the device *in situ* and can troubleshoot the system.
- Record the ICP measurement at least every hour. Alert the senior clinical staff if there are abnormal readings or sudden changes in the ICP.
- Calculate the cerebral perfusion pressure (CPP) and document it. The CPP is equivalent to the mean arterial pressure (MAP) minus the ICP— e.g. a MAP of 90mmHg – an ICP of 20mmHg = a CPP of 70mmHg.
- Ensure that the CPP is maintained within the prescribed parameters.
- Observe the pulse and trend waveforms (fibre-optic catheters), which will indicate changes in the ICP and also errors in the ICP monitoring device. A normal waveform has an upstroke that corresponds to systole, followed by three small peaks (P1, P2, and P3) believed to correspond to the a, c, and v waves of the jugular venous pulse.

Care of the bolt

- Check the entry site of the ICP bolt into the skull every 4 hours. It should be dressed with a sterile, occlusive dressing. Observe the dressing for any signs of leakage. It should be changed, using a strict aseptic technique, if it becomes soiled or loose.

Care of the patient

- Monitor the patient's level of consciousness using the Glasgow Coma Scale at least every 4 hours or more frequently if there are any changes in the patient's neurological status.
- Manage any signs of ↑ ICP immediately.
- Document the episode of care.

Practice tip
- Plan any care so that activities that cause a 'spike' in the ICP (e.g. suctioning) are not clustered together.

Pitfall
- Not assessing the patient as well as the monitoring device. Zero drift occurs in the devices the longer they are left *in situ* (i.e. they become more prone to erroneous readings). Always assess the patient first.

Assessment of fluid requirements in burns patients

Background

The ↑ capillary permeability owing to burns causes plasma loss, resulting in hypovolaemia and the potential for hypovolaemic shock. Treatment with intravenous fluids is recommended in burns >15% of the total body surface area (TBSA) in adults and >10% of the TBSA in children. The amount of fluids required is calculated on the basis of the surface area of the burns and body weight. Several formulae exist to calculate fluid requirements. These vary in the type of solution required and quantity administered. Two of the most commonly used are the Parkland and the Muir–Barclay formulae.

Equipment

- Lund and Browder chart.
- Calculator.

Procedure

- Explain the procedure and gain consent.
- Find out the patient's weight.
- Estimate the percentage surface area involved in the burn (BSA), excluding simple erythema, using the following methods:
  - A Lund and Browder (L&B) chart (Fig. 9.2).
  - The 'rule of nines' if an L&B chart is unavailable (Box 9.2).
- Calculate the fluid requirements using either the Parkland or Muir–Barclay formula:
  - Parkland: 2–4mL × weight (in kg) × %BSA during a period of 24 hours from the time of the burn. Give 50% of fluids over the first 8 hours and 50% of fluids over the ensuing 16 hours (Ringer's lactate is used).
  - Muir–Barclay: %burn × weight (in kg)/2 = one aliquot of fluid. Give six aliquots of fluid over the first 36 hours from the time of the burn in 4, 4, 4, 6, 6, and 12 hour sequences (Ringer's lactate and colloid are used).

Practice tips

- The patient's palm is ~1% TBSA and can be used for estimating patchy areas.
- The 'rule of nines' is modified in infants and children as the head makes up a larger percentage of the body surface area (📖 Box 9.2).

Pitfalls

- Adhering blindly to a derived rule from a formula can lead to over- or under-resuscitation. Regardless of the formula used, the first 24–48 hours usually require frequent adjustments in the rate of administration. Urinary output every hour and other clinical indices should be used to guide fluid management—titrating the rate of fluid administration to a urine output of 30–50mL/hour for an adult.
- Glycosuria, resulting in an artificially ↑ rate of urine output owing to osmotic diuresis. Urinalysis should be performed during the first 8 hours to screen for this.

- Inaccurate estimation of the TBSA, usually overestimation, often resulting from the incorrect inclusion of simple erythema in the estimate.

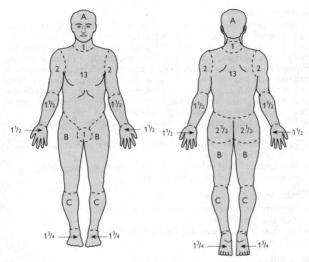

Fig. 9.2 Lund and Browder chart for the assessment of burns. Reproduced from Wyatt et al., *Oxford handbook of emergency medicine*, 3rd edn. With permission from Oxford University Press.

Box 9.2 Additional burn assessment rules

Adults rule of 9's:
Head	= 9%
Each arm	= 9%
Each leg	= 18%
Front of trunk	= 18%
Back of trunk	= 18%
Perineum	= 1%

Infants rule of 9's:
Head	= 20%
Each arm	= 10%
Each leg	= 20%
Front of trunk	= 10%
Back of trunk	= 10%

Use of a conductive water therapy system in hypo/hyperthermia

Background

Severe hyperthermia and hypothermia are life-threatening conditions. Hyperthermia ↑ oxygen consumption and metabolic rate, and puts undue strain on the cardiorespiratory system. Hypothermia slows the body metabolism and causes fluid shifts and cardiac irritability. Induced hypothermia has been shown to have beneficial effects on outcomes in patients with head injury or cardiac arrest. Dual-purpose hyperthermia and hypothermia conductive-water therapy systems are a cost-effective and convenient way of warming or cooling patients. They are used in intensive care and elsewhere for the following:

- To replace body heat lost in 1° hypothermia and after long surgical procedures.
- To lower the body temperature therapeutically in patients with head injury or post cardiac arrest.
- To counteract the ↑ in body temperature owing to heat stroke, infection, drugs, and neurological lesions.

Equipment

- Hypothermia/hyperthermia device and associated connections—e.g. a cooling blanket.
- Sterile, single-use oesophageal temperature probe.
- Cold water.

Procedure

- Explain the procedure and gain consent.
- Position the hypothermia/hyperthermia blanket either under or on top of the patient (on top is the most effective position but often the most inconvenient).
- Ensure that there is a sheet between the blanket and the patient's skin to prevent cold/heat-induced injury. Observe the skin for erythema, pallor, or discolouration.
- Fill the blanket with the required amount of cold water.
- Set the hypothermia/hyperthermia device to the desired temperature. The high flow rate enables rapid hyperthermia/hypothermia treatment and maintains a consistent water temperature throughout the warming/cooling blanket.
- Insert the oesophageal temperature probe.
- Monitor the temperature every hour to prevent excessive changes in body temperature.
- Observe and listen for any alarms. Most machines have built-in safety monitoring systems, with over- and under-temperature safety controls that give audible and visible alarms, if temperatures exceed or fall below machine temperature settings.
- Assess pressure areas and reposition the patient at least every 4 hours.

Practice tip

- The oesophageal temperature is more accurate and reflects rapid changes in body temperature more accurately than the tympanic, axillary, or rectal temperature. If the oesophageal temperature cannot be measured, the tympanic temperature should become the reading of choice.

Pitfall

- Inadvertently puncturing the water-filled hypothermia/hyperthermia device blanket, leading to an electrical fault.

Transfer of acutely unwell patients

Background
The primary goal is to facilitate the safe transfer of an acutely unwell patient between a ward or site of resuscitation and a critical care area. Many patients suffer further adverse physiological changes during transfer, many of them potentially life threatening. Transport itself causes its own complications. Meticulous preparation, resuscitation, and stabilization of the patient before transfer are the key to minimizing complications.

Equipment
- Transfer trolley.
- Oxygen tubing, oxygen source and a full oxygen cylinder (ensure you have sufficient oxygen for the transfer and the correct size of cylinder).
- Oxygen mask.
- Oral airways.
- Suction apparatus (wide-bore, rigid suction catheter) and flexible suction catheters.
- Cardiac monitor, blood pressure cuff and pulse oximeter.
- Fully charged and functioning portable ventilator and tubing.
- Self-inflating bag and reservoir/stethoscope.
- Intubation equipment/defibrillator/emergency drug box.
- Spare infusions of current medications.
- Spare intravenous fluids, infusion sets and spare infusion.
- Fully charged syringe driver and infusion devices, if being used.
- Medical and nursing notes, X-rays, observation charts, and results.

Procedure
Before a decision to transfer is made, the following should be considered:
- What is wrong with the patient and why is the transfer taking place?
- What treatments are ongoing and what treatments are needed?
- Where is the most appropriate place for the patient to be?
- Are the appropriate people involved in the decision-making process?
- Who has accepted the patient in the critical care receiving area?
- When will the bed be available?
- Has the receiving area been given a complete verbal handover, including patient details, medical history, current problem, treatment, and results?
- Are the correct personnel available for the transfer?
- Is the patient aware of the procedure and has consent been obtained?
- Have any family members/next of kin been informed?
- If the decision to transfer the patient is then made, the transfer team should reassess the patient and review the medical notes.
  In particular they should assess:

Airway
- Is the airway safe? Does it need to be secured and protected before transport? Tracheal intubation before transport is mandatory if there are concerns about the integrity of the airway.
- If the patient is intubated, the position of the endotracheal tube should be confirmed and the tube securely fastened.

Breathing
- Is ventilation adequate? Does the patient require ventilation for transfer?
- Intubated patients are often paralysed, sedated, and mechanically ventilated. Stabilize the patient on the transport ventilator and check blood gases before transfer.

Circulation
- Are the heart rate and blood pressure adequate?
- The patient should ideally have a minimum of two wide-bore peripheral intravenous cannulae if they have no central access.
- Consider an arterial line for continuous monitoring of blood pressure.

Disability
- Assess and document the Glasgow Coma Scale GCS score.
- Intubate and ventilate if the GCS score is 8 or less or is deteriorating before transfer.

Exposure
- If appropriate, expose the patient for a full examination before transfer. Then 'mummy' wrap the patient to prevent heat loss during transfer.

Other factors to consider before transfer
- Empty the urinary catheter bag, if applicable.
- Discontinue nasogastric (NG) feeds and aspirate the NG tube.
- Protect the patient's cervical spine and stabilize long-bone/pelvic fractures in trauma victims.

Just prior to transfer
- Move the patient onto the bed/transfer trolley.
- Secure all lines and infusions. Avoid trailing monitor leads.
- Ensure all documentation, charts, and notes are ready for transfer.

Practice tips
- Escorting personnel should be of appropriate seniority and trained in transferring patients.
- Send personnel ahead to open doors and call lifts.

Pitfalls
- Poor documentation of the transfer and inadequate handover can cause lack of continuity of care and harm by omission.
- Running out of oxygen during the transfer.
- Not ensuring the equipment is charged adequately before transfer.
- Inappropriate personnel (e.g. a junior nurse or doctor without advanced airway skills) involved in the transfer.
- Not resuscitating and stabilizing the patient optimally, as appropriate, before transfer.
- Spending too much time resuscitating a patient if the destination is theatre to control severe haemorrhage owing to trauma or other causes. In this situation, once immediate life-threatening airway and breathing problems have been dealt with, speed and efficiency are essential.

Respiratory system

Fiona Branch
Nurse Consultant, Critical Care Clinical Lead Specialist Support,
Nottingham University Hospitals NHS Trust, UK

Frank Coffey
Consultant in Emergency Medicine, Emergency Department,
Nottingham University Hospitals NHS Trust, Associate Professor
and Consultant in Advanced Clinical Skills, School of Nursing,
Midwifery & Physiotherapy, University of Nottingham, UK

History-taking

Background

The primary function of the respiratory system is to supply the blood with oxygen and to remove carbon dioxide from the body. Respiratory ailments are one of the commonest reasons for patients to seek health-care advice. It is important to take a thorough and systematic history. The depth and focus of the history will depend on the circumstances and the training and experience of the health care worker (HCW).

Procedure

Presenting complaint/current health

- The six cardinal presenting symptoms of the respiratory system are dyspnoea, wheeze, cough, sputum, haemoptysis and chest pain. Enquire about each of these and if any are present obtain more detail.
  - *Dyspnoea* (shortness of breath)—what is your breathing like normally? What is it like now? If more difficult than usual can you explain why? Are you ever short of breath? If so, does it occur at rest, with minimal activity (e.g. dressing yourself), moderate exertion (e.g. walking 100 yards on the flat) or more severe exertion (e.g. walking upstairs). Does anything in particular make the breathing worse? Do you awake at night struggling to breathe (paroxysmal nocturnal dyspnoea)? Does lying flat make you (more) breathless (orthopnoea)? Do you do anything to make the breathing easier (e.g. use inhalers or sleep upright using a number of pillows)? Has any deterioration in breathing been sudden or gradual?
  - *Wheeze*—are you normally wheezy? If present when did it start? Did it come on suddenly or gradually? Did anything provoke it, e.g. high pollen count or chest infection)? Do you feel breathless as well?
  - *Cough*—do you have a cough? If so, when did it start? What does it sound like? (e.g. dry, wet, barking, rasping, croupy). When does it occur? Does anything make it better or worse? Is it worse at any particular time of the day? (nocturnal cough is common in asthma).
  - *Sputum*—do you bring up phlegm? When did it start? What colour is it? Has the colour changed? How much do you cough up in a day (quantify using measurements of teaspoons, tablespoons or cups)?
  - *Haemoptysis*—have you coughed up any blood? Is it bright or dark blood? How much blood is there? Is it mixed in with the phlegm or does it occur before or after you cough? Are you sure that you're coughing it up (rather than spitting it out—oral bleeding—or bringing it from the gullet or stomach (haematemesis)?
  - *Chest pain*—what is the pain like? When did it come on? How did it come on? (Was it sudden or gradual?) Is it constant or intermittent? How long does it last when present? What makes it better or worse? Does the pain go anywhere (radiate)? Does it keep you awake at night? Is it associated with breathlessness, palpitations, sweating, nausea, vomiting?
- Ask about the presence of *ankle swelling*.

Past medical history

- Have you had any previous problems with or been in hospital for your chest, heart or breathing? Have you suffered from *asthma, chronic bronchitis, emphysema, TB* or any other respiratory condition? Enquire about other medical problems and previous hospitalizations.

Medications

- Are you on any medications for your chest including inhalers, over-the-counter remedies or alternative medicines? Enquire about the oral contraceptive pill and hormone replacement therapy in ♀.
- Have you had a flu or pneumonia vaccine?
- Are you allergic to any medications? Do you have any other allergies? Is there anything that makes you breathless, wheezy or causes you to cough?

Habits

- Do you or have you smoked? If the patient has given up smoking, note for how long. Ensure that they haven't given up a forty a day habit the previous week!
- Cigarettes are often recorded in 'pack years':

  Number of pack years = (number of cigarettes smoked per day × number of years)/20

  20 per day for a year is 1 pack year. 10 per day for 8 yrs = 4 pack yrs
- Do you drink alcohol—usually recorded in units/week. One unit is roughly equivalent to half a pint of beer, one standard glass of wine, or a standard measure of spirits.
- Do you or have you used recreational or Illicit drugs—e.g. cannabis, cocaine, and heroin.

Family history

- Is there any family history of respiratory disease such as *asthma, tuberculosis, cystic fibrosis, bronchitis, emphysema or lung cancer.* Is there any heart disease in the family?

Social history

- What kind of work do/did you do? Are you or have you been exposed to cigarette smoke, chemical fumes, asbestos, dusts, moulds or animal droppings?
- Describe your living accommodation. Who lives with you?
- Do you have any pets including birds?
- Have you travelled abroad recently? If so, where to?
- Take a sexual history and ask about risk factors for HIV.

Systems review

- Do a full systems review, in particular enquiring about *constitutional symptoms* such as weight loss, appetite, fatigue, and general well-being. Ask about night sweats.
- Enquire particularly about ear, nose and throat (ENT) and upper respiratory symptoms such as nasal blockage, nasal discharge, post nasal drip, sinus pain.

Pitfalls

- Panicking when faced with an acutely breathless patient and not asking pertinent questions that may give clues to the diagnosis e.g. presence and nature of chest pain.
- Delaying treatment to take a detailed history in an acutely unwell patient. You should be instituting emergeny treatment as you take a history.

Examination of the respiratory system 1: general observation, hands, face, and neck

Background

Examination of the respiratory system should be done in a systematic fashion. In practice it is integrated into the overall examination of the patient. The depth and focus of the examination will depend on the circumstances and the training and experience of the health care worker (HCW). All HCWs should be able to recognize a patient in respiratory distress requiring urgent attention (📖 on pages 203 and 210). A full respiratory examination includes the vital signs and examination of the hands, head, neck and lower limbs as well as the chest. Examination of the chest itself involves inspection, palpation, percussion and auscultation (📖 on p. 290–297).

Equipment

- Clock or watch with second hand.
- Sphygmomanometer.
- Pulse oximeter.
- Stethoscope.

Procedure

- Explain procedure and gain consent.

General observation

- Does the patient look unwell? Are they drowsy or distressed? Is their breathing laboured? Are they using their accessory muscles of respiration? Are they obviously tachypnoeic? Can they complete sentences? Are they cyanosed or anaemic? Listen for coughing and wheezing.
- Look at the environment for medications (e.g. inhalers), oxygen therapy, chest drains, mobility aids, cigarettes, lighters, matches, etc.
- If there is a sputum pot at the bedside? Observe the quantity and colour of the sputum and for the presence of blood.

Vital signs

- Measure the respiratory rate (📖 on p. 54). Observe the pattern, depth, regularity and uniformity of breathing.
- Measure the pulse rate and assess its rhythm. Is it bounding (strong and forceful) which can occur in hypercapnia (CO_2 retention)?
- Measure temperature and blood pressure.
- Measure SpO_2 with a pulse oximeter.

Hands

- Look at the hands for signs relevant to the respiratory system: clubbing, tar staining (often inaccurately called nicotine staining), cyanosis, tremor and flapping tremor (asterixis). Flapping tremor is best observed with the arms out stretched, wrists dorsiflexed and fingers splayed wide.
- Do the hands feel cold (peripheral vasoconstriction or heart failure) or are they warm with dilated veins (possibly due to CO_2 retention)?

Face and neck
- Is there contraction of the sternomastoid or other accessory muscles? Is there supraclavicular or suprasternal retraction?
- Is the trachea midline? Is there tracheal descent with inspiration, best felt by putting a finger on the thyroid cartilage? It can be present in any respiratory distress and is common in COPD. (Tracheal tug is also used to describe tracheal descent with inspiration, but more properly describes tracheal descent synchronous with the cardiac cycle and due to an aneurysm of the aortic arch.)
- Look for a ↑ jugular venous pulse.
- Feel for nodes in the anterior and posterior cervical chains in the neck and in the scalene area behind the clavicle.
- Look at the eyes for chemosis (swelling of the conjunctiva) and evidence of Horner's syndrome (ptosis and meiosis).
- Look at the lips and the inside of the mouth for central cyanosis.

Practice tip
- When looking for a flapping tremor in the hands, ask the patient to put their arms out straight in front of them and bend their wrists back as if they were pushing against an imaginary wall.

Pitfalls
- Not counting the respiratory rate or counting it inaccurately.
- Failing to palpate for nodes in the supraclavicular and scalene areas.

Examination of the respiratory system 2: inspection and palpation of the chest

Background

Examination of the chest starts with inspection and palpation.

Procedure

Inspection

- Inspect the chest for wounds, bruising, scars, diffuse swellings and discrete lumps. Look for scarring from radiotherapy or radiotherapy localization tattoos. Look for scars from previous surgery including old TB surgery.
- Look for abnormalities in the shape of the chest. Pectus carinatum (pigeon chest) is a prominence of the sternum and adjacent costal cartilages. It is a common sequel of chronic respiratory disease in childhood. In undernourished populations it may be caused by rickets. Pectus excavatum (funnel chest) is a depression of the sternum which is usually a benign developmental defect. Rarely it can be severe enough to restrict ventilatory capacity.
- Look at the anteroposterior diameter of the chest relative to the lateral diameter. In normal subjects the ratio is 5:7. In emphysema, the two measurements might approximate (barrel chest).
- Are both sides of the chest moving symmetrically with respiration?
- Is there any intercostal or supraclavicular retraction which can be present in severe asthma, COPD or upper airway obstruction?
- In trauma look for a flail segment (area of chest with paradoxical movement, i.e. indrawing during inspiration) which occurs when 2 or more ribs are fractured in 2 or more places.

Palpation

- Palpate the entire chest (front and back) for tenderness, lumps or crepitus.
- Test chest expansion (front and back) (Fig. 10.1). From the front, place your hands on each side of the lower lateral rib cage. Slide your thumbs medially towards the centre (at approximately the level of the lower sternum). Ask the patient to take a deep breath. Observe how much the thumbs move away from each other as the chest expands and look for symmetry. They should move at least 5 cm: <2 cm is definitely abnormal. From behind, do a similar manoeuvre with your thumbs over the spine at the level of the 10th ribs and your fingers grasping and parallel to the lateral rib cage. Chest expansion can also be measured by placing a tape measure around the lower third of the chest and measuring the maximum inspiratory/expiratory difference in the chest circumference. This however will not demonstrate the side of a unilateral ↓ in chest expansion.
- Feel for (tactile) vocal fremitus by placing the palm or ulnar aspect of your hand on equivalent areas of the chest wall and ask the patient to say 'ninety-nine' or 'one, one, one'. Vocal fremitus is a vibration felt on the chest during low-frequency vocalization. It is pathologically increased over consolidation and decreased or absent over large pleural effusions or pneumothoraces.

Practice tips

- Small flail segments can be difficult to see. It is important to look at the chest from different angles if a flail segment is a possibility.
- If you are unsure whether local pain over a rib is due to a fracture, anteroposterior chest compression ('rib spring') can be done. Exert pressure with one hand on the sternum and the other over the thoracic spine. If pain is felt away from the centre and over the rib then it is likely that there is a fracture. This manoeuvre should not be done if there is a high likelihood of a fracture as it is very painful. It is useful as a screening test.
- Tactile vocal fremitus is a crude test and only when it is absent, e.g. over a large pleural effusion, is it likely to provide useful information.

Pitfall

- Not palpating the chest systematically (particularly in trauma), and missing lumps, rib fractures or subcutaneous emphysema.

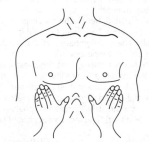

Chest expansion on inspiration: the thumbs
move apart.

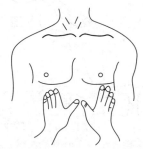

Chest expansion on expiration: the thumbs
move back.

Fig. 10.1 Assessment of chest expansion. Reproduced from Robinson and Scullion (2008) *Oxford handbook of respiratory nursing.* With permission from Oxford University Press.

Examination of the respiratory system 3: percussion of the chest

Background

Percussion is an important technique of physical examination. It helps to establish whether underlying tissues are air-filled, fluid-filled or solid. The percussion note over normal lung is resonant. When lung becomes airless due to consolidation, collapse or fibrosis the percussion note becomes dull. Pleural effusions are 'stony dull' to percussion and pneumothoraces 'hyperresonant'. The lungs are hyper-resonant all over in chronic obstructive pulmonary disease (COPD).

Technique

The technique requires practice to do effectively. You must train your ear to recognize differences in percussion notes. As well as the sounds, learn to identify the feel of the different notes under your finger. The technique as described below is for right-handed health care workers. Left-handed people can percuss with their left hand.

- Place your left hand on the patient's chest wall, palm downwards with the fingers slightly separated. The fingers should follow the ribs and lie between them ideally. The middle phalanx of the middle finger should be exactly over the area to be percussed.
- Press the left middle finger firmly against the chest wall while the thumb, index, ring and little fingers are lifted away from the chest.
- The centre of the middle phalanx is then struck with the tip of the middle finger of the right hand (Fig. 10.2). This finger should be partially flexed and relaxed. It should strike the middle phalanx at a right angle (to provide a hammer effect). The movement should come from your wrist.
- Withdraw the striking finger quickly to avoid damping vibrations.

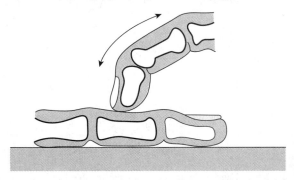

Fig. 10.2 Percussion technique. Reproduced from Thomas and Monaghan (2007) *Oxford handbook of clinical examination skills*. With permission from Oxford University Press.

Procedure

- Explain the procedure and gain consent.
- Percuss the anterior, lateral and posterior aspects of the chest in the areas demonstrated in Fig. 10.3.
- Percuss symmetrically from the top down comparing equivalent areas on each side of the chest. Percuss or strike twice in each area. Omit the areas over the scapulae.

Practice tips

- Make sure you keep the nail of your percussing middle finger trimmed.
- Practise the technique on different surfaces —e.g. walls and tables as well as on various parts of your own body.
- You can also practise by percussing the middle phalanx of your outstretched left hand without anything underneath.
- Be aware that the normal areas of dullness over the heart on the left side and the liver below the 6th rib anteriorly on the right are often diminished in hyperinflated states such as COPD or severe chronic asthma.
- Diaphragmatic excursion is sometimes measured by percussion but is crude and does not correlate well with radiological assessment.

Pitfalls

- Not pressing firmly enough on the chest with the hyperextended left middle finger. If a louder note is required it is more effective to apply more pressure with the extended left middle finger on the chest than to tap harder with the percussing digit.
- Using the pad of the striking finger rather than its tip.
- Not withdrawing the striking finger quickly after percussion leading to dampening of the sound. The right middle finger should 'bounce' off.
- Not percussing symmetrically and comparing equivalent area of the chest.
- Not being aware of the areas of normal dullness over the heart and liver.
- Not displacing large breasts to percuss and missing an abnormal percussion note as a result.

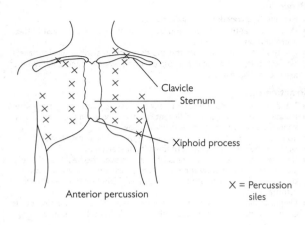

Clavicle
Sternum

Xiphoid process

Anterior percussion

X = Percussion
siles

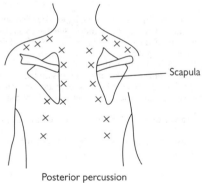

Scapula

Posterior percussion

Fig. 10.3 Key areas for chest percussion. Reproduced from Robinson and Scullion (2008) *Oxford handbook of respiratory nursing.* With permission from Oxford University Press.

Examination of the respiratory system 4: auscultation of the chest

Background

Auscultation is the most important examination technique for assessing airflow through the tracheobronchial tree. In combination with percussion and tactile fremitus it also enables the clinician to gain information about the lungs and pleural spaces. Auscultation involves listening to the quality of the *breath sounds* and listening for *added sounds*. Vocal resonance can also be tested.

Breath sounds are the result of vibrations of turbulent airflow in the proximal large airways. They are transmitted along the smaller airways and lungs to the chest wall:

- Normal breaths sounds are *vesicular*. They are soft and low-pitched. The intensity ↑ throughout inspiration, continues without a pause into expiration and fades about one-third of the way through expiration.
- *Bronchial breath sounds* are louder and can be higher or lower in pitch depending on whether they are due to consolidation (high pitch) or fibrosis (low pitch). There is a short gap between inspiration and expiration with the latter being of equal length or longer. Bronchial breathing can normally be heard over the trachea. Bronchial breathing heard over the chest is usually due to consolidation or dense fibrosis.
- *Bronchovesicular* breath sounds can sometimes be heard in the 1st and 2nd intercostal spaces (anterior chest) and between the scapulae (posterior chest). Inspiration and expiration are equal in length with no gap in between.

Added (adventitious) sounds are sounds superimposed on the usual breath sounds:

- *Crackles* are discontinuous non-musical brief sounds usually heard during inspiration. They are described as *fine* or *coarse*. Coarse crackles are louder and lower in pitch. Crackles are caused by the explosive reopening during inspiration of peripheral small airways that have become occluded during expiration. They occur in pulmonary oedema, fibrosis, bronchitis or bronchiectasis. Fibrosis crackles are fine and end inspiratory and sound like Velcro. Oedema crackles are wetter and coarser and sound like when you rub your hair together just by your ear. Bronchiectatic crackles are very coarse and are low-pitched. Crackles can also be caused by secretions. When this is the case they usually alter after asking the patient to cough.
- *Wheeze* is a high, medium or low-pitched sound produced by the passage of air through narrowed airways as in asthma or COPD or a through a bronchus partially occluded by a tumour or foreign body.
- *Stridor* is caused by large airway or tracheal obstruction. It is a loud high-pitched sound, often audible without a stethoscope.
- A *pleural rub* is a creaking sound caused by the movement of inflamed pleural surfaces over each other. It is best heard towards the end of inspiration and the beginning of expiration. A pleural rub can be present in pneumonia and pulmonary embolism.
- A *Hammond crunch* is a crunching sound heard over the heart in pneumomediastinum and pneumopericardium.

Equipment
- Stethoscope.

Procedure
- Explain the procedure and gain consent.
- Ensure that the patient is relaxed and sitting upright in a chair bed or examination couch.
- Use the diaphragm of your stethoscope to auscultate, placing it firmly against the patient's bare skin. Warm it before use.
- Ask the patient to take deep breaths in through the mouth.
- Auscultate the front and back of the patient's chest in the areas demonstrated in Fig 10.3. Start at the top and work systematically downwards. Listen for at least one full breath (inspiration and expiration) in each area.
- Always compare equivalent areas on each side of the chest.
- When auscultating the posterior chest, ask the patient to cross both arms in front of their chest.
- Listen to the quality of the breath sounds and for the abnormal added sounds described above.
- *Diminished breath sounds* are heard in the following circumstances:
  - The patient is poorly positioned or not breathing deeply.
  - There is no air entry to generate the sound, e.g. atelectasis.
  - There is air entry but insufficient turbulence to generate a sound, e.g. severe asthma ('silent chest').
  - There is air entry but transmission is hindered by an air solid interface (pneumothorax) or a fluid solid interface (pleural effusion).
- Crackles should be described as *coarse* or *fine* and also according to the phase of respiration in which they occur, e.g. the late inspiratory fine crackles of pulmonary oedema.
- Wheeze can also be described by its timing with respiration, e.g. inspiratory, expiratory or both.
- If you hear abnormally located bronchial breath sounds check vocal resonance. Ask the patient to say 'ninety-nine'. Normally sounds transmitted are muffled. In the presence of consolidation the words are louder and more distinct. The patient's whispered voice may also be heard clearly through the stethoscope over a consolidation (whispering pectoriloquay).

Practice tips
- Eliminate external noise when auscultating. Do not be afraid to ask for radios or TVs to be turned down.
- Wetting a patient's chest hair with warm water can ↓ the sounds made by friction of hair against the stethoscope.
- When auscultating ask the patient to take deep breaths through their mouth—nasal breathing produces less clear breath sounds.

Pitfalls
- Taking shortcuts and only listening to some of the chest.
- Listening through clothing.
- Failing to listen all the way through expiration.
- Being unaware that movement of the stethoscope on the chest wall can sound similar to a pleural rub.

Recording peak flow

Background

The peak-flow meter measures peak expiratory flow rate (PEFR) which is the maximum flow achievable from a forced expiration starting at full inspiration with an open glottis. It is recorded in L/minute. The peak-flow rate is lower when the airways are obstructed. It is used primarily in the assessment and management of asthma. The frequency of readings will depend on the indications for the peak flow and the patient's condition.

Equipment
- Peak-flow meter.
- Disposable mouthpiece.
- Peak-flow chart.

Procedure
- Calculate the predicted peak flow according to the age, sex and height of patient using a peak-flow chart.
- Explain the procedure and gain consent.
- Demonstrate the correct technique if the patient is not experienced in using a peak-flow meter.
- Position the patient in an upright position, ideally standing.
- Check that peak-flow meter pointer is at zero.
- Ensure that the meter is held horizontally and that the patient's fingers are out of the way of the pointer.
- Ask the patient to take in as deep a breath as possible.
- Instruct the patient to put the mouthpiece in between their teeth and to close their lips tightly around it.
- Ask the patient to blow out as hard as possible with a sudden, sharp, blow. ('Huff'—i.e. forced expiration).
- Read the position of the pointer.
- Take the best of three readings, resetting the meter to zero each time.
- Record the highest forced expiration on the peak-flow chart and note the position of the patient when it was taken (e.g. sitting or standing).
- Calculate the peak flow as a percentage of the usual or predicted peak flow for that person.
- Document the episode of care.

Practice tip
- Breathless patients might only manage one attempt at peak-flow readings.
- Don't confuse PEFR with forced expiratory volume in 1 second (see page 292). Although they may correlate well in asthma, a normal PEFR does not exclude a reduced FEV_1 in chronic obstructive pulmonary disease (COPD).

Pitfalls

- Poor technique, e.g. failure to take full inspiration or expiration.
- Patients 'preparing' themselves by taking repeated deep breaths.
- Not ensuring that you have the correct chart for the correct meter. New Mini-Wright peak-flow meters are being introduced with the new European standard; these have a distinctive yellow dial. The scale on these differs from some current peak-flow meters.

Spirometry

Background

Spirometry is a pulmonary function test (PFT) that measures how much (i.e. volume) and how fast (i.e. flow) air can be inhaled and exhaled from the lungs. It is used in the diagnosis of various lung conditions and is also useful for monitoring the natural history of diseases, for assessing pre-operative risk and for quantifying the effects of treatments. Spirometry is not advised in patients with a recent pneumothorax, unstable angina or recent eye surgery. A spirometer calculates and graphs the results which include the forced expiratory volume in one second (FEV_1), and the forced vital capacity (FVC), the total volume forced out of the lungs. Spirometry may be normal in patients with asthma between attacks.

A spirometry reading usually shows one of four main patterns:

1. Normal.
2. An obstructive pattern which is caused by narrowing of the airways e.g. asthma and chronic obstructive pulmonary disease (COPD) which results in a ↓ FEV_1 and FEV_1/FVC ratio that is lower than normal. The FVC may be raised in COPD.
3. A restrictive pattern which is caused by conditions that affect the lung tissue itself, or the ability of the lungs to expand, e.g. fibrosis or scarring of the lung, or, a physical deformity that restricts the expansion of the lungs. The FEV_1 and FVC are decreased but the ratio of FEV_1/FVC is normal.
4. A combined obstructive/restrictive pattern, e.g. asthma plus another lung disorder.

Equipment

- Spirometer.
- Disposable mouthpiece.
- Recording chart.
- Predicted values table.
- Nose clip.

Procedure

- Use the predicted values table to calculate the FVC and FEV_1 according to the age, sex and height of the patient.
- Explain the procedure and gain consent.
- Demonstrate the correct technique.
- Ensure that the patient is sitting upright with their feet firmly on the ground, or standing.
- Apply a nose clip to the patient's nose to ensure that no air escapes.
- Ask the patient to:
  - take in as deep a breath as possible.
  - seal their lips around the mouthpiece of the spirometer.
  - blow out as fast and for as long as they can until their lungs are completely empty.
  - breathe in again as forcibly and fully as possible (if an inspiratory curve is required).
- Repeat the procedure at least three times to check for consistency of recordings. Reset the machine to zero each time.
- Read and record the results.
- Document the episode of care.

Practice tips
- The patient should be rested and should not smoke, do vigorous exercise or have a heavy meal before the test.
- If the diagnosis is uncertain, reversibility testing can be carried out by recording a baseline spirometer reading as outlined above before administering medication (bronchodilator, steroids) and repeating the test. Significant reversibility is defined as an ↑ in FEV_1 that is both >200mL and 15% of the pre-test value.
- Don't confuse FEV_1 with PEFR (📖 see page 290). Although they may correlate well in asthma, a reduced FEV_1 may be present in chronic obstructive airways disease (COPD), despite a normal PEFR.

Pitfall
- Poor technique, e.g. failure to take full inspiration or expiration.

Pulse oximetry and oxygen saturation monitoring

Background

A pulse oximeter determines the percentage of haemoglobin saturated with oxygen (SpO_2). This is a close estimate of the arterial oxygen saturation. The SpO_2 is determined by a sensor, usually placed on a patient's finger or earlobe, and is given as a digital readout. Most units also display heart rate with an audible signal for each pulse beat. The normal SpO_2 is >95%. Pulse oximetry is used to identify early hypoxaemia and to evaluate the effectiveness of oxygen therapy.

Equipment

- Pulse oximeter.
- Pulse oximeter probe.

Procedure

- Explain the procedure and gain consent.
- Turn the pulse oximeter on and allow it to go through its calibration and check tests.
- Select the site for application of the probe, usually a finger. It can also be applied to an earlobe, bridge of the nose or toe.
- Ensure the finger is clean. Remove any nail varnish or synthetic nails as these can affect the readings.
- Position the probe avoiding excess force. Ensure it is placed symmetrically on both sides of the finger. Avoid taping the probe if at all possible.
- Allow up to 30sec for the pulse oximeter to detect the pulse and to calculate the oxygen saturation.
- Check that the device is detecting a satisfactory pulse by ensuring that there is an adequate plethysmograph waveform (pulse amplitude). If this is not present readings are likely to be inaccurate.
- Set the alarm limits.
- Rotate the site every 4 hours to prevent ischaemia during continuous monitoring.
- Document the episode of care and record the displayed oxygen saturation and pulse rate. The FiO_2 should also be documented, e.g. SpO_2 98% on air or SpO_2 92% on FiO_2 of 40%.
- Obtain parameters from the medical staff acceptable for that individual patient: these should be documented in the notes.
- Report any low readings, e.g. below 90%, as soon as possible, inform the medical staff, assess and review the patient.

Practice tip

- On rare occasions, tape might be required to secure the probe in agitated patients. In these circumstances, more frequent repositioning of the probe should occur and this should be written into the patient's care plan. The tape should be removed as soon as it is feasible.

Pitfalls

- Relying on pulse oximetry alone to assess the patient's cardiorespiratory status. Pulse oximetry does not tell you about the patient's ventilatory status. A patient on supplementary oxygen might have life-threatening hypoventilation/hypercapnia with a normal SpO_2. Observe the patient and the monitor.
- Not being aware that there is a lag time between a hypoxic event and the subsequent ↓ in SpO_2. Observe the patient!
- Not being aware that pulse oximetry is inaccurate when the O_2 saturation is <70%.
- Not giving due consideration to the factors that can interfere with pulse oximetry and cause false readings:
  - Low perfusion or vasoconstriction, e.g. in hypovolaemia or hypotension for other causes.
  - Peripheral vascular disease, hypothermia, or cardiac failure.
  - Motion artefact, e.g. shivering.
  - Cold peripheries.
  - Venous congestion/oedematous fingers.
  - The inflated cuff of an automatic blood pressure monitor on the same limb.
  - Excessive ambient light, e.g. theatre overhead lights.
  - Tricuspid regurgitation (causing pulsatile venous flow) especially with ear probes.
  - Certain intravascular dyes, e.g. methylene blue (used in parathyroid surgery and to treat methaemoglobinaemia).
  - The presence of abnormal haemoglobins, e.g. carboxyhaemoglobin, which will a give a spuriously high reading.

Administration of oxygen

Background

Oxygen is given to prevent or correct hypoxaemia in respiratory failure and to optimize tissue oxygenation in all forms of shock. Inspired oxygen concentration (FiO_2) can be controlled by the oxygen flow rate or the mask design. The concentration prescribed depends on the condition being treated and the patient's cardiorespiratory status. Inappropriate oxygen administration can have serious or even lethal effects. In acute hypoxic emergencies, however, high-flow oxygen should always be given until a senior practitioner arrives. Oxygen can be administered through nasal cannulae, various types of masks or through an endotracheal tube if the patient is ventilated:

- *Nasal cannulae:* deliver low oxygen concentrations (24–35%) that vary with the oxygen flow rate and the patient's inspiratory flow rate. They can be used for long periods of time. They are comfortable and allow the patient to eat and drink. They are not suitable for patients with nasal obstruction. Nasal cannuale might cause headaches and dry mucous membranes if the flow rate is >4L/minute.
- *Semi-rigid face masks (e.g. Hudson):* can deliver concentrations between 24% and 65%. They are dependent on the patient's respiratory rate and depth of breathing. They are not practical for long-term use.
- *Venturi (fixed performance) masks:* deliver a predictable oxygen concentration irrespective of respiratory pattern. They deliver a relatively low flow of oxygen through a narrow jet (Venturi barrel) which can be altered to deliver fixed oxygen concentrations (24, 28, 31, 35, 40 and 60%).
- *Non-rebreathing trauma masks:* have a reservoir bag that is filled with pure oxygen. They can deliver oxygen concentrations of >80% provided the bag has been inflated before use. These semi-rigid masks have a one-way valve that prevents accumulation of expired gases and retention of carbon dioxide. They are effective for short-term treatment of very ill patients.

Equipment

- Oxygen supply.
- Flow meter to control oxygen delivery.
- Oxygen tubing.
- Delivery system: usually mask or nasal cannulae.
- Humidification.

Procedure

- Explain procedure and gain consent. Ensure that the patient is aware of the hazards of oxygen administration, particularly of smoking when near oxygen. Visitors should also be advised.
- Decontaminate hands.
- Sit the patient upright or semi-recumbent, if possible.
- Select the appropriate oxygen delivery system.
    - *Nasal cannulae:* insert a prong into each nostril. Place the tubing over the ears and secure either under the chin or behind the head.
    - *Face masks:* place the mask over the patient's face and secure with the elastic . If using a reservoir bag inflate it with oxygen before use.
    - *Venturi mask:* adjust the barrel to deliver the required oxygen concentration.
- Connect the tubing to the oxygen flow meter and turn on to the required flow rate. Oxygen should be prescribed in *percentages* for venturi masks and by *flow rate* for nasal cannulae and non-rebreathing masks.
- Attach a humidification device if required (📖 on p. 304–307).
- Assess the patient's appearance, respiratory rate and oxygen saturations. If hypoxaemia persists the patient may require invasive or non-invasive respiratory support.
- Monitor for signs of carbon dioxide narcosis (tremor, asterixis, confusion, drowsiness, fast bounding pulse).
- Encourage oral hygiene and an adequate fluid intake to prevent dry lips and mouth.
- If the mask or nasal canulae become grossly contaminated with secretions they should be replaced.
- Document the episode of care.

Practice tips

- Readjust the delivery device straps at least 2-hourly to prevent any tissue damage, particularly around the ears and the bridge of the nose.
- If using a reservoir bag, the flow rate must be kept sufficient to keep the bag at least a third to half full at all times.

Pitfalls

- Not keeping the oxygen cylinder in an upright position, particularly when transporting patients. This makes it difficult to see the flow meter and check that it is functioning. An appropriate oxygen cylinder holder should be used.
- Withholding oxygen in patients in severe respiratory distress or hypoxaemic in order to do arterial blood gases on room air.
- Failing to remove oxygen therapy when defibrillating in a cardiac arrest situation, which is a fire hazard.

Humidification with cold water

Background

When oxygen is delivered in high concentration or for prolonged periods it can dry the mucous membranes of the upper respiratory tract, causing soreness, and make lung secretions stickier and more difficult to expectorate. Humidification of a gas means adding moisture to it. Gases can also be heated. The main indications for humidification and heating of gases are the use of high-flow oxygen, mechanical ventilation and CPAP (📖 on p. 332). There are 3 main categories of humidification: cold water humidification which is adequate for most patients on wards and at home, hot water humidification and heat and moisture exchange (📖 on p. 308).

Equipment

- Oxygen supply.
- Sterile water.
- Humidifier.
- Oxygen mask or nasal cannulae.
- Corrugated aerosol ('elephant') tubing.

Procedure

- Cold water humidifiers deliver ~50% normal moisture; they act like large-volume nebulizers. They cannot be relied upon as a sole source of humidification and should be used in conjunction with a nebulizer and adequate hydration. Most systems in use involve an adaptor which screws into the oxygen supply and a bottle of sterile water.
- Explain the procedure and gain consent.
- Decontaminate hands.
- Connect the corrugated oxygen tubing at one end to the adaptor and at the other end to a face mask/tracheostomy mask.
- Set the correct % of oxygen, as prescribed and adjust the flow meter, as directed on the adaptor. When running you can hear the oxygen 'bubbling' through the system.
- Ensure that there is a visible stream of aerosol at the patient end of the circuit.
- Observe the system hourly to ensure correct functioning.
- Change the bottle of sterile water when it is empty or after a 24-hour period to minimize the risk of infection. Decontaminate hands before doing this and avoid touching connections directly. Most systems (tubing, adaptor and mask) also need to be changed between 1–7 days depending on which brand is used.

Practice tips
- If oxygen is discontinued and then recommenced the whole system should be renewed.
- Be aware that cold water humidification might cause bronchospasm.

Pitfall
- Not changing the whole circuit as recommended by the manufacturer.

Heated humidification

Background

Hot water humidifiers will deliver 100% moisture provided the temperature is maintained. They come with specific humidification sets and chambers that are heated to a preset temperature according to whether the patient is self ventilating or intubated. Heat and moisture exchangers (HMEs) trap the heat and moisture from an exhaled breath, allowing heating and humidification of the inhaled breath to 75% normal moisture.

Equipment

- Oxygen supply.
- Sterile water.
- Humidifier.
- Oxygen mask or nasal cannulae.
- Corrugated aerosol ('elephant') tubing.
- Appropriate adapter.

Procedure

Hot water humidification

- Explain the procedure and gain consent.
- Decontaminate your hands.
- Plug in the humidifier.
- Open the circuit with the oxygen tubing and water chamber and insert into the humidifier.
- Connect the sterile water to the chamber.
- Connect the temperature probes, one by the heater chamber and one as close to the patients mouth as possible (into the ventilator circuit at the Y connector the T-piece of a CPAP circuit).
- Attach the oxygen supply to the heater chamber. Connect the tubing from the heater chamber to the patient.
- Select the heater mode, usually 'intubated' or 'non-intubated', and switch on.
- Observe the system regularly to ensure that it is functioning correctly and record the heater temperature hourly. Overheating can cause burning. Underheating carries the risk of infection. The system should have inbuilt safety alarms.
- Change the sterile water when it is empty or after a 24-hour period
- Change the heated circuit every 5–7 days dependent on which brand of system is used.

Heat–moisture exchangers

- Open the HME and insert either between the corrugated oxygen tubing and the mask/tracheotomy mask or between the ventilator circuit and the endotracheal tube/tracheotomy tube.
- Check for patency hourly or if the patient appears to have difficulty in breathing. Copious secretions or a sputum plug might block the HME, in which case another form of humidification might be required.
- Change every 24 hours or if wet.

Practice tip
- If oxygen is discontinued and then recommenced, the whole system should be renewed.

Pitfall
- Not changing the whole circuit as recommended by the manufacturer.

Oral suction

Background

Oral suction removes excessive secretions and keeps the mouth and airway clear. Its primary indication is an inability on the part of the patient to clear the airway or mouth by cough or huff. It is used extensively in emergency departments, critical care areas and theatre for patients with a ↓ Glasgow Coma Score. Oral suctioning is performed using a Yankauer device (tonsil-tip suction apparatus) or a catheter. The large opening of the Yankauer sucker enables suctioning of thick or copious secretions. It is angled to follow the contours of the oral cavity along the palate and facilitates suction of the posterior oropharynx and buccal pouches in where secretions might collect.

Equipment

- Functional suction unit: 15–20kPa, 100–150mmHg, and 150–200cmH$_2$O.
- Sterile multi-eyed suction catheters, sizes 12 and 14FG.
- Wide-bore rigid suction tube (Yankauer sucker).
- Sterile gloves.
- Oxygen therapy and humidification administration equipment.
- Jug or bowl of water.
- Protective eyewear.

Procedure

- Explain the procedure and gain consent.
- Pre-oxygenate, if required.
- Decontaminate your hands.
- Put on disposable gloves and apron.
- Don protective eyewear.
- Turn on the suction apparatus and set the suction pressure to a maximum of 20kPa/200cmH$_2$O/150mmHg.
- Attach the sterile catheter or wide-bore sucker to the suction apparatus.
- Open the patient's mouth or ask the patient to open their mouth so that you are able to see where the secretions are.
- Insert the catheter/sucker into one side of the mouth, inside the cheek without applying suction.
- Then apply suction and gently withdraw the catheter. Repeat on the other side of the mouth and if visible secretions can be localized.
- Evaluate the colour, consistency, and amount of secretions removed.
- Dispose of the used equipment and gloves in the clinical waste.
- Rinse suction tubing by sucking sterile water through the tubing until clear.
- Ensure that the patient is comfortable after suctioning.
- Assess respiratory role, colour and oxygen saturation.
- Assess the patient's requirements for further suctioning.
- Document the episode of care.

Practice tips

- Oral suctioning can be a traumatic process and ∴ should only be used where other methods are ineffective. In conscious patients other methods should be considered such as deep breathing, nebulizers, or self-percussion.
- Ensure wide-bore suction catheters are changed very 24 hours or more frequently if secretions adhere to them.

Pitfalls

- Inserting the suction apparatus too deep and/or with excessive force, causing vomiting and the risk of aspiration.
- Forceful suctioning causing injury to the tongue, teeth or buccal mucosa.
- Not checking that the apparatus is functioning correctly before needing it in an emergency.

Nasal suction

Background

Nasal suction is used in patients who have ↓ level of consciousness, tiredness, muscle weakness or paralysis and might not have a strong enough cough to clear secretions or to maintain a clear airway. This will result in ↑ work of breathing and ↓ oxygenation. Suctioning might be necessary to prevent secretion build-up and to preserve dignity in a patient who is unable to cough or swallow. Nasal suction should not be carried out in patients with basal skull fractures, CSF leakage, severe epistaxis, occluded nasal passage or deranged clotting, as suctioning might cause further damage. It is an unpleasant procedure and should only be used when necessary.

Equipment

- Functional suction unit: 15–20kPa, 100–150mmHg, and 150–200cmH$_2$O.
- Sterile multi-eyed suction catheters: sizes 8 and 10FG.
- Sterile gloves.
- Nasopharyngeal airway: optional.
- Oxygen therapy and humidification administration equipment.
- Jug or bowl of water.
- Sterile lubricant.
- Protective eye wear.
- Bag–valve–mask device.
- Oxygen supply.

Procedure

- Explain the procedure and gain consent.
- Insert a nasopharyngeal airway if required (📖 on p. 208).
- Decontaminate your hands.
- Put on clean disposable gloves and apron.
- Pre-oxygenate, if required.
- Turn on the suction apparatus and set the suction pressure to a maximum of 20kPa/200cmH$_2$O/150mmHg.
- Attach the correct sized sterile catheter to the suction apparatus ensuring the catheter remains in the sterile packaging.
- Put a sterile glove on the dominant hand.
- Hold the exposed catheter in the dominant hand while removing packaging with the other hand. Ensure the sterile catheter does not touch anything else.
- Dip tip of catheter into sterile gel and insert into nostril with no suction pressure.
- Advance the catheter gently towards the back of the nose until resistance is felt.
- Rotate the catheter gently between the thumb and index finger until the resistance is overcome.
- Continue to advance the catheter while asking the patient to take a deep breath this enables the catheter to pass into the trachea. A cough is then stimulated.
- Apply continuous suctioning whilst withdrawing the catheter slowly and steadily for a maximum duration of 10–15sec.

- Release the suction and wrap the catheter in the dominant hand.
- Invert the glove and discard the catheter and glove in the clinical waste.
- Evaluate the colour, consistency and amount of secretions removed.
- Assess the patient's respiratory rate, colour and oxygen saturation to ensure they have not been compromised by the procedure.
- If further suction is required fresh gloves and a new sterile catheter will be needed. The process is then repeated following the same steps.
- Document the episode of care.

Practice tip
- If you put the suction tubing with the suction catheter attached but still in its packaging under your armpit it is easier to hold it and remove the packaging.

Pitfall
- Spending too much time performing suction leading to hypoxia and bradycardia.

Obtaining a nasopharyngeal aspirate

Background
Nasopharyngeal aspiration (NPA) is the preferred method for collecting specimens for viral culture in patients with respiratory tract infections and suspected influenza. The results might be important to direct antiviral treatment or might inform infection control measures.

Equipment
- Functional suction unit, 15–20kPa, 100–150mmHg, and 150–200cmH$_2$O.
- Appropriate size of sterile multi-eyed suction catheter.
- Sterile gloves.
- Sputum/mucous trap.
- 20mL of 0.9% sodium chloride solution.
- Sterile gallipot.
- Protective eyewear.
- Oxygen specimen form.
- Specimen form.

Procedure
- Explain the procedure and gain consent.
- Decontaminate your hands.
- Put on clean disposable gloves and apron.
- Open the gallipot and tip the 0.9% sodium chloride into it.
- Turn on the suction apparatus and set the suction pressure to a maximum of 20kPa/200cmH$_2$O/150mmHg.
- Attach the suction catheter to the sputum trap, and connect it to the suction apparatus, ensuring the catheter remains in the sterile packaging.
- Put a sterile glove on the dominant hand.
- Hold the exposed catheter in the dominant hand while removing the packaging with the other hand. Ensure that the sterile catheter does not touch anything else.
- Measure the distance from the tip of the patient's nose to the external opening of the ear (this depth is necessary to reach the posterior pharynx). Hold the tubing at that distance. Do not move your fingers or advance the tube further than that point.
- Ask the patient to tilt their head back slightly.
- Pre-oxygenate, if required.
- Pass the catheter along the base of one nostril into the nasopharynx and apply suction.
- Hold the sputum trap upright to prevent secretions from going into the suction apparatus.
- Repeat with the same suction catheter into the other nostril for a maximum duration of 10sec.
- Release the suction and remove the catheter.
- Flush the catheter with 3mL of transport medium (0.9% sterile sodium chloride solution).
- Disconnect the sputum trap and seal.
- Invert the glove and discard the catheter and glove in the clinical waste.

- Assess the patient's respiratory rate, skin colour +/– oxygen saturation, to ensure they have not been compromised by the procedure.
- Label the sample. Ensure that the request form is correctly filled in with patient details, clinical information and investigation request.
- Send to the laboratory for processing immediately.
- Document the episode of care.

Practice tip

- Ensure the sputum trap is held upright. Otherwise secretions will be lost into the suction apparatus.

Pitfalls

- Not delivering the specimen to the microbiology lab within 1–2 hours of obtaining the specimen. Deliver the specimen by hand, not through a tube or shoot system.
- Forgetting to sample from both nostrils.

Obtaining a sputum sample

Background

Sputum is made up of secretions, mucus and other matter coughed up from the lungs and large airways. It can be examined and cultured to aid diagnosis in conditions such as pneumonia, TB, lung abscess, lung cancer and asbestosis. Sensitivity to antibiotics can also be ascertained. The simplest way to obtain sputum is by asking the patient to cough it up. Nasotracheal suctioning can be used in patients who are obtunded or who have a weak cough (📖 on p. 318). Sputum samples can also be obtained by bronchoscopy or rarely by trans-tracheal aspiration.

Equipment

- Sterile gloves.
- Protective eyewear.
- Sterile 0.9% saline solution if required.
- Sterile sputum specimen collection container.

Procedure

- Explain the procedure and gain consent. Emphasize to the patient the importance of bringing up sputum, the thick secretions from the lungs, rather than saliva from the mouth. Explain that deep breathing before coughing helps to loosen secretions and bring them to the back of the throat (📖 on p. 360).
- Ensure privacy because sputum production is potentially embarrassing for the patient.
- Sit the patient upright.
- Remove dentures, if present.
- Decontaminate your hands.
- Put on disposable gloves and apron
- Don protective eyewear.
- Uncap the container. Avoid touching the inside of the container.
- Encourage the patient to take at least three deep breaths and then to force out a deep cough.
- Ask them to 'spit' their secretions into the sputum container.
- Ask them to continue to cough until you have a sample, ideally of at least 15mL (although this may not always be possible).
- Seal the sputum container securely.
- Remove and discard your gloves in clinical waste.
- Decontaminate your hands.
- Label the sample and send to the laboratory immediately.
- If the patient is having trouble bringing up secretions administer nebulized saline or water and consider physiotherapy.
- Document the episode of care.

Practice tip
- Sputum specimens should ideally be collected first thing in the morning when secretions are most plentiful.
- With appropriate education, that patient should be able to produce the sputum sample independently.

Pitfalls
- Obtaining an insufficient sputum sample. At least 15mL should be collected if possible.
- Delaying transport of the sample to the laboratory.

Collecting sputum using nasotracheal suction

Background

Sputum is made up of secretions, mucus and other matter coughed up from the lungs and large airways. It can be examined and cultured to aid the diagnosis in conditions such as pneumonia, TB, lung abscess, lung cancer and asbestosis. Sensitivity to antibiotics can also be ascertained. Nasotracheal suctioning is used in patients who are obtunded or who have a weak cough.

Equipment

- Functional suction unit, 15–20kPa, 100–150mmHg, and 150–200cmH$_2$O.
- Appropriate sized sterile multi-eyed suction catheter.
- Water-soluble lubricant.
- Sterile gloves.
- Protective eyewear.
- Sterile water in a container.
- Inline sterile specimen trap.
- Monitoring equipment including pulse oximeter.
- Resuscitation equipment nearby.

Procedure

- Explain the procedure and gain consent. Warn the patient that they might cough, gag or feel like they can't breathe during the procedure. Explain that these are normal responses.
- Position the patient upright in a chair or bed, if possible.
- Decontaminate your hands.
- Administer high-flow oxygen by face mask.
- Open the equipment, being careful not to contaminate items.
- Connect one end of the suction tubing to the suction port and the other to the adapter in the inline specimen trap.
- Don protective eyewear.
- Put on sterile gloves.
- Attach the free end of the suction catheter to the specimen trap.
- Hold the exposed catheter in the dominant hand while removing the packaging with the other hand. Ensure the sterile catheter does not touch anything else.
- Test the suction by briefly dipping it into the sterile water and applying suction.
- Instruct the patient to tilt their head back or extend head slightly if patient obtunded and no contraindications.
- Dip the tip of the catheter into lubricant and gently insert it into one of the nares. The patient might cough when the catheter reaches the back of the throat.
- As the patient coughs, advance the catheter gently but rapidly into the trachea. Ask the patient to take deep breaths through their mouth to help insertion.
- Ask the patient to give you a deep cough and apply suction pressure for 5–10sec (never >15sec).

- If you are unsuccessful on your first attempt, stop the suction and pull back the catheter slightly.
- Let the patient rest for a 4–6 breaths before trying again.
- Stop the procedure immediately if the patient becomes distressed or cyanosed.
- When you have collected a sample stop the suction and gently remove the catheter.
- Hold the specimen trap upright to prevent secretions going into the suction apparatus.
- Administer oxygen to the patient.
- Detach the suction catheter from the inline trap and discard it and the gloves in the clinical waste.
- Seal the in line specimen trap.
- Evaluate the colour, consistency and amount of secretions removed.
- Label the trap and send it to the laboratory immediately with an appropriate request form.
- Ensure that the specimen from the patient corresponds with the details on the request form. The request form that accompanies the specimen must be completed fully to include:
  - Patient's name and hospital number.
  - Date of birth.
  - Ward/department.
  - Consultant.
  - Specimen.
  - Date specimen was taken and the correct request for the required investigation.
  - Clinical details.
  - The practitioner's name must be clearly identifiable and appropriately signed.
  - Document the episode of care.

Practice tips
- Putting the suction tubing with the suction catheter attached but still in its packaging under your armpit makes it easier to remove the packaging.

Pitfalls
- Not holding the specimen trap upright, resulting in the secretions being lost in the suction apparatus.
- Not delivering the specimen to the microbiology laboratory within 1–2 hours of obtaining the specimen.

Obtaining sputum using endotracheal and tracheostomy tubes

Background

Sputum is made up of secretions, mucus and other matter coughed up from the lungs and large airways. It can be examined and cultured to aid diagnosis in conditions such as pneumonia, TB, lung abscess, lung cancer and asbestosis. Sensitivity to antibiotics can also be ascertained. Patients in critical care areas with endotracheal tubes and tracheostomies are at high risk of nosocomial infections and accurate culture is vital.

Equipment

- Functional suction unit, 15–20kPa, 100–150mmHg, and 150–200cmH$_2$O.
- Suction tubing.
- Appropriate size of sterile multi-eyed suction catheter:

    The suction catheter size required = the size of the endotracheal tube (ETT) x 3 divided by 2

    Example: For an 8 mm ETT tube, a size 12 suction catheter is required.

- Sterile and non-sterile gloves.
- Eye protection.
- Sterile water.
- Sterile sputum trap.
- Monitoring equipment including pulse oximeter.
- Resuscitation equipment nearby.

Procedure

- Assemble the necessary equipment.
- Explain the procedure to the patient, if conscious.
- Ensure privacy.
- Decontaminate your hands.
- Pre-oxygenate the patient.
- Select the correct size suction catheter.
- Open the sterile gloves, sterile suction packaging and sterile sputum trap.
- Attach the suction tubing to the sputum trap.
- Attach the suction catheter to the sputum trap.
- Put a sterile glove on the dominant hand.
- Hold the exposed catheter with the dominant hand while removing the packaging with the other hand. Ensure the sterile catheter does not touch anything else.
- Disconnect the patient from the ventilator with the non-gloved hand.
- Insert the catheter gently into the airway with **no** suction applied until resistance is met.
- Withdraw the suction catheter 1–2cm.
- Apply suction for ~10sec (not >15sec).
- If the patient is conscious, ask the patient to take a deep breath while the catheter is being inserted. When a cough is stimulated, apply suction for ~10sec.

- Withdraw the catheter.
- Reconnect the patient to the ventilator.
- Hold the sputum trap upright to prevent secretions from going into the suction apparatus.
- Remove the suction catheter from the sputum trap. Invert the sterile glove over the catheter and discard them both in clinical waste.
- Seal the sputum trap with the sterile cap provided.
- If repeat suctioning is required to obtain an adequate sample, wait for several minutes before repeating. Fresh gloves and a new sterile catheter will be needed. The process is then repeated following the same steps. Do not do >2–3 suction passes at any one sampling episode.
- Monitor the patient throughout the procedure. If any signs of distress, hypoxia or cardiac dysrhythmia occur the procedure should be stopped immediately and the patient observed.
- Evaluate the colour, consistency and amount of secretions removed and assess for the presence of blood.
- Decontaminate your hands.
- Label the sputum trap and send to the laboratory as soon as possible with an appropriate request form.
- Ensure that the specimen from the patient corresponds with the details on the request form. The request form that accompanies the specimen must be completed fully to include:
  - Patient's name and hospital number.
  - Date of birth.
  - Ward/department.
  - Consultant.
  - Specimen.
  - Date specimen was taken and the correct request for the required investigation.
  - Clinical details.
  - The practitioner's name must be clearly identifiable and appropriately signed.
- Document the episode of care.

Practice tips

- If you put the suction tubing with the suction catheter attached but still in its packaging under your armpit it is easier to hold it and remove the packaging.
- You might not need to disconnect the patient from the ventilator if you have a catheter mount with a removable cap. Simply open the cap during the procedure and close it at the end.

Pitfalls

- Not holding the sputum trap upright results in the secretions being lost in the suction apparatus.
- Not delivering the specimen to the microbiology lab within 1–2 hours of obtaining the specimen.

Types and use of inhalers 1

Background

Inhalers deliver medications directly to the lungs with fewer side-effects than medication taken by mouth or injection. They usually contain bronchodilator or corticosteroid medication. Several types of inhaler are used in the treatment of asthma and other chronic obstructive airway diseases. *Pressurized metered dose inhalers (MDIs)* use a chemical propellant to emit a 'puff' of the medication from the inhaler. This type of inhaler is quick to use, small and convenient but many patients find co-coordinating their breathing with delivery difficult. *Spacer devices* are large plastic containers (often in two halves that click together) that are used with the pressurized aerosol inhalers to improve and facilitate delivery. The patient doesn't have to co-ordinate breathing with activation of the inhaler device. The spacer holds the drug like a reservoir when the inhaler is pressed. A valve at the mouth end ensures that the drug is kept within the spacer until the patient breathes in. When the patient breathes out, the valve closes. *Breath activated inhalers* and *dry powder inhalers (DPIs)* are discussed later (📖 on p. 322, 324, and 326). The choice of inhaler depends on the drug to be administered and the patient's age, coordination, dexterity and lifestyle. The commonest side-effect of inhaled medication is hoarseness. Oropharyngeal candidiasis is particularly associated with steroid inhalers.

Equipment

- Inhaler device of choice.
- Medication.
- Glass of water.

Procedure

- Explain the procedure and gain consent.
- Decontaminate your hands.
- Check the medication is as prescribed and in date.

Instructions for use of a standard MDI

Instruct the patient as follows:

- Remove the cap from the mouthpiece and make sure that there is nothing in the mouthpiece.
- Shake the inhaler to mix the medication and the propellant.
- Have the mouthpiece facing you holding the rest of the inhaler facing upwards.
- Sit upright with your head tilted slightly backwards.
- Breathe out slowly and as completely as possible.
- Place the mouthpiece in your mouth and seal your lips around the mouthpiece without biting it. Keep your teeth apart and tongue flat on the floor of the mouth to allow the medication to enter your lungs.
- Take a deep breath in slowly through your mouth. Just after the beginning of the breath, press down on the inhaler canister to release the medicine.
- Continue to breathe in as fully as possible.

- Remove the inhaler and hold your breath for as long as possible up to 10sec.
- Breathe gently out through your nose.
- Before another puff, wait for ~1 minute. Shake the inhaler again and repeat the technique as above.
- Replace the cap on the mouthpiece when finished.
- Rinse your mouth out with water and clean your teeth (particularly after steroid inhalers).

Instructions for use of a spacer device and MDI

Instruct the patient as follows:
- Remove the cap from the mouthpiece of the inhaler, check the mouthpiece and shake the inhaler.
- Insert the inhaler into the spacer.
- Sit upright with your head tilted slightly backwards.
- Breathe out slowly and as completely as possible.
- Place the mouthpiece of the spacer in your mouth and seal your lips around it without biting it. Keep your teeth apart and tongue flat on the floor of the mouth to allow the medication to enter your lungs
- Press down on the inhaler canister to release the medicine.
- Start breathing in from the spacer mouthpiece as soon as possible after firing the 'puff' into the device.
- Breathe in slowly and deeply through your mouth and hold for 10sec.
- Breathe out through the mouthpiece and breathe in again. Repeat this for up to 4–5 breaths (without pressing the MDI) to ensure that as much as possible of the medication has been received.
- If you need more than one puff, wait for 30–60sec, shake the inhaler again and then repeat the technique as above, pressing on the canister again to release another puff of medication.
- When you are finished remove the inhaler from the spacer and replace the cap.
- Rinse your mouth out with water and clean your teeth (particularly after steroid inhalers).

Cleaning the spacer device
- The device should be rinsed daily in soapy water.
- Allow to air dry. Rubbing creates static electricity.
- Replace the device every 6 months.

Practice tips

- Check new inhalers or ones that haven't been used for >1 week by spraying into the air.
- Calculate how long the inhaler will last, using the number of metered inhalations it contains and the doses required. Patients should have a spare inhaler in case of emergency, particularly when on holidays.

Pitfalls

- Using poor inhaler technique or a device inappropriate for the patient.
- Using a spacer device incompatible with the MDI. Make sure that the model of spacer is compatible with the MDI canister.

Types and use of inhalers 2: breath activated inhalers

Background

Breath activated (or actuated) metered dose inhalers (MDIs) use the patient's inspiration to activate delivery of the medication. This eliminates the need for hand coordination with the inspiration. They have a chemical propellant to 'squirt' the drug out of the canister. The *Autohaler®* and *Easi-Breathe®* are examples of breath activated inhalers.

Equipment

- Inhaler device of choice.
- Medication.
- Glass of water.

Procedure

Instructions for breath-activated MDI *(e.g. Autohaler® and Easi-Breathe®)*[1]

- Explain the procedure and gain consent. Explain to the patient that the release of the medication is triggered by their breath in rather than pressing down on the canister.
- Decontaminate your hands.
- Check the medication is as prescribed and in date.

Instruct the patient as follows:

- Shake the inhaler several times.
- Prime the device. (The method of priming will depend on the type of breath activated inhaler. *Autohalers®* are primed by pushing the priming lever completely up and holding the inhaler upright. *Easi-Breathe®* has a tight cap on the mouthpiece that needs to be levered open.)
- Sit upright with your head tilted slightly backwards.
- Breathe out slowly and as completely as possible.
- Place the mouthpiece in your mouth and seal your lips around the mouthpiece without biting it. Keep your teeth apart and tongue flat on the floor of the mouth to allow the medication to enter your lungs.
- Breathe in slowly and deeply through your mouth. Do not stop when the canister dispenses medication (clicks or puffs). Continue taking a deep breath.
- Remove the inhaler and hold your breath for as long as possible up to 10sec.
- Breathe gently out through your nose.
- If you need more than one puff, wait for 30–60sec, shake the inhaler again and then repeat the technique as above.
- When you are finished, for the Autohaler® push the lever down and replace the cap and in the case of *Easi-Breathe®* close the cap with the inhaler upright.
- Rinse your mouth out with water and clean your teeth (particularly after steroid inhalers).

---

1. This topic is adapted with permission from the *Oxford handbook of clinical examination skills.*

Practice tips

- Calculate how long the inhaler will last, using the number of metered inhalations it contains and the doses required. Patients should have a spare inhaler in case of emergency, particularly when on holidays.
- The lever or lid on the breath activated MDI can be quite stiff, press against a table for leverage.
- A patient changing from a pressurized MDI to a breath-activated inhaler might notice a lack of sensation in the throat when the dose is delivered. Explain that this is normal.

Pitfalls

- Using poor inhaler technique or a device inappropriate for the patient.
- Storing the inhaler in a valve-down position for a few hours might affect delivery of the medication.

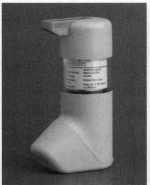 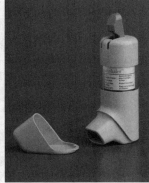

Fig. 10.4 Autohaler®. Note the lever on the top. Remember that the inhaler must be primed for each dose. Reproduced from Thomas and Monaghan (2007) *Oxford handbook of clinical examination skills*. With permission from Oxford University Press.

Types and use of inhalers 3: dry powder inhalers

Background

Dry powder inhalers (DPIs) deliver medication in a powder form. Unlike the MDIs they do not have a chemical propellant to 'squirt' the drug out of the canister. Instead the patient inhales the powder. Various devices on the market have different methods of providing the correct amount of powder for each dose. The *Turbohaler*® and the *HandiHaler*® are described here. The *Turbohaler*® is preloaded whereas the *HandiHaler*® requires a dose to be inserted into the inhaler via a capsule each time it is used.

Equipment

- Inhaler device of choice.
- Medication.
- Glass of water.

Procedure

Instructions for dry powder inhalers (e.g. Turbohaler® and HandiHaler®)[2]

- Explain the procedure and gain consent.
- Check the medication is as prescribed and in date.
- Decontaminate your hands.

Instruct the patient as follows:

- Prime the dose.
- For the *Turbohaler*® (which is preloaded):
  - Unscrew and remove the white cover
  - Hold the inhaler upright
  - Twist the grip clockwise and then anticlockwise as far as it will go until a click is heard.
- For the *HandiHaler*® (which is not preloaded):
  - Open the cap by pulling it upwards exposing the mouthpiece
  - Open the mouthpiece by pulling it upwards exposing the chamber
  - Take a capsule from the blister-pack and insert it into the chamber
  - Replace the mouthpiece making sure it clicks and leave the cap open.
  - Press the side button a few times to pierce the capsule which you can see through a small window in the chamber).
- Sit upright with your head tilted slightly backwards.
- Breathe out slowly and as completely as possible.
- Seal your lips around the mouthpiece of the inhaler.
- Breathe in deeply through your mouth (You should hear the capsule vibrate in the *HandiHaler*® variety)
- Remove the inhaler and hold your breath for as long as is comfortable up to 10sec.
- Remove the used capsule from a *HandiHaler*® and replace the cap.

---

2. This topic is adapted with permission from the *Oxford handbook of clinical examination skills*.

Practice tips
- A patient changing from a pressurized MDI to a DPI might notice a lack of sensation in the throat when the dose is delivered. Explain that this is normal.
- Calculate how long the inhaler will last, using the number of metered inhalations it contains. Patients should have a spare inhaler in case of emergency, particularly when on holidays.

Pitfalls
- Using poor inhaler technique or a device inappropriate for the patient. Patients with hand diseases or deformities may find it difficult to use DPIs as they require a degree of manual dexterity to prime or load.
- Not having a powerful enough inspiration for DPIs. Some patients also find the sudden puff of medication off-putting whilst trying to concentrate on breathing. There are devices which can calculate whether a patient had sufficient inspiratory flow to deliver the drug into their airways.
- Breathing out into a DPI. This can clog the inhaler.

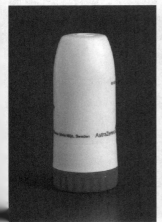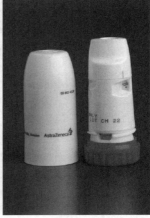

Fig. 10.5 Turbohaler®. Note the tiny dose-indicating window. Reproduced from Thomas and Monaghan (2007) *Oxford handbook of clinical examination skills*. With permission from Oxford University Press.

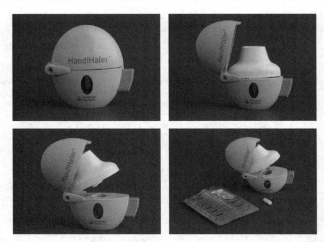

Fig. 10.6 HandiHaler®. Note the button at the side for piercing the capsule and the small window at the front. Reproduced from Thomas and Monaghan (2007) *Oxford handbook of clinical examination skills.* With permission from Oxford University Press.

Nebulizers

Background

A nebulizer converts a solution of drug into an aerosol for inhalation. The drug is delivered to the airways through a mouthpiece or face mask. Nebulizers are mainly used to treat asthma, chronic obstructive pulmonary disease (COPD) and cystic fibrosis. Bronchodilators and steroids are the most commonly used medications. Indications include acute attacks or where compliance with metered dose inhalers or spacer devices is poor. Nebulizers can be used in the home setting.

Equipment

- Oxygen supply.
- Electrical compressor/compressed air.
- Nebulizer chamber and mouthpiece or face mask set.
- Connection tubing (straight/semi-rigid tubing must be used to maintain the correct flow and to avoid disconnection).
- Prescribed medication.
- Prescription chart.
- Ampoules of 0.9% sodium chloride solution, if required as a diluent.
- Peak-flow meter and peak-flow chart.

Procedure

- Explain the procedure and gain consent.
- Assist patient into a comfortable position, preferably sitting upright.
- Plug the compressor unit into the mains if using compressed air to drive the nebulizer.
- Decontaminate your hands.
- Connect one end of the tubing to the gas delivery system (air or oxygen) and the other end to the nebulizer chamber.
- Prepare the prescribed medication. Check the drug and its expiry date.
- Unscrew the top of the nebulizer chamber and insert the medication.
- If required, dilute the drug solution with the required amount of 0.9% sodium chloride. 4–5mL is the optimum amount of solution in the nebulizer chamber.
- Screw the top of the nebulizer chamber back on.
- Attach the face mask or mouthpiece to the top of the chamber. Face masks should be close fitting. Mouthpieces are recommended when steroids, antibiotics or antimuscarinic bronchodilators (anticholinergics) are being nebulized.
- If a mouthpiece is used, advise the patient to place it between their teeth and to seal their lips around it. They should take slow deep breaths through their mouth and if possible hold each one in for 2–3sec.
- Ensure the nebulizer chamber is upright to enable maximum delivery of medication.
- Switch the compressor on or set the oxygen/ compressed air flow to 6–8L/minute.
- Observe the patient during the procedure for any change in their condition.

- Switch off the compressor or flow meter when the nebulizer starts to 'splutter' as this indicates that the treatment has finished. This usually takes ~7–10min.
- Discard the small amount of liquid that remains in the nebulizer chamber.
- After use wash the nebulizer chamber. Then reconnect it to the tubing and blow air from the gas supply through it for a few seconds to dry it. Disconnect the tubing from the compressor unit and store for next use.
- Nebulizer chambers, masks and tubing should only be used for a maximum period of 24 hours before being replaced.

Practice tips

- Drugs should only be added to the nebulizer chamber immediately before administration, as most medications do not contain preservatives.
- Owing to the viscosity of steroids and antibiotics, nebulizing time might need to be ↑ and ideally a nebulizer system with a mouthpiece used.
- Drops of drug solution might form on the sides of the nebulizer chamber. Gently tap on the side of the chamber to knock these droplets back into the drug solution.
- Nebulized solutions can be used for a range of indications, e.g. nebulized adrenaline is used in anaphylactic reactions involving the upper airways. Nebulized salbutamol is one of the treatments for hyperkalaemia.

Pitfalls

- Using water for injection as a diluent because it might cause bronchoconstriction in nebulized form.
- Using high-flow oxygen to drive a nebulizer for a patient with COPD unless specifically prescribed. Oxygen can blunt the hypoxic ventilator drive in these patients leading to life-threatening hypercapnia.
- Domiciliary oxygen cylinders may not be suitable for driving nebulizers and advice should be sought from the oxygen contractor.

Continuous positive airway pressure (CPAP)

Background

A CPAP device provides constant positive pressure throughout the respiratory cycle. It prevents alveolar collapse, and ↑ functional residual capacity and lung compliance. It helps to rectify ventilation perfusion mismatches. The effect of CPAP is to ↓ the work of breathing and to improve oxygenation. It can be delivered by mouth, nose, or through an endotracheal tube or tracheostomy. CPAP is often used out of hospital in the treatment of obstructive sleep apnoea (OSA). The positive pressure prevents the upper airways from collapsing in this condition. In hospital, CPAP is used in acute respiratory failure, pulmonary oedema and as an aid to weaning from a ventilator. CPAP is contraindicated if the patient is very drowsy, unable to protect their airway or if there is a pneumothorax. They must also possess adequate respiratory muscle strength and be haemodynamically stable. Bilevel (or biphasic) positive airway pressure (BiPAP) delivers CPAP but also senses when an inspiratory effort is being made and delivers a higher pressure during inspiration. When flow stops, the pressure returns to the CPAP level. This positive pressure wave during inspiration unloads the diaphragm, decreasing the work of breathing. BiPAP has been used for years in patients with chronic respiratory failure due to neuromuscular problems or chest wall abnormalities. In patients with respiratory failure a common technique with BiPAP is to begin with the expiratory level at 5cm H_2O and the inspiratory level at 15cmH_2O. The levels are adjusted based on patient comfort, tidal volume and blood gases. Both BiPAP and CPAP are effective in preventing intubation and decreasing mortality in patients with acute respiratory failure in properly selected patients.

Equipment

- CPAP delivery device/flow meter.
- CPAP circuit.
- Oxygen analyzer.
- PEEP valves 2.5, 5, 7.5, 10, 15, and 20cm.
- CPAP face/nasal mask.
- T-piece.
- CPAP head straps.
- Humidification device.
- Oxygen supply.
- Pulse oximetry.
- HME/filter (see p. 308).

Procedure

- Explain the procedure and gain consent.
- Explain to the patient that it takes 20–30min to build up the pressure again every time the mask is removed.
- Set up the CPAP circuit and connect the flow meter and oxygen analyser and humidifier.
- Obtain a baseline set of observations.

- Place the patient in an upright position.
- Hold the facemask over the patient's face.
- Gradually ↑ the pressure until the patient gets used to the device, then attach the head straps.
- Readjust to ensure there are no leaks and the straps are not pushing against the ears.
- Adjust the flow to ensure the PEEP valve is partially open and moving with the patient's breaths and is displaying the correct value.
- The usual starting level is 5cmH$_2$O. The pressure should be ↑ in increments of 3–5cmH$_2$O up to 10–15cmH$_2$O, although >10cmH$_2$O is rarely used.
- Adjust the oxygen to the required concentration.
- If the flow meter does not have an inbuilt safety valve, a PEEP valve of a higher value must be present in the circuit in case of failure of the prescribed valve.
- Reassess the patient's observations to check for any change in respiratory or cardiovascular function.
- Monitor and record fluid balance carefully to prevent dehydration.
- A nasogastric tube might be needed to prevent gastric distension and encourage adequate dietary intake.
- Loosen mask every 4 hours to relieve conjunctival oedema.
- Reposition the patient regularly to prevent pressure sore development.
- Document the episode of care.

Practice tips
- Communication is essential to reassure the patient, relieve anxiety and promote cooperation.
- Explain to the patient that talking may be difficult while wearing the mask.
- Medication might be required to maintain compliance.
- Be aware that CPAP can cause hypotension by ↓ cardiac output and venous return.

Pitfall
- Not giving adequate explanation of the procedure to the patient, resulting in poor compliance.

Measurement of end-tidal carbon dioxide

Background

Capnometry is the measurement of end tidal carbon dioxide (ET CO_2). It is a reflection of metabolism, circulation and ventilation. Capnography is the graphic display of CO_2 concentration against time. The shape of the waveform (see below) is more important clinically than the concentration displayed numerically. A photo detector measures the amount of infrared light absorbed by airway gas during inspiration and expiration. A monitor converts this data to a numeric measurement of CO_2 tension in mmHg or % CO_2 and produces the waveform. The normal end-tidal value is about 40mmHg or 5%. It is used continuously or intermittently to confirm that an endotracheal tube is in the trachea, to assess the effectiveness of resuscitation and in non-intubated patients to assess the severity of asthma/COPD and response to treatment. There are two main methods for obtaining gas samples for analysis: mainstream and sidestream.

The normal capnograph has four distinct phases (see Fig. 10.7 opposite).

- Phase 1 (A–B) contains no exhaled CO_2 and represents exhalation of anatomic dead space gas.
- Phase 2 (B–C) has a sharp upstroke corresponding to the appearance of ↑ alveolar CO_2 in expired gas.
- Phase 3 (C–D) or the plateau phase reflects exhalation of gas from uniformly ventilated alveoli. The highest point D is the end tidal CO_2 concentration, i.e. the maximal concentration of expired CO_2.
- Phase 4 (D–E) is the rapid descent of CO_2 concentration to baseline during inspiration.

Equipment

- Capnograph module, sensor cable, airway adaptor—mainstream only.
- Capnograph, water trap and sampling line—sidestream only.
- Battery—if not mains powered.

Procedure

- Explain the procedure and gain consent, if applicable.
- Prepare the equipment.

Using a mainstream adaptor (inline)
- Insert the CO_2 module into the monitor housing device.
- Connect the sensor cable to the module.
- Connect the airway adaptor to the sensor cable and calibrate according to the manufacturer's instructions.
- Place the adaptor in line at the end of the patient's endotracheal tube. A waveform and CO_2 values should be displayed.
- Select alarms limits and set according to prescribed values.
- Select time for averaging of CO_2—i.e. single breath, 10sec, or 20sec.
- Observe the waveform.

Using a sidestream system (aspiration)
- Connect the water trap between the sample line and analyser to protect the optical equipment.
- Connect the sampling tube to a T-piece inserted at the endotracheal tube in intubated patients or to the nostril or mask in non-intubated patients.
- Switch on. The tiny aspiration pump will then aspirate 150–200mL/minute of gas from the breathing circuit and transport the gas sample through the sampling tube to the CO_2 analyser.
- Water vapour from the circuit condenses on its way to monitor.

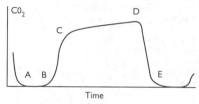

Fig. 10.7 The normal capnograph.

Assisting with pleural aspiration

Background

The pleural space can be aspirated for therapeutic or diagnostic purposes. The site of aspiration can be detected by percussion but is more accurately ascertained by ultrasound. A needle biopsy of the pleura can be performed at the same time as a diagnostic pleural aspiration.

Equipment

- Sterile IV cut-down pack.
- Sterile drape/dressing towel.
- Sterile gloves.
- 2% chlorhexidine in 70% isopropyl alcohol.
- Sterile gauze swabs.
- Sharps box.
- 2, 5, 20, and 50mL syringes.
- 1% or 2% lidocaine solution.
- Selection of needles.
- Specimen container.
- Sterile dressing.
- Cannula.
- Biopsy equipment if a pleural biopsy is to be performed.

Procedure

- Ensure that the procedure has been explained and consent gained.
- Obtain baseline observations before the procedure.
- Prepare the equipment, wash hands and open pack.
- Place the patient in an upright position. They may lean forward with their arms and head supported on a pillow.

The person carrying out the procedure will

- Wash their hands and put on sterile gloves.
- Clean and drape the area around the intended insertion site.
- Administer 2–3mL of 1% or 2% lidocaine solution into the surrounding skin with a narrow guage needle (25 guage).
- Use a larger bore (21 guage) needle to infiltrate the chest wall down to the pleura with local anaesthetic (avoiding the intercostal nerves and vessels which run on the underside of the rib). When the pleura has been pierced, the operator can aspirate fluid into the syringe to confirm the presence of an effusion.
- For a diagnostic tap, insert a large bore needle attached to a 20 or 50mL syringe and aspirate 20–50mL of fluid. The operator will then syringe the fluid into sterile containers for transport to the laboratory for analysis.
- For a therapeutic tap, insert a plastic cannula size 14 or 16 into the pleural space attached to a syringe. When fluid is aspirated the operator will then advance the cannula a further 0.5–1cm to ensure that it is in the pleural space. When the central needle and stylet are removed a 50mL syringe is attached through a three-way tap. Up to 1–1.5L of fluid or blood can then be aspirated, 50mL at a time, turning the tap off to the environment when the syringe is removed to be emptied between aspirations.

When the aspiration has been completed the assistant will:
- Place a firmly applied sterile dressing over the wound.
- Ensure that the operator has placed all sharps in the sharps container and discard clinical waste.
- Wash hands.
- Reassess the patient and repeat observations.
- Reposition the patient, if required.
- Ensure that the specimen bottles and request cards have been labelled properly and dispatched to the laboratory.
- Document the episode of care.

Practice tip
- Stop the aspiration and re-evaluate if the patient starts to cough, feels giddy or light-headed or has chest discomfort.

Pitfall
- Aspirating fluid too rapidly or aspirating >1.5L in an adult. This can lead to pulmonary oedema.

Chest drain insertion: Seldinger technique

Background

Chest drains are inserted into the pleural space of the chest to remove air (pneumothorax), fluid (pleural effusion), blood (haemothorax), chyle or pus (empyema). The size and type of chest drain used depend on the indication and patient characteristics. The Seldinger technique is the commonest method now used to drain simple pneumothoraces and pleural effusions. There will be minor differences in the technique depending on the equipment, which may vary slightly between institutions. The open technique is used when large-bore drains are required (📖 on p. 338). In either technique, the free end of the tube is usually attached to an underwater seal kept below the level of the chest. It could also be attached to a flutter valve. Either method allows air and fluid to pass in only one direction.

Equipment

- Seldinger chest drain pack (containing chest drain, chest drain needle, syringe, scalpel, 3-way tap and guide wire).
- 2% chlorhexidine in 70% isopropyl alcohol.
- Sterile gown, mask and gloves x 1.
- Sterile towel, dressings and gauze swabs.
- Incontinence pad.
- Non-dissolvable suture and needle x 1.
- 10 mL syringe.
- 1 orange needle, 1 green needle.
- 1% lidocaine solution (at least 10mls).
- Sterile chest-drain bottle, tubing and two clamps.
- 500mL of sterile water—if underwater seal is used.
- Suitable dressing (e.g. Hypafix® or Drainfix®)/tape.
- Monitoring equipment.
- Sterile suction tubing and low-suction unit.

Procedure

- Explain the procedure and gain consent.
- Ensure that the patient has had adequate pain relief.
- Monitor the patient's pulse, respiratory rate, blood pressure, oxygen saturation and pain.
- Check the history and re-examine the patient and the CXR to be certain of the side of insertion.
- Position the patient semi recumbent with the arm on the side of insertion above their head.
- Ensure that an incontinence pad is placed on the bed or couch to mop up spillage.
- Put on an apron and decontaminate your hands.
- Mark the insertion site with a pen, explaining to the patient what you are doing. The usual site for insertion is the 5th intercostal space just anterior to the mid axillary line and just above the 6th rib (to avoid the neurovascular bundle running on the underside of the 5th rib).
- Sterilise the area with 2% chlorhexidine in 70% isopropyl alcohol on cotton balls. Work in a spiral pattern outwards from the insertion site.
- Administer local anaesthetic (1% lidocaine) into the skin using a syringe and orange needle.

- Change the orange needle for a green one and administer local anaesthetic into the subcutaneous tissues, muscle and pleura (remember to withdraw the plunger each time prior to injecting to ensure that you are not in a blood vessel).
- Advance the needle through the pleura and aspirate air (pneumothorax) or pleural fluid (effusion). If you aspirate air when draining an effusion it is likely that you have inserted the needle into the lung. Withdraw the needle and assess for a pneumothorax.
- Allow a few minutes for the anaesthetic to work.
- Use the scalpel to make a small incision in the skin.
- Take the needle with the curved tip and attach it to a syringe (there may be a central stilette in the needle which should be removed). The curved tip should point up for a pneumothorax and down for an effusion. There is a corresponding mark on the hub so that you know which way it is facing when it is in.
- Advance the needle into the chest through the anaesthetized tissues until you are in the pleural cavity and aspirate air or fluid depending on whether you are aspirating a pneumothorax or a pleural effusion.
- Disconnect the syringe, holding the needle in place in the chest.
- Straighten the curved tip of the guidewire and then thread the guidewire through the needle into the pleural cavity.
- When the guidewire is halfway in the chest discard the guidewire cover.
- Withdraw the needle from the chest ensuring that the guidewire is held in place. When the needle has been threaded off the guidewire only the wire remains in the chest.
- Thread the introducer over the guidewire and into the pleural cavity to make a tract for introduction of the chest drain, holding onto the guidewire at all times. A rotational movement of the introducer aids insertion.
- Remove the introducer back off the wire, again ensuring that the guidewire is held in place in the chest.
- Then thread the chest drain (with its central stiffner in place) over the guidewire. Ensure that some of the wire is protruding from the proximal end of the drain *before* you push the drain into the chest. It may be necessary to pull the wire slightly out of the chest to do this.
- Hold the guidewire as you push the chest drain over it into the pleural cavity.
- When the chest drain is in the pleural cavity, withdraw the wire and the chest drain stiffner.
- Attach the 3-way tap with all the ports closed.
- Attach the chest drain to tubing and connect the tubing to the chest drainage bottle already filled with 500mls sterile water.
- Secure the drain with a non-absorbable suture. Do a simple skin suture above the drain and wrap the ends tightly around the drain, knotting it a number of times.
- Apply a suitable dressing such as Hypafix® or Drainfix®.
- Open the 3-way tap. Air should start to bubble in the chest drain bottle in the case of a pneumothorax, or fluid should flow into it if there is an effusion.
- Ask the patient to take deep breaths. The water level in the tubing should rise and fall ('swing') with respirations.
- Discard all sharps in the sharps bin and waste in the clinical waste disposal
- Request a post-insertion chest X-ray (CXR).
- Document the episode of care.

Chest drain insertion: open technique

Background

The indications for chest drain insertion are outlined on p. 338. The 'open technique' is used in the setting of blunt trauma and cardiothoracic surgery or for other situations where a wide bore drain (28Fr or larger in an adult) is indicated, e.g. extensive surgical emphysema overlying a pneumothorax. The Seldinger technique, now commonly used for drainage of pneumothoraces and pleural effusions is described 📖 on p. 338.

Equipment

- Chest-drain insertion pack.
- 2% chlorhexidine in 70% isopropyl alcohol.
- Sterile gown, mask and gloves x 1.
- Sterile towel, dressings and gauze swabs.
- Incontinence pad.
- Sterile scalpel and blade.
- Non-dissolvable suture and needle x 1.
- Selection of needles and syringes.
- 1% lidocaine solution.
- Sterile chest-drain bottle, tubing and two clamps.
- 500mL of sterile water if underwater seal is used.
- Tape.
- Monitoring equipment.
- Sterile suction tubing and low-suction unit.

Procedure

- Explain the procedure and gain consent.
- Check the history, re-examine the patient and the CXR to be sure of the side of insertion.
- Position the patient in a semi recumbent position with the arm on the side of insertion above their head. In trauma where spinal injury is a concern and in unconscious patients the procedure is performed with the patient supine (📖 see fig10.8, p. 342).
- Place the incontinence pad on the bed/couch to mop up any spillage.
- Decontaminate your hands and put on a sterile gown.
- Clean and drape the area around the intended insertion site. The usual site of insertion is just anterior to the mid-axillary line in the 5th intercostal space (see fig. 10.8).
- Administer local anaesthetic into the skin, subcutaneous tissues, muscle, and pleura, and allow time for it to take effect.
- After infiltrating the pleura with local anaesthetic, advance the needle slightly the needle into the pleural cavity. This should confirm free air, blood or other fluid on aspiration. If you aspirate air when draining an effusion it is likely that you have inserted the needle into the lung. Withdraw the needle and assess for a pneumothorax.
- Use the scalpel to make a 2cm incision in the skin (above the 6th rib to avoid the neurovascular bundle running on the underside of the 5th rib).
- Dissect bluntly through the intercostal muscles down to pleura using a forceps and a gloved finger.
- Pass a finger or forceps through the pleura.

- Sweep around inside the thoracic cavity feeling for lung or any other structures (e.g. abdominal contents in trauma) and for adhesions.
- Pass the chest tube into the thoracic cavity (the metal trochar should be removed before insertion). A clamp can be attached to the proximal end of the tube to guide it into place.
- Advance the tip of the tube towards the apex for a pneumothorax or base if draining an effusion.
- Attach the tube to the underwater or flutter valve system, aided by your assistant. The collection bottle should always be below the level of the patient's chest to prevent reflux into the chest.
- Look for condensation or fluid in the tube as a sign of correct placement.
- Ask the patient to take deep breaths. The water level in the tubing should rise and fall ('swing') with respirations.
- Suture the tube into position with e.g. a large silk suture attached to the skin and then firmly around the tube.
- Suture across the incision (with plain or mattress 3.0 nylon sutures) if there is a gap between the tube and the wound ends that could cause leakage.
- Apply a sterile dressing to the drain site and apply tape to secure the drain and tubing.
- Discard all sharps in the sharps bin and waste in the clinical waste disposal.
- Order a post-insertion CXR.
- Document the episode of care.

Practice tips

- Warn the patient that they will feel the pressure of the tube being inserted.
- The procedure can be extremely uncomfortable, particularly if there are rib fractures. Administer analgesia, e.g. morphine 10mg IV, at least 15min before the procedure if time allows. Sedation can also be employed by personnel trained in its use.
- Purse string sutures can cause puckered unsightly scars and should not be used.

Pitfalls

- Not having the bottle primed with water before the tube is inserted.
- Not ensuring that the tube is underwater in the bottle.
- Using trocars to aid insertion of the drain leading to damage to intrathoracic and intra-abdominal structures.
- Using the entire safe dose of local anaesthetic early in the procedure. Some should be kept to infiltrate the deeper muscles and pleura after dissecting down.
- Using 2% lidocaine local anaesthetic, which ↑ the chances of not having sufficient volume to fully anaesthetize the area. It is preferable to use 1% when using the dissection technique.
  Not securing the drain to the chest, or poor connections in the system leading to the drain becoming disconnected or leaking.

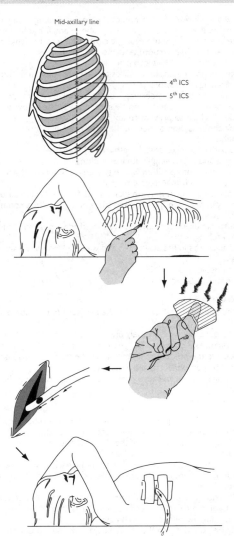

Mid-axillary line

4th ICS

5th ICS

Fig. 10.8 Insertion of a chest drain—open technique. Reproduced from Wyatt et al. (2006) *Oxford handbook of emergency medicine*, 3rd edn. With permission from Oxford University Press.

Assisting with insertion of a chest drain

Background

The indications for chest drain insertion and the different types of drain are outlined on p. 338 and 340.

Equipment

- Chest-drain insertion pack (open or Seldinger depending type).
- 2% chlorhexidine in 70% isopropyl alcohol.
- Sterile gown, mask and gloves.
- Sterile towel, dressings and gauze swabs.
- Sterile scalpel and blade.
- Non-dissolvable suture and needle x 1.
- Selection of needles and syringes.
- 1% lidocaine solution.
- Sterile chest-drain bottle, tubing and two clamps.
- 500mL of sterile water if underwater seal is used.
- Incontinence pad.
- Tape.
- Monitoring equipment.
- Sterile suction tubing and low-suction unit if required.

Procedure

- Ensure that the procedure has been explained and consent gained.
- Ensure that adequate pain relief has been given.
- Monitor the patient's pulse, respiratory rate, blood pressure, oxygen saturation and pain levels before and during the procedure.
- Prepare the equipment.
- Position the patient to facilitate insertion of the chest drain.
- Place the incontinence pad on the bed/couch to mop up any spillage.
- Decontaminate your hands.
- Open the sterile packs.
- Open all equipment onto the sterile field.
- Prepare the chest-drain tubing and bottle or flutter valve. The bottle should be primed with sterile water, the baseline level equating to zero on the bottle.
- Needles, syringes and 1% lidocaine (up to 20mL) will be required for local anaesthetic.
- Elevate the patient's arm above their head on the side of insertion.

The health care worker (HCW) carrying out the procedure will:

- Decontaminate their hands and put on a sterile gown with your help. Ideally they should also wear a mask.
- Clean and drape the area around the intended insertion site. The usual site of insertion is just anterior to the mid-axillary line in the 5th intercostal space.
- Anaesthetize the area.
- Insert the chest drain (📖 on p. 338, 340).
- Attach the drain to the tubing and chest drain bottle (or flutter valve) with your help.

Assisting with insertion of a chest drain

Background

The indications for chest drain insertion and the different types of drain are outlined on p. 338 and 340.

Equipment

- Chest-drain insertion pack (open or Seldinger depending on drain type).
- 2% chlorhexidine in 70% isopropyl alcohol.
- Sterile gown, mask and gloves.
- Sterile towel, dressings and gauze swabs.
- Sterile scalpel and blade.
- Non-dissolvable suture and needle × 1.
- Selection of needles and syringes.
- 1% lidocaine solution.
- Sterile chest-drain bottle, tubing and two clamps.
- 500mL of sterile water if underwater seal is used.
- Incontinence pad.
- Tape.
- Monitoring equipment.
- Sterile suction tubing and low-suction unit if required.

Procedure

- Ensure that the procedure has been explained and consent gained.
- Ensure that adequate pain relief has been given.
- Monitor the patient's pulse, respiratory rate, blood pressure, oxygen saturation and pain levels before and during the procedure.
- Prepare the equipment.
- Position the patient to facilitate insertion of the chest drain.
- Place the incontinence pad on the bed/couch to mop up any spillage.
- Decontaminate your hands.
- Open the sterile packs.
- Open all equipment onto the sterile field.
- Prepare the chest-drain tubing and bottle or flutter valve. The bottle should be primed with sterile water, the baseline level equating to zero on the bottle.
- Needles, syringes and 1% lidocaine (up to 20mL) will be required for local anaesthetic.
- Elevate the patient's arm above their head on the side of insertion.

The health care worker (HCW) carrying out the procedure will:

- Decontaminate their hands and put on a sterile gown with your help. Ideally they should also wear a mask.
- Clean and drape the area around the intended insertion site. The usual site of insertion is just anterior to the mid-axillary line in the 5th intercostal space.
- Anaesthetize the area.
- Insert the chest drain (📖 on p. 338, 340).
- Attach the drain to the tubing and chest drain bottle (or flutter valve) with your help.

- Ensure that the tube in the underwater seal bottle is under water at a depth of 2–3cm with a side vent open to allow escape of air (unless suction is in progress).
- Observe for swinging of the fluid level. If the drain is not swinging, check for kinks loops or blockages. It might, however, mean that the lung is fully expanded. Positive end expiratory pressure (PEEP) and one-way valve systems can also dampen oscillations.
- Observe for bubbling in the underwater seal bottle. If there is continuous bubbling try and identify the source of the air leak (☐ see page 346).
- If there is a persistent air leak around the drain site consider low-pressure suction.
- Record the volume and character of the drainage. The frequency of recording will vary depending on the circumstances. Mark the drainage bottle each time. If drainage stops, check the tubing for kinks or bends and ensure that it is low enough for gravity to assist drainage. Report if there is sudden cessation of drainage, excessive drainage or a worrying change in the nature of the drainage (e.g. straw-coloured becoming bloody).
- Change the bottle if it is more than three-quarters full (☐ on p. 354).
- Drain site dressings should be changed when soiled or if there are signs of infection.
- Ensure that chest drain clamps are by the bed in case of an emergency. Drains should not be routinely clamped because this might cause a tension pneumothorax.
- Document the episode of care.

Practice tip
- Remind patients if they need to mobilize that they must take the drain with them.

Pitfalls
- Changing a bottle and forgetting to put sterile water in it leading to a tension pneumothorax.
- Not checking that low suction (if required) is at the prescribed level, usually 15–20cmH$_2$O/5kPa/~35mmHg, and attached.

Management of non life-threatening chest drain complications

Background

Chest-drain complications may be discovered on routine assessment (📖 see p. 346) or if the patient seeks advice or assistance. The health care worker (HCW) looking after chest drains should know how to assess and manage complications. Life-threatening complications are addressed on p. 350.

Equipment

- Dressing pack/sterile dressing.
- Sterile chest drain bottle and tubing.
- 500mL of sterile water if underwater seal is used.
- Tape.
- Chest-drain tubing, clamps × 2.
- Monitoring equipment—pulse oximeter, BP cuff, and cardiac monitor.
- Sterile suction tubing and low-suction unit.

Procedure

- **If the drain has fallen out of the chest and there is a pleural air leak:** apply pressure with a gauze swab over the chest-drain wound and oppose edges. Release the pressure periodically or if there is any sign of respiratory distress. Call for senior medical help and organize preparation for a replacement tube.
- **If there is accidental disconnection of the drainage tubing from the chest drain:** clamp the tube immediately and attach a new drainage system. Remove the clamp and ask the patient to cough. If the patient shows any sign of respiratory compromise call a doctor immediately.
- **If the drainage tube is disconnected and becomes contaminated:** submerge the chest tube ~3cm below the surface of a 250mL bowl of sterile saline or water until a new chest drainage unit is set up.
- **If drainage stops:** check the tubing for kinks or bends and ensure that it is low enough for gravity to assist drainage.
- **If the drain (fluid level) is not swinging:** check for kinks loops or blockages. It might, however, mean that the lung is fully expanded. PEEP and one-way valve systems can also dampen oscillations.
- **If there is persistent bubbling:** try to identify its source. Fluctuation of the bubbling with respiration suggests the lung as the source. Pinch or clamp momentarily near the chest wall. If the bubbling continues there is a loose connection or leak hole in the tubing. If it stops there is a leak at the insertion site or in the lung. Check the insertion site for position of the drain and for a leak. Make sure that the catheter 'eyelets' are not outside the chest wall. Inform the clinician looking after the patient if there is new, ↑ or unexpected air leak.

Pitfall

- Clumping a bubbling chest drain longer than "momentarily".

Management of life-threatening chest drain complications

Background

Patients with chest drains *in situ* need careful observation. They have the potential to deteriorate rapidly if complications arise. The deterioration might be a fault with the drainage system or related to a recurrence or worsening of the condition for which the chest drain was inserted. It might be owing to a pathological process not directly related to the chest drain, e.g. a pulmonary embolus or myocardial infarction. The major hazard in pleural chest drainage is tension pneumothorax. Massive bleeding from a drain could also occur for a variety of reasons and require surgical intervention. Health care workers (HCWs) should have a systematic approach to assessing the patient and the chest drainage system to identify the cause of any life-threatening complications and to take appropriate action.

Equipment

- A spare set of equipment should always be available in case of emergency.
- Chest drain tubing clamps × 2.
- A large bore venflon (14G).
- IV fluids.

Procedure

- All patients with chest drains should be closely observed. If they experience new onset chest pain, difficulty in breathing or a sudden change in cardiovascular status they require immediate attention.

Assess the patient

- Firstly rapidly assess the patient using the ABCDE approach (🕮 on p. 202). Record vital signs (🕮 on p. 42).
- Look for the symptoms and signs of a tension pneumothorax:
  - Patient complaining of worsening breathlessness—'I can't breathe'.
  - Tachypnoea, use of accessory muscles.
  - Chest not moving on the affected side.
  - Hyperresonant to percussion.
  - ↓ or absent breath sounds.
  - Tracheal deviation to the opposite side.
  - Cardiovascular compromise—tachycardia ± hypotension.
  - Cyanosis.
  - Hypotension as the condition progresses.
  - The most common cause of tension pneumothorax in a patient with a chest drain *in situ* is obstructed tubing.
- Look for signs of hypovolaemic shock, which combined with massive blood loss into the drain is an indication for immediate surgery.

Assess the chest drain and drainage system

- Start at the insertion site unless there is an obvious problem elsewhere.
- Is the chest tube still in the pleural cavity? Chest tubes can fall out or be pulled out if not properly secured.
- Is there any subcutaneous emphysema (crepitus) on palpation around the tube?
- Is the tube obstructed anywhere?
  - Look for kinking or blockage of the tube with clot.
  - Ensure that the tube has not been clamped.
- Is there water in the drainage bottle? Is the bottle full?
- Is there a sudden ↑ in blood loss into the chest drain bottle? This occurs most commonly in the context of trauma or post cardiothoracic surgery. 1000–1500mL of blood or ongoing loss of >200mL/hour is significant and almost certainly will require the patient to go to theatre.

Pitfalls

- Panicking and not assessing the patient and the drainage system in a systematic manner.
- Failing to summon senior help early.

Management of suction in chest drains

Background

If there is persistent air leakage or a large collection of fluid, continuous suction can be used to enhance drainage and to extract air from the pleural space to restore negative pressure. Suction can be applied through an independent suction pump or low-pressure piped wall suction using a low-pressure suction unit. Too little suction might prevent lung expansion and ↑ the risk of infection, atelectasis, and tension pneumothorax. Too much suction might cause damage to the lung tissue or perpetuate existing leaks. The usual amount of suction used is 5kPa or $-20cmH_2O$. There are two types of suction used: wet or dry. In wet suction the height of a column of water in the suction control chamber controls the amount of suction transmitted to the pleural cavity. In dry suction, the suction is controlled by a self-compensatory regulator.

Equipment

- Needle and syringe.
- Water.

Procedure

- Explain procedure and gain consent.

Dry suction

- Connect the suction tubing to the suction unit and switch on. You should be able to hear the suction, if not apply to a gloved finger to 'feel' the suction.
- Check that the dial is set to the prescribed suction ($-20cmH_2O$ is the most common for adults).
- Connect the free end of the suction tubing to the chest-drain bottle.
- Ensure the suction tubing is not disconnected or occluded.

Wet suction

- Check that there is continuous gentle bubbling which indicates that the suction is working. If there is no bubbling, make sure that the suction tubing is connected and not occluded. If there is vigorous bubbling, it might be that the patient has a large leak with air flow greater than the suction can handle.
- Check the water level in the suction control chamber. Discontinue the suction momentarily to do this. If the chamber is underfilled add fluid. If it is overflowing withdraw fluid from the self-sealing chamber diaphragm on the suction chamber.

Practice tip

- If you suspect the suction has stopped working but are unsure if the problem is with the chest drain or the suction unit, temporarily clamp/kink the chest drain above the connection between the suction tubing and the drainage tubing from the patient. Disconnect and listen for a 'slurp': this will confirm that the suction is functioning but the chest drain might be blocked.

Pitfall

- Not using a low-pressure suction unit.

Changing an underwater drain bottle

Background

A chest-drain bottle that is too full results in impaired drainage. When drainage approaches the three-quarters level, the bottle should be changed as a matter of routine. Bottles should also be replaced if they have been in use for >5 days or if a clot is blocking the system.

Equipment

- Sterile chest-drain bottle and tubing.
- 500mL of sterile water.
- Chest-drain tubing clamps × 2.
- Sterile suction tubing and low-pressure suction unit.
- Gloves and apron.
- Solidifying agent (optional).

Procedure

- Explain the procedure and gain consent.
- Prepare the equipment.
- Decontaminate your hands and put on an apron and gloves.
- Check the sterile integrity of the replacement bottle and tubing.
- Remove the bottle and tubing set and from its packaging.
- Fill the bottle with sterile water to the 'prime level' on the label.
- Insert the tubing set into the replacement bottle taking care not to contaminate the end to be inserted into the chest drain.
- Twist to lock the tubing into place.
- Clamp off the chest drain using both chest drain clamps to prevent any backflow of air or fluid.
- Disconnect the old tubing and bottle and attach the new one.
- Release the clamps as soon as the new tubing is attached.
- Ensure that there is oscillation (swinging) of the fluid in the underwater tube.
- If suction is used, transfer it to the replacement bottle.
- Lift the old tubing above the level of the old bottle to expedite any excess fluid entering the bottle. Disconnect the tubing from the bottle and discard it in clinical waste.
- Add a solidifying agent to the chest-drain bottle to solidify the contents, seal the old bottle with the seal provided and place in clinical waste.
- Document the episode of care.

Practice tips

- It is easier to change the bottle if two people are present, one to remove the old tubing and one to attach the new.
- If the seal to cover the old bottle is mislaid, do not remove the tubing set. Cut through the tubing and place the end of it over the suction port on the lid of the bottle to create a seal.

Pitfalls

- Not unclamping as soon as the bottle has been changed.
- Omitting to put sterile water in the new bottle with the potential of developing a tension pneumothorax.

Removal of a chest drain

Background

The timing of removal of a chest drain is dependent on the original reason for insertion and the clinical and radiological progress of the condition. In the case of pneumothorax, the drain should not usually be removed until bubbling has ceased and chest radiography demonstrates lung reinflation. Clamping of the drain before removal is generally unnecessary. Removal of a chest drain is a two-person procedure.

Equipment

- Dressing pack.
- Sterile dressing pack.
- Sterile gloves.
- Sterile stitch cutter.
- Suture pack.
- Suture (3/0) nylon.
- 2% chlorhexidine in 70% isopropyl alcohol.
- 1% or 2% lidocaine solution.
- Sachet of 0.9% saline solution.
- Sharps container.

Procedure

- Explain the procedure and gain consent.
- Place the patient in an upright position.
- Prepare the equipment.
- Decontaminate your hands and put on sterile gloves and an apron.
- Remove the dressing from the drain site.

The health care worker (HCW) carrying out the procedure should perform the following:

- Clean the area around the drain site with normal saline.
- Insert local anaesthetic if a suture will be required to close the chest drain wound.
- Cut the suture securing the drain with the sterile stitch cutter or scissors.
- Instruct the patient (if awake) to breathe in to the maximum and to hold their breath.
- Remove the chest drain with a fast firm movement on expiration.

The second HCW should perform the following:

- Immediately hold the wound edges opposed. The wound is then sutured by the first person with simple or mattress sutures (usually 3/0 nylon).
- Place a dressing over the wound.
- Place sharps in the sharps container.
- Discard clinical waste.
- Wash your hands.
- Re-position the patient, if required.
- Arrange a post-drain removal chest X-ray.
- Document the episode of care.
- Monitor patient post-procedure.

Practice tip

- An airtight seal can be created over the hole in the chest when the drain is removed by placing a piece of gauze with aquagel over it. Fold over a piece of gauze twice. Place a blob of aquagel about the size of a 50p piece on the middle of it. Hold the gel at the skin/drain interface during removal. When the drain is out, the blob of gel on the gauze covers the hole.

Pitfall

- Allowing air to enter the chest when removing the drain.

Assisting with bronchoscopy

Background

Bronchoscopy involves endoscopic examination of the upper airways and bronchial tree using either a flexible fibre optic or a rigid bronchoscope. The procedure is used to evaluate and diagnose suspicious lesions, to take tissue and sputum samples for examination, to remove secretions, plugs and foreign bodies from the airways, to control bleeding and to assist with difficult intubations. It is usually performed under sedation with local anaesthetic, although rigid bronchoscopy generally requires a general anaesthetic. Complications include larygospasm, bronchospasm, pneumothorax, haemorrhage, hypotension and hypoxaemia.

Equipment

- Bronchoscope—the type will depend on the purpose of the bronchoscopy.
- Functioning light source.
- Sterile suction tubing.
- Biopsy forceps—optional.
- Sterile specimen containers/sputum traps.
- Sterile gloves and gown.
- Sterile bowl/jug.
- Sterile water x 500mL.
- Bronchoscope swivel connector and cap.
- Sterile lubricant.
- Airway/mouthguard.
- Sedative agent, if required.
- Local anaesthetic spray.

Procedure

- Ensure that the procedure has been explained and consent gained.
- Prepare the equipment. Check that the light source is functioning and that the bronchoscope has been sterilized.
- Monitor the patient's pulse, respiratory rate, blood pressure, oxygen saturation and pain levels before and during the procedure.
- Position the patient in a flat supine position (if their condition allows).
- Assist with the administration of sedation and local anaesthetic as requested.
- Administer 100% oxygen, if requested by the medical practitioner.
- If an endotracheal tube is *in situ* (e.g. in an intubated patient in intensive care), the assistant should ensure that it is kept secure throughout the procedure.
- Open the sterile packs and equipment.

The health care worker (HCW) carrying out the procedure will perform the following:

- Wash their hands and put on gloves and apron.
- Prepare the equipment and connect the light source and suction.
- Place a mouth guard around the scope, if required.
- Lubricate the bronchoscope.

- Introduce the scope gradually into the airway observing the trachea, carina and the bronchi.
- Remove secretions and take specimens and biopsies, as appropriate. Physiotherapy and lavage can be performed to aid the process.
- Remove the bronchoscope.

The assistant should then perform the following:

- Help to reposition the patient appropriately following removal of the scope.
- Reassess the patient and repeat observations, including pulse oximetry.
- ↓ the oxygen to normal levels as soon as the patient's condition allows.
- Ensure that all specimens and forms are correctly filled in and labelled before dispatch to the laboratory.
- Ensure that the person carrying out the procedure has cleaned the bronchoscope and checked its integrity after use before sterilizing.
- Document the episode of care.
- The patient should be observed for 2–4 hours after the procedure or until the effects of the sedation wear off.

Pitfall

- Failing to secure and protect an endotracheal tube adequately before and during the procedure, resulting in dislodgement.

Chest physiotherapy

Background

Chest physiotherapy is a broad term describing physical treatments which help to remove excess secretions from the lungs, expand collapsed alveoli and on occasions reinflate collapsed lung, lobe or lobar segments. It is predominantly used for patients with ↑ amounts of mucus, weak respiratory muscles or ineffective coughs for whatever reason. Some of the techniques can be performed by any health care worker (HCW) with appropriate training. Others should only be done by physiotherapists. The treatment should be discontinued immediately if the patient complains of pain, or has dyspnoea, hypoxia, heamoptysis or tachycardia. Physiotherapy is critical in some chronic lung diseases such as cystic fibrosis. Patients should be educated in self-physiotherapy if possible.

Equipment
- Sputum cup.
- Tissues.
- Pillows.
- ± suction.

Procedure
- Explain procedure and gain consent. The patient should wear one layer of soft comfortable clothing or a towel.

The active cycle of breathing techniques (ACBT)
- Sit the patient in a comfortable position. Ensure that they have adequate pain relief.
- Thoracic expansion deep breathing—first, encourage the patient to take deep inspirations keeping expiration quiet and relaxed. Following this they should attempt a deep cough. Tightening stomach muscles ↑ the power of the cough.
- Forced expiration: ask the patient to inhale deeply and then forcefully exhale (huff). A huff from a high lung volume (when a deep breath has been taken in) will clear secretions from the upper airways and a huff from mid to low lung volume will clear secretions from the lower more peripheral airways.

Incentive spirometry
- An incentive spirometer is a device that can be used to encourage patients to do deep breathing.

Percussion
- Position the patient supine or prone depending on area to be treated.
- Hold your hand in a rigid dome shape. This traps air in the hand, softening the strikes.
- Gently strike the area over the lobes to be drained in a rhythmic pattern. It should be performed for ~20sec at a time with pauses for 5sec or longer. This minimizes the risk of desaturation in patients with moderate or severe lung disease. Percussion can be used in short bursts combined with ACBT techniques. More tenacious secretions might need up to 5min percussion.

Vibration
- Place flattened hand over section of chest wall, tense upper arm and shoulder muscles at a rate of up to 200/minute. This method essentially involves shaking the area of lung being treated. Ask the patient to exhale as slowly and completely as possible making a 'sss' or 'fff' sound.

Postural drainage
- Position the patient so that the trachea is inclined downwards and below the affected area. It allows gravity to assist drainage of secretions.
- Remain in position for ~15–20min.
- Repeat two to three times daily.
- Ask the patient to spit out any secretions loosened.

Practice tips
- ↑ activity as tolerance to the procedure improves. The manoeuvres can be uncomfortable and tiring.
- Administer water or saline nebulizer before physiotherapy to ↓ thickness of sputum.
- Early in the morning before the patient gets out of bed is a good time to perform physiotherapy. The chest is more relaxed and secretions easier to remove.
- Physiotherapy before bedtime can be beneficial in reducing night time coughing.
- Postural drainage can be used effectively in conjunction with percussion.
- Place pillows under the pelvis, not the chest, to achieve the position for drainage.
- Involve relatives in the care, techniques can be taught to enable them to continue care in the home setting.

Pitfalls
- Performing physiotherapy after a meal. Wait for at least one hour after food and half an hour after drinks.
- Wearing rings, which can cause damage to the patient's skin.

Cardiovascular system

Kate Johnson
Formerly Senior Lecturer in Cardiac Nursing, City University,
London, UK

Martyn Bradbury
Clinical Skills Network Lead, School of Nursing and
Community Studies, Faculty of Health and Social Work,
University of Plymouth, UK

History-taking and assessment

Background

A comprehensive assessment of the cardiovascular system will allow the health care worker (HCW) to determine the patient's signs and symptoms and, consequently, the most appropriate treatment. A number of generic skills, such as communication, observation, and technical skills are used.

A variety of assessment formats are used. In deteriorating or unstable patients, a more rapid assessment using the airway, breathing, circulation, disability, and exposure (ABCDE) approach may be adopted. Alternatively, in stable patients, a more complete physical assessment using a top-to-toe approach may be more useful. The assessment should also include establishing relevant risk factors, past medical history, social history, family history, and medication history.

Equipment

- Electrocardiogram (ECG) machine.
- Assessment sheet (or other suitable documentation).
- Sphygmomanometer.
- Stethoscope.
- Pulse oximeter.

Procedure

- Explain the procedure and gain consent.

Airway

Assess for signs of partial or complete airway obstruction. This might include:
- No sound—this could indicate complete obstruction.
- Snoring, gurgling, and gasping.
- Any visible airway obstruction.
- Laryngeal oedema.
- Evidence of swelling e.g. tongue.
- Bleeding.

Breathing

- Rate, rhythm, and depth of respiration (<10 breaths/minute or >30 breaths/minute indicates a problem).
- Use of accessory muscles to help breathing, e.g. sternomastoids.
- Breath sounds—listen for any gurgling, wheezes, and crackles.
- Equal air entry—the right and left chest wall should rise symmetrically. Asymmetric chest movement may be indicative of pneumothorax or lung disease on that side.
- Position of the trachea. This should lie in the midline and be equidistant from the sternomastoids.
- Evidence of peripheral or central cyanosis.
- Complaints of shortness of breath or difficulty with breathing.
- Number of pillows required to sleep.
- Smoking history.
- Presence and appearance of sputum, e.g. quantity, colour, consistency.
- Shortness of breath on exertion.
- Oxygen saturation levels (SpO_2)📖 on p. 302.

Circulation
- Palpate central and peripheral pulses noting heart rate, rhythm, and pulse volume (it is not possible to palpate peripheral pulses if systolic blood pressure is <80mmHg).
- Check blood pressure 📖 on p. 56, 58.
- Record 12 lead ECG 📖 on p. 370.
- Observation of neck veins to see if they are full or collapsed and central venous pressure (CVP) 📖 on p. 244, if available.
- Urine output—should be >0.5mL/kg body weight/hour—and fluid balance.
- Evidence of bruising, swelling, redness, bleeding, or pain.
- Capillary refill—assess by applying pressure to the fingertip for 5sec. When the pressure is removed, normal skin colour should return within 2sec.
- Colour, appearance, and temperature of the skin.
- Observation of wound sites, if present.

Disability
Neurological status is assessed initially using the alert, responsive to voice, responsive to pain, or unresponsive (AVPU) scale 📖 on p. 596. A more in-depth assessment, such as the Glasgow Coma Scales (GCS) 📖 on p. 582, can follow. In the pre hospital setting the FAST stroke screening tool can be used to assess for **F**acial weakness, **A**rm weakness and **S**peech problems and determine that it is **T**ime to transfer the patient to hospital. Also, assess the blood sugar level 📖 on p. 66 and consider any other factors that could affect level of consciousness, for example hypoxia, poor perfusion, and the effects of any drugs taken.

Exposure
At this point, consider any other factors that could cause the patient's condition to deteriorate. If not already recorded, take the patient's temperature. Check the body for any rashes and oedema.

Pain assessment
- Location, severity, duration, precipitating, and relieving factors—description of pain.
- A pain assessment tool should be used 📖 on p. 108.

Other
- Look for xanthelasma (small, raised, yellowish plaques on and around the eyelids) or corneal arcus (a whitish arc seen just inside the cornea at the periphery of the iris), which are suggestive of hyperlipidaemia.
- Nail and hand assessment—look for splinter haemorrhages and clubbing of the nails (loss of nail-bed angle, ↑ curvature of nail, and bulbous ends of fingers). Rarely, Osler's nodes (red tender nodules on the finger pulps or radial palm) and Janeway lesions (non-tender erythematous or haemorrhagic lesions on the palms and finger pulps) may be seen in infective/bacterial endocarditis.
- Calculate the body-mass index (BMI) 📖 on p. 416

  BMI = weight (kg)/height^2 (m).

- Check for allergies.

Cardiac monitoring

Background

Cardiac monitoring provides continuous tracing of the patient's heart rate and rhythm through leads that are attached to electrodes placed on the patient's chest. It allows the health care worker (HCW) to observe for changes in the rate, rhythm and pattern of the electrocardiogram (ECG) and to initiate early treatment as appropriate. Many cardiac monitors also have the facility to simultaneously monitor oxygen saturation (SpO_2), non-invasive blood pressure (NIBP), and respiration. A rhythm strip can usually be printed from the monitor for further analysis.

Procedure

The normal ECG waveform (see Fig. 11.1) comprises a number of clearly distinct waves which represent the changes in electrical activity that occur within the heart during the cardiac cycle.

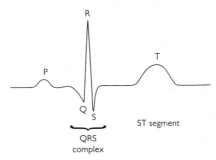

Fig. 11.1 A normal ECG waveform. Reproduced from Thomas and Morgan (2007) Oxford handbook of clinical examination and practical skills. With permission from Oxford University Press and the authors.

- P wave: this precedes the QRS complex and represents depolarization of the atria
- QRS complex: this comprises three distinct waves and represents depolarization of the ventricles
- Q wave: the first downward (negative) deflection
- R wave: the first upward (positive) deflection
- S wave: a downward (negative) deflection that occurs after the R wave
- T wave: this follows the QRS and represents ventricular repolarization.

When observing the ECG it is therefore important to begin by determining if there is electrical activity. If not, check the patient, leads, electrodes, and gain (the size of the ECG display) on the monitor. Next ensure that the ECG trace is running at 25mm per second and begin ECG interpretation:

- Check the rate—each large square (5 small squares) = 0.2sec and each small square = 0.04sec. To calculate the rate, count the number of QRS complexes within a 6-second strip (30 large squares) and multiply this number by 10 (this will = the heart rate).
- Check the rhythm—is the distance between the QRS complexes regular? If not is there any pattern to the irregularity?
- Look for atrial activity—is there a P-wave before each QRS complex? Check the PR interval (the time from the beginning of the P-wave to the start of the QRS complex). This should normally be less than 0.2sec (5 small squares).
- Look at the QRS complex and check its duration. Normally this should be <0.12sec (3 small squares).
- Report any abnormalities.

Practice tip

- The interpretation of the ECG is a complex skill and beyond the scope of this book. As such, the reader is directed to refer to HCWs who have experience in ECG interpretation, and to the numerous texts that explain this clinical skill in detail.

Pitfalls

- Failing to palpate the patient's pulse when the pulse rate is displayed on the cardiac monitor. Remember that in pulseless electrical activity (PEA) arrest the ECG might display a normal cardiac rhythm even though there is no cardiac output.
- Not recognizing the limitations of your own knowledge and failing to seek expert advice early enough.

Applying and positioning of electrodes

Background

Both 3-lead and 5-lead monitoring systems can be used. The principles of monitoring are the same for each system.

Equipment

- Cardiac monitor.
- Disposable monitor electrodes.
- Razor or clippers.
- Alcohol impregnated swab.

Procedure

- Check that the monitor is working.
- Explain procedure and gain consent.
- Decontaminate your hands.
- Ensure that the patient's skin is dry—an alcohol swab can be used to remove excess oil.
- Excess hair will lead to poor electrode contact—shave or clip hair, if necessary.
- Check the expiry date of the electrodes.
- Attach a monitoring electrode to the right shoulder just below the clavicle and attach the red electrode, the second monitoring electrode should be placed on the left shoulder just below the clavicle and attached to the yellow electrode; the third monitoring electrode should be placed on the skin on the left-hand side of the abdomen and attached to the green electrode. If a 5-lead system is used, the first 3 leads are positioned, as outlined above, and then the black lead is placed on the right-hand side of the abdomen and the white lead is placed in the middle of the patient's chest.
- Select the ECG lead to monitor—this would usually be lead 2, but leads 1 or 3 can be used if they provide a better trace.
- Set the alarm parameters on the monitor and ensure these are switched on.
- Check all connections and quality of the ECG trace.
- Decontaminate your hands.
- Document episode of care.

Practice tips

- Modified chest lead 1 can be recorded by placing the black electrode on the right shoulder, the yellow electrode on the left shoulder, and the red electrode in the middle of the abdomen.
- Change electrodes every 24–72 hours to prevent the gel from drying out and the patient's skin from becoming sore.
- If the patient is mobile, a telemetry system can be used. The telemetry system is attached by the method outlined above, but the patient carries the telemetry box with them. The rhythm can be observed on a monitor, either on the same ward or on a ward nearby.
- ▶ Be aware of safety aspects of telemetry, for example, although the rhythm can be observed, the patient might not always be within view of the HCW.
- Telemetry unit batteries should be changed regularly.

Pitfalls

- Siting electrodes in areas where defibrillation pads or paddles might be placed during cardiopulmonary resuscitation (CPR) 📖 on p. 377.
- Shivering and electrical pumps can cause electrical interference and affect the ECG trace. Ensure that the patient is warm and comfortable and that pumps are moved as far from the monitoring equipment as possible.
- Siting monitoring electrodes over bone rather than muscle.

Performing a 12-lead electrocardiogram

Background

The 12-lead ECG gives a more complete three-dimensional view of the heart when compared with standard cardiac monitoring. The ECG measures the changes of electrical current within the heart and is a valuable diagnostic tool in establishing the cardiac rhythm and if there has been injury, ischaemia or infarction within the heart. When an electrode is placed on the skin surface overlying the heart and attached to an ECG machine, the trace will show an upwards deflection as a cardiac impulse is travelling towards it and a downwards deflection if the impulse is travelling away from it. This is because the heart muscle has different directions of force (or vectors). The electrical current predominantly flows from the base to the apex of the heart.

Equipment

- ECG machine.
- ECG electrodes.

Procedure

- Explain the procedure to the patient and gain consent.
- Check that the ECG machine is stocked with paper.
- Check the expiry date of the electrodes.
- Decontaminate your hands.
- Position patient, ideally recumbent, and ensure that they are comfortable and relaxed.
- Remove excess hair and moisture from the patient's skin.

Limb leads

- Place an ECG electrode and red lead on the right arm at the wrist or shoulder.
- Place an ECG electrode and yellow lead on the left arm at the wrist or shoulder.
- Place ECG electrode and green lead on the left leg—normally at the ankle, but also at the top of the leg if required.
- Place ECG electrode and the black lead on the right leg.

Chest leads

The chest /precordial leads (see Fig. 11.2) are attached to ECG electrodes placed as follows
- V1 4th intercostal space at the right sternal border.
- V2 4th intercostal space at the left sternal border.
- V3 midway on the diagonal line formed between V2 and V4.
- V4 5th intercostal space on the midclavicular line.
- V5 anterior axillary line in the same horizontal plane as V4.
- V6 mid-axillary line in the same horizontal plane as V4 and V5.
- Ask patient to remain still and not talk while ECG is recorded.
- Check that the machine is calibrated correctly and then press start.
- Check the tracing for movement or artefact and, if necessary, repeat.
- Remove electrodes, unless serial ECGs are being recorded.

- Record the patient's name, hospital number, date, and time on the ECG. If the patient is experiencing chest pain then this should also be noted on the ECG.
- Ensure the patient is comfortable.
- Dispose of clinical waste and put equipment away.
- Decontaminate your hands.
- Document episode of care.
- Analyse the ECG.

Practice tips

- A posterior ECG can be recorded by moving the chest leads around to the patient's back (5th intercostal space).
- A right-sided ECG can be recorded by putting V3 to V6 in the same anatomical position on the right-hand side of the chest and swapping the position of V1 and V2.

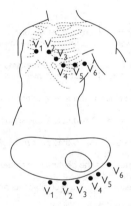

Fig. 11.2 Positions of the chest leads. Adapted with permission from Chikwe J, Beddow E and Glenville B (2006) *Cardiothoracic surgery*, Oxford University Press.

Transcutaneous external cardiac pacing

Background

Transcutaneous external cardiac pacing (TECP) involves passing an electrical current through the heart from electrical pads placed on the skin surface in an anterior lateral or anterior posterior configuration. Its use is usually reserved for the emergency situation for the treatment of conditions such as profound bradycardia, ventricular standstill, complete heart block, and during or immediately after cardiac arrest. TECP is normally used as a temporary measure until other, more sustainable interventions, e.g. transvenous pacing can be undertaken 📖 on p. 374.

Equipment

- Defibrillator with external pacing facility.
- Pacing pads (in some cases, the pads might be the same as those used for cardiac defibrillation).
- Scissors or hair clippers.

Procedure

- Explain the procedure and gain consent as appropriate. Conscious patients should be warned that the procedure might be uncomfortable or painful.
- Ensure the patient's skin is dry and remove excess chest hair. (Cutting/clipping the patient's body hair is better than shaving as it helps to prevent microburns).
- Set the defibrillator to pacing mode—refer to the manufacturer's guidelines.
- Apply the anterior (negative) pad below the left nipple in a V3 position along the left sternal border.
- Place the lateral (positive) pad so that the centre of the pad is located in the mid-axillary line (V6 position).
- Connect the pacing leads of the defibrillator to the pacing pads.
- Check all connections and cables.
- Set the preferred heart rate (usually 60-80 beats per minute) to demand pacing.
- Observe ECG monitor and gradually ↑ the pacing voltage until there is electrical capture—normally between 60 and 100 milliamperes (mA).
- Check for a pulse (central and peripheral).
- Assess response to treatment, i.e. obtain rhythm strip for patient records, check blood pressure, monitor level of consciousness and degree of any pain.
- Document episode of care.

Practice tips

- If an anterior lateral pad position is unsuccessful in establishing cardiac capture then an anterior/posterior pad position might be more successful with the posterior pad placed in the left infra scapula position.
- TECP is often painful and the patient may require sedation or analgesia.

- When there is failure to obtain cardiac capture it is usually due to poor positioning of the electrode, poor pad contact (sweat, hair, and electrode), or battery failure (note that battery depletion can be rapid).
- Some older defibrillators may also require the use of monitoring electrodes to obtain an ECG.

Assisting with transvenous cardiac pacing

Background

There are a number of indications for cardiac pacing which include atrio-ventricular block and bradycardia with inadequate cardiac output.

The transvenous route can be used to establish either a temporary or a permanent cardiac pacing system. Permanent pacing is usually undertaken in a designated cardiac catheter laboratory. In temporary pacing, the pacing wire is usually inserted through the subclavian, internal jugular, or external jugular vein, with the pacing electrode(s) positioned in the right atria, right ventricle, or both (dual-chamber pacing). The pacing wire is then attached to an external pacing box. The procedure is normally performed in a designated pacing theatre because local anaesthetic and fluoroscopic imaging are usually required. The pacing wire is inserted by the medical staff using an aseptic technique. A defibrillator and resuscitation equipment should be readily available.

Equipment

- Sterile pacing set.
- Skin-cleansing, agent e.g. chlorhexidine, povidine iodine (as per local policy).
- Sterile towel/drapes.
- Selection of 25, 23 and 21 gauge needles and 5 + 10 mL syringe.
- Local anaesthetic, e.g. lidocaine 1%.
- Pacing wire.
- Sterile dressing.
- Pacing box and leads.
- Cardiac monitor.
- Trolley.
- Imaging equipment and personal protective equipment as required.

Procedure

- The doctor should explain the procedure to the patient and gain consent before he/she inserts the pacing wire.
- Where fluoroscopic X-ray screening is used ensure all staff are wearing x-ray shielding personal protective equipment (PPE).
- Ensure the patient is attached to a cardiac monitor.
- Wash hands and put on sterile gloves, gown and mask.
- Ensure an aseptic technique is used throughout the procedure.
- Cleaning solution should be poured into the appropriate container.
- The pacing wire should be opened and placed on the sterile field.
- The area chosen for venous access should be cleaned and a sterile drape placed around the site.
- Local anaesthetic, e.g. lidocaine 1%, is usually injected.
- The introducer and pacing wire is inserted using a Seldinger technique. This usually involves inserting an introducer into the right internal jugular, external jugular or subclavian vein. The pacing wire is then passed into the vein through the introducer and advanced into the chamber(s) of the heart that are to be paced.

- Attach pacing wire to the pacing box leads.
- Check the pacing threshold (see 📖 p. 376).
- Set an appropriate pacing rate—demand pacing.
- Secure pacing wire, clean off any remaining skin preparation solution and cover site with sterile dressing.
- Dispose of sharps and other clinical waste.
- Remove gloves and decontaminate hands.
- Make the patient comfortable.
- Document the procedure, including the pacing rate and pacing threshold.
- A chest X-ray should be performed to confirm pacing wire position and exclude pneumothorax.

Practice tips

- All leads should be secured and the patient should be educated to ensure that they do not accidentally disconnect them.
- The threshold should be checked daily.
- The patient should remain monitored.
- The site should be observed for signs of infection and the dressing changed, as required.

Pitfalls

- Potential complications of transvenous pacing include haemorrhage, infection, haemo/pneumothorax, failure to pace, failure to sense, failure of ventricular capture, disconnection, arrhythmia and pericardial effusion/tamponade.

External pacemaker threshold testing

Background
The pacing threshold should be checked daily. Inflammation and displacement of the pacing wire can lead to an ↑ voltage being required to ensure effective pacing is achieved. Two health care workers (HCWs) should be involved in checking the pacing threshold.

Equipment
- The patient should be on a cardiac monitor.
- Emergency resuscitation equipment should be close by.

Procedure
- Explain the procedure to the patient and gain consent.
- Decontaminate your hands.
- Identify the previous threshold level and underlying rhythm from the patient's notes.
- The patient should be in bed and attached to a cardiac monitor.
- If the patient is not pacing all the time, the sensing rate should be ↑ to 10 beats above the intrinsic heart rate—a continuous pacing rhythm should now be seen on the cardiac monitor.
- One HCW should be responsible for changing the voltage and the other for watching the monitor and observing the patient.
- ↓ output slowly in increments of 0.1 volts (V), until loss of ventricular capture is observed.
- ↑ output slowly, until ventricular capture returns. The point at which capture returns is the pacing threshold and is measured in volts (this should be <1.0V).
- The threshold, underlying cardiac rhythm and final output set should be clearly documented in the relevant patient records.
- Ensure the patient is comfortable.
- Decontaminate your hands.

Practice tips
- The output is usually set between two and three times the threshold level.
- Any significant ↑ in pacing threshold and any change or deterioration in the underlying rhythm should be reported immediately to medical staff because further intervention might be required.

Cardiopulmonary resuscitation

National guidelines on resuscitation are published by the Resuscitation Council (UK) and include guidance and treatment algorithms for both adult and paediatric resuscitation in the following circumstances:

- Basic life support.
- In-hospital resuscitation.
- Advanced life support.

Further reading

Comprehensive guidance can be accessed at http://www.resus.org.uk.

Basic life support: adult

Cardiopulmonary arrest in the adult is predominantly due to a cardiac cause. As such, the emphasis during basic life support (BLS) is on preventing hypoxic cerebral damage by applying effective cardiac compression and secondary ventilation.

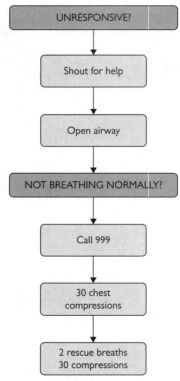

Fig. 11.3 Algorithm for adult BLS. Reproduced with kind permission from the Resuscitation Council UK © 2005.

Basic life support: paediatric

Cardiopulmonary arrest in the infant or child is usually asphyxial in origin. As such, the emphasis is on airway management and the application of effective ventilation prior to obtaining emergency medical assistance and applying cardiac compression.

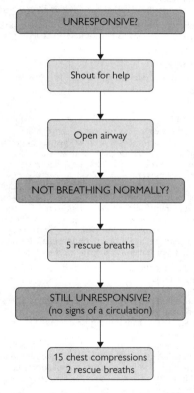

After 1 minute call resuscitation team then continue CPR

Fig. 11.4 Algorithm for paediatric BLS. Reproduced with kind permission from the Resuscitation Council UK © 2005.

In-hospital resuscitation

Background

In the event of a cardiac arrest, the following are vital:

- Immediate recognition of patient collapse.
- Initiate basic life support as soon as possible, in particular chest compressions.
- Call for help.
- Defibrillation (if indicated) should be applied as early as possible.

Several health care workers (HCWs) will usually assist, but a coordinated approach is important to ensure that resuscitation is initiated quickly and effectively.

Equipment

- Resuscitation trolley.
- Oxygen.
- Suction.

Procedure

- Check the area for any hazards or dangers.
- Assess the patient's level of consciousness by gently shaking them by the shoulders and shouting in both ears.
- If there is no response, call for help—this might require pulling an emergency buzzer.
- Open the airway using a head-tilt, chin-lift manoeuvre.
- Open mouth and observe for signs of airway obstruction.
- Use suction or forceps and attempt to remove any obstruction.
- While maintaining an open airway, assess for the absence of normal breathing by looking at the movement of the chest, listening for breath sounds, and feeling for breath on the cheek for up to 10sec.
- If trained, simultaneously palpate for the presence of a carotid pulse.

Where the patient is not breathing and does not have a pulse, perform the following actions:

- Delegate someone to call the cardiac arrest team using the local cardiac arrest procedure (usually by dialling 2222) and collect defibrillator and other resuscitation equipment.
- Perform cardiopulmonary resuscitation (CPR) at a ratio of 30 compressions to 2 ventilations.
- Place the heel of one hand along the middle of the lower half of the sternum. Place the heel of the other hand on top of the first hand and link the fingers so that pressure is applied to sternum rather than the ribs. Ensure that the shoulders are directly over the sternum with the elbows locked and the arms straight.
- Compress the sternum 4–5cm at a rate of 100 compressions per minute.
- After 30 chest compressions, perform ventilations using a pocket mask or airway adjunct and bag–valve–mask system as available. (If using a bag–mask–valve system, connect to oxygen with a flow rate of 15L/minute.)

- When defibrillator arrives, apply adhesive defibrillator pads, initiate cardiac monitoring and briefly interrupt chest compression to analyse cardiac rhythm.
- If trained and rhythm is ventricular fribillation (VF) or ventricular tachycardia (VT) attempt defibrillation: 📖 on p. 386.
- Recommence CPR immediately.
- Once the cardiac arrest team arrives assist with advanced life support.

Practice tips
- Put on gloves as soon as possible.
- There are a variety of airway adjuncts available, including oropharangeal airway (OPA) and laryngeal mask airway (LMA). HCWs should be familiar with those available in their local practice area and have received appropriate training before using them.
- The use of bag–valve–mask system is best achieved by two people—one person to hold the mask in place and ensure an airtight seal and a second person to squeeze the bag and provide ventilation.
- Performing cardiac compression is tiring. As such, change the person performing the compressions every 2min.
- Check the contents of the cardiac arrest trolley on a regular basis and ideally daily, replacing items as necessary and ensuring all equipment is in good working order.
- If relatives are present, they might wish to stay with the patient during resuscitation. This should be handled sensitively and a HCW should remain with them.
- If the patient's next of kin is not present, they should be contacted as soon as possible.

Pitfalls
- Interpreting the presence of agonal breathing (occasional gasping, laboured, noisy or slow breathing) as a sign of life. Agonal breathing, which can occur for several minutes following the onset of cardiac arrest, should be regarded as the absence of normal breathing and an indicator of cardiorespiratory arrest.
- Using excessive shoulder shaking and head tilt in patients with suspected cervical spine injury. In these cases, open the airway using the jaw-thrust technique and stabilize the neck using manual inline stabilization.
- Failing to attend to the needs of other patients during a cardiac arrest. This can be a distressing and anxiety-provoking experience for them.

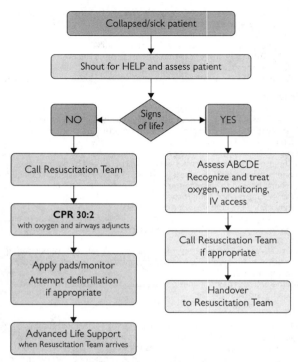

Fig. 11.5 In-hospital resuscitation. Reproduced with kind permission from the Resuscitation Council (UK) © 2005.

Advanced life support: adult

Advanced life support (ALS) includes the use of defibrillation for VF/VT arrest, advanced airway management techniques, e.g. endotracheal (ET) intubation, Intravenous (IV) drug administration, and the identification and treatment of the reversible causes of arrest.

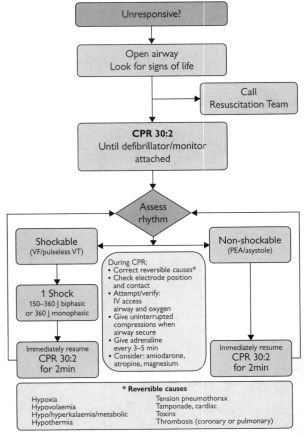

Fig. 11.6 Adult ALS. Reproduced with kind permission from the Resuscitation Council (UK) © 2005.

Advanced life support: paediatric

The presenting cardiac rhythm in cardiorespiratory arrest in the infant or child is usually asystole or pulseless electrical activity (PEA). As such, paediatric ALS places an emphasis on advanced airway management and ventilation, intravenous (IV) or intraosseous (IO) drug administration and the identification and treatment of reversible causes.

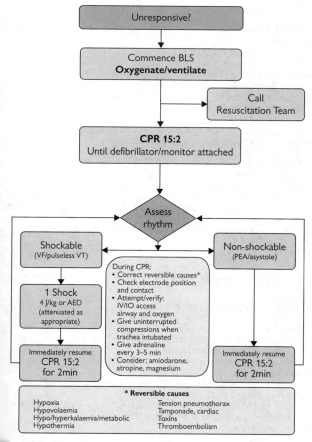

Fig. 11.7 Paediatric ALS. Reproduced with kind permission from the Resuscitation Council (UK) © 2005.

Defibrillation

Background

Early cardiac defibrillation is vital in improving survival from ventricular fibrillation (VF) and ventricular tachycardia (VT) arrest. Cardiac defibrillation can be performed using either a manual or an automated external defibrillator (AED). Defibrillation aims to stop arrhythmia and allow the sino-atrial (SA) node to re-establish a normal cardiac rhythm. The procedure must only be carried out by health care workers (HCWs) who have received appropriate training.

Manual defibrillation

Procedure
- Follow the ALS algorithm 📖 on p. 384.
- Ensure the patient's skin is dry.
- Remove chest hair from defibrillator pad sites. However, do not delay defibrillation if this cannot be done quickly.
- Apply defibrillator pads—one below the clavicle to the right of the sternum (sternal pad), and an apical pad on the mid-axillary line (in the same position as V6). If defibrillator paddles are used, apply water-based gel pads to chest, in same position as above.
- Remove any transdermal nitrate patches.
- Remove oxygen.
- If a shockable rhythm is observed (VT/VF), charge defibrillator, following manufacturer's instructions, ensure everyone stands clear and deliver charge, using the paddles or pads, to the patient's chest. The amount of energy required will depend on the type of defibrillator being used (monophasic or biphasic), the manufacturer's guidelines and the ALS algorithm.
- Check that everyone is standing clear before delivering the shock.
- Replace the paddles, if used.
- Immediately resume 2min of CPR before reassessing the patient.
- Follow ALS algorithm.

Defibrillation using an AED

Procedure
- Follow AED algorithm (see Fig. 11.8).
- Turn the AED on and follow voice prompts.
- Ensure the patient's skin is dry.
- Remove chest hair from defibrillator pad sites. However, do not delay defibrillation if this cannot be done quickly.
- Remove any transdermal nitrate patches.
- Remove oxygen.
- Apply defibrillation pad to the right upper chest to the right of the sternum and below the clavicle.
- Apply second defibrillation pad vertically over the apex of the heart in the mid-axillary line (same position as V6).
- Connect pads to the AED.

- AED will analyse the cardiac rhythm and decide if a shock is required (Ensure no one is touching the patient while the AED is analysing the cardiac rhythm.)
- Follow voice prompt commands.
- If a shock is required, ensure everyone is clear before delivering the shock.
- Recommence CPR immediately following delivery of the shock.
- Reassess the patient after 2min.
- Follow AED algorithm.

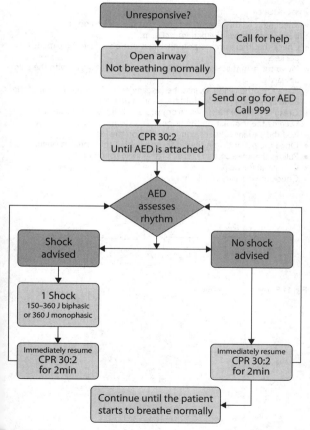

Fig. 11.8 AED algorithm. Reproduced with kind permission from the Resuscitation Council (UK) © 2005.

Recovery position

Background
The recovery position is a safe position in which to place an unconscious patient. The airway should remain patent and obstruction should not occur if the patient vomits.

Equipment
No specific equipment is required.

Procedure
- Kneel next to the patient, ensuring that it is safe to do so.
- If present, remove the patient's glasses.
- Check that there are no potential injurious objects in the patient's pockets.
- Move the arm that is nearest to you out at a right angle, with the palm upwards.
- Place the other hand against the casualty's cheek, with the back of the hand against the cheek. Hold the hand in position.
- Grasp the leg furthest away from you and bring the knee up while keeping the foot flat on the floor.
- Roll the patient towards you by pulling on the leg.
- Once the patient is on their side, ensure that the airway is open.
- Pull up the knee so that it is at a right angle to the body.
- Go or call for help.
- Check the casualty regularly.

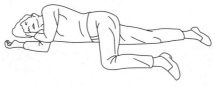

Fig. 11.9 The recovery position.

Ankle–brachial pressure index (ABPI)

Background
This is a crucial assessment tool for determining the arterial blood flow into the lower limbs and for establishing the presence of peripheral vascular disease (see Table 11.1).

Equipment
- Sphygmomanometer.
- Appropriately sized cuff.
- Stethoscope.
- Hand-held Doppler scanner.
- Conducting gel.
- Paper towel.
- Non-sterile gloves (where skin is broken).

Procedure
- Explain the procedure to the patient and gain consent.
- Decontaminate your hands and put on non-sterile gloves as required.
- Position the patient—supine/semirecumbent.
- Allow the patient to rest for several minutes before taking readings.
- Palpate and note the position of the brachial artery.
- Apply the blood pressure cuff to the patient's arm.
- Apply conducting gel over the brachial or radial artery and obtain the best Doppler sound.
- Inflate the cuff until the pulse sound disappears.
- Deflate the cuff slowly (2mm/sec) and note the systolic blood pressure, as indicated by the return of the first Doppler sound.
- Repeat the procedure in the other arm and record the highest reading.
- Locate the posterior tibial and dorsalis pedis (pedal) pulses.
- Position the cuff around the patient's calf, immediately above the ankle.
- Apply conducting gel over the posterior tibial artery.
- Inflate the cuff to 30mm/Hg above the highest systolic blood pressure reading obtained in the arm.
- Deflate the cuff slowly and record the systolic blood pressure, as indicated by the return of the first Doppler sound.
- Repeat the procedure for the pedal pulse and note the highest reading.
- Repeat the procedure for the other leg and note the highest reading.
- Remove any excess gel and make the patient comfortable.
- Calculate the ABPI for each leg by dividing the highest ankle pressure by the highest systolic brachial pressure. (Example: 160mm/Hg ÷ 166mm/Hg = ABPI of 0.96.)
- Document findings.
- Decontaminate your hands.

Practice tips
- Follow the general recommendations for obtaining systolic blood pressure 📖 on p. 56 when taking readings.
- Position the Doppler probe at an angle to the artery to obtain the best sound (usually at 50°).

Pitfall
- Applying high-compression bandaging without first obtaining the ABPI. Compression bandaging should not be used if the ABPI is <0.8.

Table 11.1 ABPI values and implications

ABPI	Implication
>0.9	Normal
≤0.89 but >0.5	Peripheral vascular disease (PVD) present. May be associated with intermittent claudication
<0.5	Severe PVD present. Requires urgent vascular referral. May be associated with ulceration, rest pain and gangrene.

Jugular venous pressure

Background
The jugular venous pressure (JVP) is an important, non-invasive aspect of the cardiovascular examination. Changes in atrial pressure are transmitted into the superior vena cava and jugular veins as a pressure wave that can be observed within the jugular veins. By measuring the maximum vertical height of the observed pressure wave, it is possible to obtain a measurement that reflects the pressure (normal $\leq$8cm H_2O) within the right side of the heart.

Equipment
- Moveable light source.
- Ruler.

Procedure
- Explain the procedure and gain consent.
- Decontaminate your hands.
- Ensure there is a good light source.
- Position the patient at 45°, with their neck supported so the neck muscles and sternomastoids, in particular, are relaxed.
- Ask the patient to tilt their head slightly upwards and away from the side of the neck that is being observed.
- Note the position of the internal jugular vein and position the light source so that it illuminates at a tangent to the vein.
- Measure the maximum vertical height, in centimetres, of the column of blood from the manubristernal angle (See Fig. 11.10.)
- Record the findings and make the patient comfortable.
- Decontaminate your hands.

Practice tips
- The normal JVP is <3cm, which equates to a right atrial pressure of $\leq$8 cm H_2O because the manubristernal angle is ~5cm above the right atria . As such, 5cm is always added to the measured JVP when calculating the atrial pressure.
- The JVP is best observed in the right internal jugular vein.
- Observation of the JVP can be aided by looking along the sternomastoids.
- Palpation of the carotid artery can help in distinguishing between venous and arterial pulsations—under normal circumstances, you cannot feel venous pulsation.
- The JVP is ↑ in conditions such as right-sided heart failure (RHF), superior vena cava (SVC) obstruction, and secondary to ↑ circulating volume (e.g. nephritis and intravenous fluid overload).
- Compression of the abdomen over the liver for 15sec leads to an ↑ in venous return and atrial pressure, consequently leading to ↑ JVP (hepatojugular reflex).
- The JVP should normally fall on inspiration.
- In constrictive pericarditis and severe RHF, the JVP ↑ on inspiration (Kussmaul's sign).

- The jugular venous waveform comprises various components that reflect various aspects of the cardiac cycle—experienced clinicians can use these as part of a more advanced cardiovascular assessment.

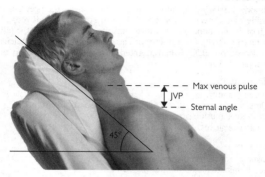

Max venous pulse

JVP

Sternal angle

45°

Fig. 11.10 Measuring the JVP. Reproduced from Thomas and Monahan (2007) *The Oxford handbook of clinical examination and practical skills.*

Pulmonary artery wedge pressure (PAWP)

Background
A pulmonary artery (PA) catheter is used to measure the pressure in the right side of the heart. If the tip of the catheter is inflated/wedged in a branch of the pulmonary artery, it reflects the pressure within the left side of the heart (PAWP). The catheter can also be used to facilitate calculation of cardiac output (CO) when inserted into the right subclavian or the internal jugular vein.

Equipment
- Cardiac monitor.
- 500mL of heparinized 0.9% sodium chloride solution.
- Intravenous infusion pressure bag.
- Non-sterile gloves.

Procedure
- Explain procedure and gain consent.
- Decontaminate hands and put on gloves.
- Keep the PA catheter line continuously flushed, using a pressure-bag system inflated to 300mm/Hg.
- Zero the system each time the patient changes position.
- Inflate the balloon slowly, according to the manufacturer's guidelines.
- Observe the monitor for a change in the waveform.
- With the balloon inflated, allow the trace to run for ~15sec.
- Freeze the monitor and deflate the balloon.
- Align the monitor cursor with the end of expiration on the waveform.
- Read and document the results.
- Unfreeze the monitor.
- Obtain a chest X-ray to check the placement and for any complications.

Practice tips
- Use the attached syringe and inflate the balloon slowly, according to the manufacturer's guidelines—usually not >1.5mL air.
- A sharp ↑ in the trace indicates the balloon is over-wedged.
- Observe the tracing regularly to ensure that the catheter is not wedged accidentally, because this causes damage to the pulmonary artery. The PA catheter entry site is a potential source of infection. As such, it should be cleaned and the dressing changed daily using an aseptic technique 📖 on p. 80. Observe the site for bleeding, swelling, redness, and signs of infection. Take care not to disconnect the lines and clearly label all lines to prevent mixing of infusions. Also observe for the following complications:
  - Pneumothorax—might occur on insertion.
  - Air embolism.
  - Thrombus formation.
  - Arrhythmias.
  - Heart block.

- Balloon rupture.
- Formation of vegetation.
- Sepsis.

Normal values

- Right atrial pressure: 0–8mmHg.
- Right ventricular systolic pressure: 15–25mmHg.
- RV diastolic pressure: 0–8mmHg (usually only seen during catheter insertion).
- PA systolic pressure: 15–25mmHg.
- PA diastolic pressure: 8–15mmHg.
- Causes of ↑ PA pressure include left ventricular failure (LVF), pulmonary hypertension, and fluid overload.
- Hypovolaemia causes ↓ PA pressure.
- PAWP: 6–12mmHg.
- Causes of ↑ PAWP include fluid overload, LVF, and Mitral Valve (MV) problems.
- Hypovolaemia causes ↓ PAWP.

Gastrointestinal system

Louise Stayt
Senior Lecturer in Professional Practice Skills, School of Health
& Social Care, Oxford Brookes University, Oxford, UK

Jacqueline Randle
Associate Professor, Clinical Skills Lead for Masters of Nursing
Science, School of Nursing, Midwifery & Physiotherapy,
University of Nottingham, UK

Frank Coffey
Consultant in Emergency Medicine, Emergency Department,
Nottingham University Hospitals NHS Trust, Associate Professor
and Consultant in Advanced Clinical Skills, School of Nursing,
Midwifery & Physiotherapy, University of Nottingham, UK

History-taking

Background

The gastrointestinal system ingests and digests food and eliminates waste products. Interruption to these processes could result in a range of signs and symptoms, e.g. pain, heartburn, nausea, vomiting, or altered bowel habits. A full evaluation of gastrointestinal symptoms and signs is essential in the assessment process.

Past health

Investigate the patient's past gastrointestinal illnesses to assess whether the current problem is new or recurring. Significant problems include:

- Inflammatory bowel disease.
- Liver, pancreas, and gall bladder diseases.
- Gastric and duodenal ulceration.
- Rectal or gastrointestinal bleeding.
- Indigestion.
- Acid reflux.
- Diverticular disease.
- Gastrointestinal cancers.
- Abdominal trauma.
- Previous abdominal surgery.
- Urinary tract surgery.
- Hepatitis vaccine.
- Previous blood transfusions.

Current health

Assess for the following:

- General health state, including general symptoms, e.g. tiredness or lethargy.
- History of specific symptoms, e.g.:
  - Abdominal pain.
  - Nausea and vomiting.
  - Heartburn / acid reflux.
  - Difficulty swallowing.
  - Altered bowel habit.
  - Rectal bleeding.
  - Bloating.
  - Flatulence.
- Assess symptoms:
  - Onset and duration.
  - Character and location (where appropriate).
  - Associated symptoms
  - Exacerbating factors
  - Relieving factors
  - Any changes over time
- Drug history and current medications, to include the following drugs:
  - Non-steroidal anti-inflammatory drugs.
  - Antibiotics.
  - Opioid analgesics.
  - Laxatives.

- Social history:
  - Alcohol intake.
  - Cigarettes.
  - Illegal drug habits.
  - Living conditions.
  - Occupation.
  - Recent holidays and travel.
  - Exercise.
  - Diet.
  - Oral hygiene.
  - Exposure to infectious diseases.
  - Psychological stress.
  - Sleep pattern.

Family health

Some gastrointestinal disorders are hereditary or have a familial link; it is essential to ascertain whether anyone in the family has had a gastrointestinal disorder. Specifically check for the following:
- Ulcerative colitis.
- Crohn's disease.
- Peptic ulcers.
- Diabetes.
- Gastrointestinal cancers.

Cultural considerations

Some gastrointestinal disorders are affected by ethnicity and cultural background—gastric cancers are more common in patients from Japan, Iceland, Chile, and Austria. Crohn's disease is more common in Ashkenazi Jewish patients from Eastern Europe.

Examining the mouth

Background

A physical assessment of the gastrointestinal system should include a thorough examination of the patient's mouth. Examine the mouth using visual observation and palpation.

Equipment

- Non-sterile gloves.
- Disposable apron.
- Disposable tongue depressor.
- Pen torch.
- Tissues or facial cloth.

Procedure

- Explain the procedure and gain consent.
- Ensure the patient is in a comfortable position.
- Decontaminate your hands.
- Put on a pair of gloves and an apron.
- Examine the jaw and observe for mobility, symmetry.
- Examine the lips and observe for:
  - Cracking
  - Bleeding
  - Ulceration
  - Oedema
  - Colour
  - Movement
  - Pain.
- Ask the patient to poke out their tongue and inspect it for:
  - Coating
  - Blisters
  - Dryness
  - Redness
  - Tremors and movement
  - Swelling
  - Ulceration
  - Tenderness.
- Ask the patient to open their mouth wide.
- Note the presence of halitosis.
- Gently place the tongue depressor on the patient's tongue.
- Using the pen torch, shine the light into the patient's mouth.
- Inspect the interior of the patient's mouth and observe the following:
  - Mucous membranes for coating, bleeding, cracking, ulceration, and redness.
  - Gums for soreness, redness, bleeding, ulceration, oedema, recession.
  - Teeth for plaque, caries, looseness, missing teeth, broken teeth, colour and debris.
  - Dentures for fit.
  - Pharynx for uvular deviation, tonsillar abnormalities, lesions, plaques and exudates.

- Remove the tongue depressor and ask the patient to close their mouth.
- Offer the patient a tissue to wipe their mouth or wipe the patient's mouth, if necessary.
- Discard the equipment using clinical waste disposal.
- Ensure the patient is comfortable.
- Decontaminate your hands.
- Document the episode of care.

Examining the abdomen – inspection

Background

Examination of the abdomen involves inspection, palpation and auscultation. Inspection involves a knowledge of what to look for. Additional training and assessment are required to be able to undertake the advanced skills of palpation and auscultation. The abdomen is traditionally divided into 4 quadrants for the purposes of description (see figure 12.1).

Procedure

- Explore the procedure and gain consent.
- Decontaminate your hands.
- Lie the patient flat.
- Expose the patient's abdomen, ensuring their upper torso and lower body remain covered.
- Inspect the abdomen for:
  - Shape, size, and symmetry.
  - Skin changes—texture and colour.
  - Scars—position, size and colour.
  - Lumps, bulges and distension.
  - Stretch marks (striae) indicative of recent weight loss, current or previous pregnancy, or steroid therapy.
  - Dilated veins.
  - Spider naevi (can also be looked for on the face, chest and arms).
- Unless proceeding to palpation, replace the patient's clothing and ensure the patient is comfortable.
- Decontaminate your hands.
- Document the episode of care.

Practice tips

- Ask the patient to elevate their head to tense the abdominal muscles. This may demonstrate divarication of the rectus abdominis muscles or hernial swellings.
- Ask the patient to cough and observe particularly the umbilical, inguinal and femoral regions for herniae. Observe for pain on coughing which may occur in peritonism.

Pitfall

- Not elevating skin folds in obese patients and missing abnormalities particularly in the groin region.

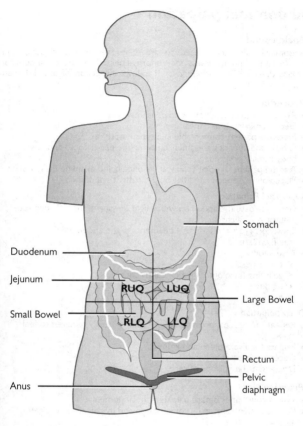

Fig. 12.1 Abdominal quadrants.

RUQ   Right Upper Quadrant
LUQ   Left Upper Quadrant
RLQ   Right Lower Quadrant
LLQ   Left Lower Quadrant

Abdominal palpation

Background
Abdominal palpation is used to assess for tenderness, masses, fluid accumulation and to assess for abnormalities of the major abdominal organs (liver, spleen and kidneys). It follows inspection of the abdomen (📖 on p. 392).

Procedure
- Explain the procedure and gain consent.
- Decontaminate your hands.
- Make the patient comfortable in a supine position.
- Expose the patient's abdomen, ensuring the upper torso and lower body remain covered.
- Ask the patient to point to any areas of pain and examine these last.
- Place your extended hand flat on the patient's abdomen.

Superficial Palpation
- Gently palpate the abdomen with a light dipping motion, flexing your metacarpophalangeal joints.≠
- Slowly progress around the 4 quadrants of the abdomen (see fig. 12.1).
- Assess for:
  - tenderness
  - guarding (involuntary reflex contraction)
  - rigidity
  - masses

Deep palpation
- Repeat the process pressing deeper (this is usually required to feel masses).
- Palpate the liver, spleen and kidneys.
- Decontaminate your hands.
- Document the episode of care.

Practice tips
- Warm your hands before palpating the abdomen.
- Put the patient at ease by conversation and by palpating very gently at first.
- When palpating watch the patient's face for signs of pain.
- Distract the patient while palpating.

Pitfalls

- Failing to examine all area of the abdomen.
- Assuming a normal abdominal examination means that there is no pathology. Elderly patients particularly if they are on steroids may not manifest classical abdominal signs. 50% of patients with significant intra-abdominal injuries may have a normal initial examination.

Abdominal auscultation

Background

Auscultation of the abdomen with a stethoscope provides information about bowel motility. It may also reveal *bruits* over the aorta or other arteries in the abdomen which suggest vascular disease. The frequency, pitch and intensity of the bowel sounds can vary. Normal bowel sounds consist of rumbling or gurgling noises that occur at a frequency of about 5-30 per minute. *Borborygmi* are prolonged rumbles ("growling") and are a normal finding. Bowel sounds may be increased in diarrhoea and early intestinal obstruction. They are markedly decreased or absent in adynamic intestinal ileus or in peritonitis. High pitched tinkling sounds are typical of intestinal obstruction.

Equipment

• Stethoscope

Procedure

• Explain the procedure and gain consent.
• Decontaminate your hands.
• Make the patient comfortable in a supine position.
• Decontaminate the stethoscope,
• Expose the patient's abdomen, ensuring the upper torso and lower body remain covered.
• Place the diaphragm of the stethoscope gently onto the abdomen. The right lower quadrant is the optimum position to hear bowel sounds.
• Listen until bowel sounds are heard or for at least one minute
• Listen over the aorta (centrally) and over the renal arteries for *bruits*
• Listen for *bruits* over the iliac arteries and the femoral arteries in the groin if you suspect arterial insufficiency in the lower limbs.
• Decontaminate your hands.
• Decontaminate your stethoscope.
• Decontaminate your hands.
• Document the episode of care,

Practice tips

• Auscultatation may be done before palpation and percussion as these manoevres may change the frequency of bowel sounds.
• Bruits confined to systole may not necessarily signify vascular disease.

Pitfall

• Not listening for long enough. Bowel sounds may occur at gaps of up to approximately one minute.

Examining the rectum and anus

Background
Examining the rectum and anus is essential in a comprehensive gastroin-testinal assessment. This procedure is required to detect haemorrhoids, polyps, fissures, faecal impaction, masses, and prostate enlargement.

Equipment
- Non-sterile gloves.
- Disposable apron.
- Lubricant gel.
- Disposable protective pad.
- Disposable wipes.

Procedure
- Explain the procedure and gain consent.
- Decontaminate your hands.
- Help the patient into the left lateral position, with knees flexed.
- Place a protective pad underneath the patient.
- Put on a pair of gloves and an apron.
- Remove the patient's clothing, as required, ensuring privacy and dignity.
- Inspect the perianal area looking for:
  - Fissures
  - Scars
  - Inflammation
  - Discharge
  - Rectal prolapse
  - Haemorrhoids
  - Polyps
- Lubricate your gloved index finger with lubricating gel.
- Slowly insert your gloved finger into patient's rectum.
- Rotate your gloved finger clockwise and anti-clockwise, palpating the walls of the rectum.
- Feel for masses, faecal impaction, and tenderness.
- In the ♂ palpate the prostate for size, consistency and the presence of nodules or tenderness. In benign prostatic hyperplasia the central sulcus is preserved and may be exaggerated. In prostatic cancer, the gland may be hard, irregular and nodular and there is often loss or distortion of the central sulcus.
- Clean the patient's peri-anal area.
- Inspect your gloved finger for colour and consistency of any faeces and the presence or absence of blood.
- Replace the patient's clothing and ensure the patient is comfortable.
- Discard the equipment using clinical waste disposal.
- Decontaminate your hands.
- Document the episode of care.

Practice tips
- Keep your fingernails short.
- To relax the anal sphincter apply gentle firm pressure for a few seconds just in front of the anal opening with the pulp of the examining finger.

As the sphincter relaxes with continued pressure, gently advance the finger into the anal canal.

- If there is severe pain with pressure at the anal opening there may be an anal fissure, ulcer, abscess or thrombosed haemorrhoid. Look for these conditions, seek advice and consider the use of local anaesthetic gel before proceeding.
- If the patient has had any of the following, caution should be taken:
  - Active inflammation of the bowel.
  - Pelvic radiotherapy.
  - Tissue fragility.
  - A known history of sexual anal abuse.
  - Spinal injury because of autonomic dysreflexia (abnormally increased or decreased response to physiological stimuli).
  - Known latex allergies.
  - Cardiac conditions, specifically angina, cardiac failure, and arrhythmias.
  - Pancytopaenia (abnormal depression of the cellular blood components).
  - Neutropaenia (diminished number of neutrophils in the blood).
  - Coagulopathy (blood coagulation disorder).
  - Low platelet count.

Pitfalls

- Not doing a rectal examination when it is indicated, to save you or the patient embarrassment; hence the aphorism "If you don't put your finger in it, you put your foot in it!"
- Performing a rectal examination when it will not change your management e.g. in a patient with suspected appendicitis, who will definitely be going to theatre. It is an unpleasant examination to undergo.
- Not being aware of the possible adverse consequences of the examination, such as:
  - Rectal trauma.
  - Rectal bleeding.

Nausea and vomiting – assessment of vomitus

Background
Nausea is a sensation of unease and discomfort associated with an urge to vomit. Nausea and vomiting are symptoms that can be caused by a variety of conditions (see table 12.1). A detailed history and examination should be undertaken to ascertain the underlying cause. If possible the health care worker should collect, measure and inspect the character of vomitus, or at least obtain a detailed description of it from the patient.

Equipment
- Non sterile gloves,
- Disposable apron.
- Disposable receiver.

Procedure
- Put on a pair of gloves and an apron.
- If possible collect a sample of vomitus in a disposable receiver.
- Inspect the vomitus and note its colour, consistency and the presence of fresh or altered blood.
  - *Coffee ground* due to old blood in the vomitus. This has the appearance of the dregs of a cup of coffee.
  - *Bright red blood (haematemasis)* – the presence of fresh blood indicates fresh bleeding from the upper gastrointestinal tract.
  - *Yellow-green vomitus (bilious)* – results from the vomiting of bile and upper bowel contents in the presence of obstruction.
  - *Faeculent vomiting* – brown offensive material. It is a late sign of small intestinal obstruction.
  - *Brown-black fluid in large volumes* may be vomited in acute dilatation of the stomach which may occur following surgery or diabetic ketoacidosis. (It requires urgent insertion of an NG tube 📖 on p. 436).
- Ascertain the approximate volume of vomitus and the amount of blood if present.
- Discard the vomitus and container in clinical waste disposal.
- Offer mouth care (📖 on p. 420) and ensure the patient is comfortable
- Document the episode of care.

Practice tips
- The ingestion of iron tablets, red wine and coffee can give vomitus an appearance that may be mistaken for coffee ground.
- Recently ingested tea can have the same appearance as faecal vomiting but does not have the offensive smell.

Pitfall
- Describing any dark vomitus as coffee ground. Coffee ground has a very distinctive colour. This reinforces the value of personal inspection by a healthcare worker.

Table 12.1 Important causes of nausea and vomiting

Side effects of drugs e.g. antibiotics, opioids
Food poisioning / gastroenteritis
Gastritis
Labyrinthine disorders e.g. viral labyrinthitis
Migraine
Pregnancy
Gastrointestinal obstruction
Appendicitis / cholecystitis / peritonitis / pancreatitis
Peptic ucler disease
Acid reflux
Urinary tract infection
Other infections – e.g. pneumonia, meningitis
Head injury
Raised intracranial pressure
Renal / cardiac / hepatic failure
Myocardial infarction
Drug overdose / poisoning
Allergy / anaphylaxis
Metabolic eg. diabetic ketoacidosis, hypercalcaemia
Chemotherapeutic agents and radiotherapy
Overeating
Excess alcohol
Cannabis
Excessive coughing
Exercise or stress

Management of nausea and vomiting

Background

Nausea is a sensation of unease and discomfort associated with an urge to vomit that commonly precedes vomiting. Problems associated with vomiting include the following:

- Loss of fluid and electrolytes.
- Interference with nutrition.
- Exhaustion.
- Soreness.
- Aspiration.
- Patient distress.

Non-pharmacological management

Non-pharmacological management includes advising patient to do the following:

- Avoid large meals—promote the eating of several small meals.
- Eat slowly.
- Drink liquids 30min before the meal.
- Eat dry foods, e.g. crackers.
- Avoid greasy foods.
- Avoid unpleasant odours, e.g. smoking and heavy perfume.
- Relax after eating.
- Remain seated, if possible.
- Elevate the head if they need to lie down.
- Avoid wearing tight, constricting clothing.
- Avoid alcohol.
- Take deep breaths when feeling nauseas.
- Comply with anti-nausea medications and techniques.
- Use mouth-care facilities 📖 on p. 420.

Pharmacological management

There are four main neurotransmitters involved in sending stimuli to the emetic chemoreceptor trigger zone and vomiting centre in the medulla:

- Dopamine
- Histamine
- Acetylcholine
- Serotonin (5-HT)

Drug therapy targets the transmission and receptor sites of these neurotransmitters.

Anti-dopaminergics

These drugs act on the emetic chemoreceptor trigger zone. They are particularly useful in relieving nausea and vomiting associated with chemotherapy, radiotherapy, surgery, and toxins, but not motion sickness. Examples are phenothiazines, metoclopramide and domperidone Common side-effects include tardive dyskinesia (involuntary movements) and sedation.

Antihistamines

Antihistamines act on the emetic chemoreceptor trigger zone, vomiting centre, and the middle ear. They are effective in treating motion sickness. An example is cyclizine. Common side-effects include dizziness, tinnitus, incoordination, fatigue and tremors.

Anti-cholinergics

These drugs work on the vomiting centre and are also good for motion sickness. An example is hyoscine. Common side-effects include dry mouth, blurred vision, urinary retention and exacerbation of acute angle glaucoma. Contraindicated in prostatic hypertrophy, untreated glaucoma and paralytic ileus.

5-HT$_3$ receptor antagonists

These drugs work on the emetic chemoreceptor trigger centre, the vagus nerve and serotonin receptors in the small bowel and are effective in the treatment of chemotherapy-associated and postoperative nausea and vomiting. Examples are ondansetron and granisetron. Common side-effects include headache, diarrhoea, fatigue and hypersensitivity reactions.

Practice tips

- Ideally, the cause of nausea and vomiting should be identified before choosing an anti-emetic agent.
- A combination of agents can be used, but two drugs from the same group must be avoided.
- Monitor the effectiveness of any anti-emetic regime and be alert for any adverse effects.
- Measure and record the volume of any vomit.
- Give mouth care 📖 on p. 420.
- Inform the medical staff if vomiting persists despite anti-emetic therapy.
- Consider pregnancy in women of childbearing age.

Pitfall

- Treating the symptoms *without* trying to elucidate and treat the underlying cause of the nausea and vomiting.

Stool assessment

Background

Bowel habit is a good indicator of overall gastrointestinal function. Ask the patient about the following:

- Frequency of defaecation.
- Time of day of defaecation.
- Flatulence.
- Constipation and diarrhoea.
- Associated pain or discomfort.
- Urgency.
- Presence of faecal incontinence.

The quality of stool can be classified using the Bristol Stool Form scale (Fig. 12.2).

Equipment

- Non-sterile gloves.
- Disposable apron.
- Disposable bedpan.

Procedure

- Explain the procedure and gain consent.
- Decontaminate your hands.
- Put on a pair of gloves and an apron.
- Ask the patient to defaecate into the disposable bedpan, advising the patient to avoid urinating at the same time (if possible).
- Inspect the patient's stool for colour, odour, consistency, and volume.
- Discard the equipment using clinical waste disposal.
- Decontaminate your hands.
- Ensure the patient is comfortable.
- Decontaminate your hands.
- Document the episode of care.

Practice tip

While examining the patient's stool, assess it for:

- Blood
- Mucus
- Undigested food
- Texture.

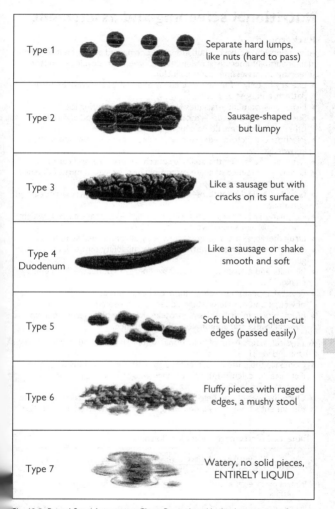

Type 1		Separate hard lumps, like nuts (hard to pass)
Type 2		Sausage-shaped but lumpy
Type 3		Like a sausage but with cracks on its surface
Type 4 Duodenum		Like a sausage or shake smooth and soft
Type 5		Soft blobs with clear-cut edges (passed easily)
Type 6		Fluffy pieces with ragged edges, a mushy stool
Type 7		Watery, no solid pieces, ENTIRELY LIQUID

Fig. 12.2 Bristol Stool Assessment Chart. Reproduced by kind permission of Dr KW Heaton, Reader in medicine at the University of Bristol. © 2000 Norgine Pharmaceuticals Ltd.

Nutritional screening and assessment

Background

All patients should have a nutritional screening and assessment to identify malnutrition. Numerous screening tools have been developed; nutritional screening and assessment should include:

- Dietary history—frequency of eating and habits, preferences, meal pattern, and portion sizes.
- Living environment—facilities for storing and preparing food.
- Socio-economic status—resources for purchasing food and reliance on other people for mealtime support.
- Psychosocial factors—depression, anxiety, bereavement, and dietary knowledge.
- Disability—affecting the ability to purchase, prepare, and eat food.
- Disease—presence of acute or chronic disease, which might influence diet, appetite, energy expenditure, or swallow.
- Gastrointestinal symptoms—anorexia, nausea, vomiting, diarrhoea, and constipation.
- Calculation of any significant weight change—compare current weight with the patient's usual weight (Table 12.2).
- Drug therapy—many drugs can induce gastrointestinal symptoms.
- Dental health—poor dentition, denture suitability, mouth ulceration, or gum disease.
- Mobility and activity level—compare energy expenditure with energy intake.
- Physical appearance—emaciation, cachexia (physical wasting with loss of weight and muscle wastage), obesity, or loose clothing.
- Blood biochemistry—plasma proteins, haemoglobin, serum vitamin and mineral levels, and immunological competence.

A physical assessment of nutritional status should include the patient's height and weight 📖 on p. 70.

- Compare the patient's current weight with their previous weight and, if applicable, calculate the percentage weight loss or gain using the formula in Table 12.2.
- Once the weight and height measurements have been taken, calculate the patient's body mass index using the formula detailed in Table 12.3.

Table 12.2 Percentage weight loss formula

$$\% \text{ weight loss} = \frac{\text{usual weight} - \text{actual weight}}{\text{usual weight}} \times 100$$

Unintentional weight loss of 10% over a period of 6 months represents malnutrition.

Unintentional weight loss of 20% over a period of 6 months represents severe malnutrition.

Table 12.3 Body-mass index (BMI) formula

Indicator of nutritional state in patients >18 years.

$$BMI = \frac{weight\ (kg)}{(height\ [m])^2}$$

BMI <20	Underweight
BMI 20–24.9	Desirable range
BMI 25–29.9	Grade I obesity (overweight)
BMI >30	Grade II obesity (obese)
BMI >40	Grade III obesity (morbidly obese)

Feeding patients

Background

Factors affecting feeding a patient include social, psychological, physical and environmental factors:

Social factors
- Religion.
- Cultural issues.
- Special diets.
- Social activity.
- Eating times.
- Family traditions or habits.
- Likes and dislikes.

Psychological factors
- Emotional well-being.
- Anxiety.
- Confusion or dementia.
- Personal beliefs.
- Embarrassment.
- Choice.

Physical factors
- Mobility and dexterity.
- Disability.
- Pain.
- Nausea and vomiting.
- Appetite.
- Bowel habits.
- Dentition.
- Availability of food.

Environmental factors
- Comfort.
- Situation.
- Nurse and patient proximity.
- Nurses' workload.
- Food presentation.
- Organization.
- Smell.
- Noise.

Feeding

Nurses now have a minor role in the preparation and serving of food to patients: in most clinical areas there is a necessary delegation of feeding to students, qualified health care assistants, or unqualified staff. However, it is the nurse who is responsible for ensuring appropriate food is provided.

Equipment
- Eating utensils.
- Plate or bowl of food to be served.

- Condiments
- Serviette.

Procedure

- Explain the procedure and gain consent.
- Decontaminate your hands.
- Help the patient into an upright sitting position.
- Sit down adjacent to the patient, in a position that enables feeding.
- Place small quantities of food onto the eating utensil (fork or spoon).
- If appropriate, encourage the patient to feed themselves.
- Ask the patient to open their mouth and gently place food into their mouth.
- Wait enough time for the patient to chew and swallow the food and repeat until the meal is complete or the patient states that they have eaten enough.
- Discard the waste.
- Decontaminate your hands.
- Document the episode of care.

Practice tips

- Time should be spent with the patient choosing from the menu.
- Hand-cleaning facilities should be offered to the patient before and after the meal.
- The patient should be consulted about the size of mouthfuls, if feeding is too slow or quick, and the temperature of the food throughout the procedure.
- Offer the patient a drink throughout feeding.
- Mouth care should be offered to the patient.
- Administration of prescribed anti-emetics before feeding might be helpful for patients with nausea.
- Feeding patients offers the registered health care worker (HCW) an opportunity to carry out a full patient assessment. If this task is allocated to a HCW, it is essential that they are adequately trained in the appropriate assessment skills so that they can report back to registered HCWs.

Mouth care

Background

The aim of mouth care is to keep the oral mucosa and lips clean and moist, prevent infection, remove food debris, and ensure the patient's mouth feels fresh and clean. A number of factors can affect the need for mouth care (Table 12.4).

Equipment

- Disposable cardboard receiver.
- Disposable tongue depressor.
- Small-headed soft toothbrush.
- Non-sterile gloves.
- Disposable apron.
- Mouth foam sticks.
- Denture pot.
- Plastic cup.
- Tissues.
- Toothpaste.
- Small torch.
- Drinking water.

Procedure

- Explain the procedure and gain consent.
- Decontaminate your hands.
- Put on a pair of gloves and an apron.
- Inspect the patient's mouth using a disposable tongue depressor and small torch.
- If the patient wears dentures, ask them to remove the dentures or remove them using paper tissues or gauze swabs and place them in a denture pot. Clean all surfaces of the removed dentures using a toothbrush or denture brush and toothpaste. Rinse thoroughly and return them to the patient.
- Brush the patient's natural teeth, gums, and tongue using a small-headed soft toothbrush and toothpaste.
- Hold the toothbrush bristles at a 45° angle to the teeth. Move the toothbrush back and forth firmly using a vibrating motion from the sulcus to the crowns of the teeth until all tooth surfaces have been cleaned.
- Bring a plastic cup filled with drinking water to the patient and ask them to rinse their mouth out, voiding the contents into a disposable cardboard receiver.
- Apply lubricant to the patient's lips, if appropriate.
- Clean and dry the toothbrush.
- Discard the equipment using clinical waste disposal.
- Remove the gloves and apron.
- Decontaminate your hands.

Practice tips
- If gums and oral mucosa are ulcerated or damaged, clean teeth, gums, and tongue using wet mouth foam sticks in a rotating motion.
- If patient cannot rinse and void, use a wet toothbrush to rinse teeth and moistened foam sticks to rinse gums, tongue, and oral mucosa.

Table 12.4 Factors influencing oral hygiene

Mouth care is an important consideration if any of the following factors are present:
Nausea and vomiting
Oxygen therapy
Nil by mouth
Dehydration
Physical disability
Antibiotics or steroids
Endotracheal intubation
Immunosupression

Enteral feeding

Background

Patients who cannot meet their nutritional requirements orally need nutritional support. If the patient has a functioning gastrointestinal tract, enteral feeding is the preferred choice of nutritional support owing to its safety of administration, ↓ cost, enhanced nutritional use, and maintenance of gut integrity. Selection of an access route for enteral nutrition depends primarily on the anticipated duration of enteral feeding:

- Short-term enteral feeding can be administered through a fine-bore nasogastric tube.
- Long-term enteral feeding is more appropriately delivered through a percutaneous endoscopic gastrostomy (PEG 📖 page 426).

Enteral feeds can be administered as a continuous infusion, an intermittent infusion, or bolus.

General observations should include:

- Temperature, pulse, respiration, and blood pressure.
- Body weight.
- Blood glucose.
- Urea and electrolytes, and full blood count.
- Fluid balance.
- Tolerance to feed.
- Bowel function.
- Enteral tube position.
- Stoma insertion site.

Complications do arise (Table 12.5).

Equipment

- Commercially prepared feed (in a pack or reservoir bottle) and enteral feeding solution.
- Giving set.
- Drip stand.
- Feed pump.
- Enteral feeding regimen.
- Fluid-balance chart.
- Additive labels.
- Label for the giving set.

Procedure

- Explain the procedure and gain consent.
- Decontaminate your hands.
- Collect equipment.
- Decontaminate the drip stand.
- Wash and dry your hands.
- Check the prescription regimen.
- Check the packaging and expiry date of the feed.
- Check the patient's details.
- If using a commercially prepared pack of feed:
  - Shake the pack.
  - Hang the pack on the drip stand.

- Close the roller clamp of the giving set.
- Unscrew and remove the protective cap on the pack of feed.
- Connect the giving set to the pack of feed.
- If using reservoir feed:
  - Shake the enteral feeding solution.
  - Fill the reservoir (empty bottle) with the desired amount of feed and replace the lid.
  - Fix the additive label to the reservoir.
  - Open the cap on the reservoir.
  - Close the roller clamp on the giving set.
  - Screw the giving set onto the reservoir.
  - Hang the reservoir on the drip stand.
- Place the drip chamber of the giving set into the pump.
- Loosen the end cap of the giving set.
- Open the roller clamp and prime the line, ensuring all of the air is expelled.
- Close the clamp and tighten the end cap.
- Stretch the silicone section of the giving set around the motor.
- Connect the end of the giving set to the feeding tube.
- Label the giving set with the date and time.
- Open the clamp and turn on the pump at the required rate to commence the feed.
- Ensure the patient is comfortable.
- Discard the equipment using clinical waste disposal.
- Decontaminate your hands.
- Document the episode of care.

Practice tip

- Monitoring enteral feeding is essential for recognizing and avoiding complications and ensuring optimal nutritional support.

Table 12.5 Complications of enteral feeding

Complication	Potential cause	Action
Dumping syndrome	Occurs if hyperosmolar solution enters the small intestine too quickly, causing a fluid shift. Can result in ↓circulating fluid volume. Signs and symptoms include tachycardia, hypotension, dizziness, abdominal pain, and diarrhoea	Stop feed immediately Treat hypotension Report to medical colleagues
Aspiration Regurgitation	Incorrect tube position	Check tube placement
		Ensure the patient is positioned at a 45° angle
		Consider a prokinetic agent
Constipation	Dehydration	Review fluid balance
	Drug side-effects	Administer laxatives
	Bowel obstruction	Discontinue feed
Diarrhoea	Drug side-effect	Consider anti-diarrhoeal agent
	Infection	Collect stool sample for microbiology, culture, and sensitivity
Nausea and vomiting	Poor gastric emptying Malabsorbtion	Consider an anti-emetic
	Rapid administration of feed	↓ rate
Blocked tube	Inadequate flushing	Flush regularly
	Administration of medicine	Use the correct preparation, e.g. liquids and suspensions

Care of percutaneous endoscopic gastrostomy tubes

Background

A percutaneous endoscopic gastrostomy (PEG) is a medical device that is placed endoscopically and delivers nutrients directly to the stomach through a tube passing through the abdominal wall (Fig. 12.3). A PEG is used for both short-term and long-term feeding. The administration of enteral feed through a PEG tube can be as a bolus or an intermittent or continuous infusion using a feeding pump.

Equipment

- Sterile dressing pack.
- Sterile 0.9% saline solution.
- Dressing trolley.
- Sterile gloves.
- Alcohol hand rub.
- 2% chlorhexidine gluconate in 70% isopropyl alcohol application.
- Disposable apron.

Procedure

- Explain the procedure and gain consent.
- Wash and dry your hands.
- Ensure the dressing trolley is clean. If visibly dirty, clean it using detergent and water.
- Assemble the equipment and put it on the bottom shelf of the trolley.
- Put on an apron.
- Decontaminate your hands.
- Commence aseptic non-touch technique 📖 on p. 80.
- Observe the peristoma site for signs of infection, inflammation, irritation, or tenderness.
- Note the length of tubing protruding from the patient's skin.
- Using one piece of moistened gauze per wipe, clean the peristoma (using a circular motion), PEG fixator, and tube.
- Dry the area using dry, sterile gauze swabs.
- Discard the equipment using clinical waste disposal.
- Decontaminate your hands.
- Document the episode of care.

Practice tips

- Do not cover stoma site with a dressing unless there is leaking or exudates.
- Rotate the PEG tube through 360° every 24 hours, to prevent epithelization on the PEG tube.

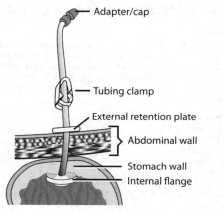

Fig. 12.3 Percutaneous endoscopic gastrostomy. © Burdett Institute, 2008.

Care of jejunostomy feeding tubes

Background

Jejunostomy feeding tubes are used when a patient has undergone upper gastrointestinal surgery and has delayed gastric emptying or pyloric obstruction. Enteral feeds through a jejunostomy tube are administered by continuous or intermittent infusion. Jejunostomy feeding tubes should be cleaned daily to maintain skin integrity and enable the early detection of problems.

Equipment

- Sterile dressing pack.
- Sterile 0.9% saline solution.
- Dressing trolley.
- Sterile gloves.
- Alcohol hand rub.
- 2% chlorhexidine gluconate in 70% isopropyl alcohol application.
- Disposable apron.
- 20mL syringe.

Procedure

- Explain the procedure and gain consent.
- Wash and dry your hands.
- Ensure the dressing trolley is clean. If visibly dirty, clean it using detergent and water.
- Place the equipment on the bottom shelf of the trolley.
- Put on a clean disposable apron.
- Decontaminate your hands.
- Commence aseptic non-touch technique 🕮 on p. 80.
- Observe the peristoma site for signs of infection, inflammation, irritation, or tenderness.
- Note the length of tubing protruding from the skin.
- Using one piece of moistened gauze per wipe, clean the peristoma (using a circular motion), stoma site, fixator device, and tube.
- Dry the area using dry, sterile gauze swabs.
- Ensure sutures are intact on the fixator device.
- Loop a large, single coil of jejunostomy tube once around the insertion site.
- Cover the coil and insertion site with a transparent, hypoallergenic, waterproof, and breathable dressing.
- Discard the equipment using clinical waste disposal.
- Decontaminate your hands.
- Document the episode of care.

Practice tips

- Administration of enteral feed, flushing, drug administration, and care of the tube should occur under aseptic conditions.
- Only use sterile water to flush a jejunostomy tube.

Fine-bore nasogastric feeding tubes

Background

Nasogastric feeding is usually the first route to be considered if the gastrointestinal tract is functioning but the oral route is contraindicated or oral intake is inadequate. Use of a fine-bore nasogastric tube is the most common route and is suitable for feeding for 4–6 weeks.

Equipment

- Fine-bore nasogastric tube (6–8Fr).
- 50mL syringe.
- Receptacle.
- Lubricating jelly.
- Glass of water.
- Clean spigot.
- Dressing trolley.
- Tissues.
- Hypoallergenic tape.
- Scissors.
- Water for flushing.
- Non-sterile gloves.
- Disposable apron.

Procedure

- Explain the procedure and gain consent.
- Agree a signal by which the patient can communicate if they want the procedure to stop.
- Stop the procedure immediately if the patient shows signs of distress, respiratory difficulties, coughing, or pain.
- Decontaminate your hands.
- Put on a pair of gloves and an apron.
- Assist the patient to sit in an upright position, with their head supported in the neutral position.
- Assess the patency of each of the patient's nostrils in turn by asking them to sniff with the other nostril closed. Choose the nostril that sounds the clearest.
- Measure the distance on the tube from the patient's earlobe to the bridge of the nose and add this to the distance from the bridge of the nose to the base of the xiphisternum. Make a note of the total distance.
- Put on a pair of gloves and an apron.
- Lubricate the proximal end of the fine-bore nasogastric tube.
- Insert the rounded end of the tube into the chosen nostril and slide it along floor of the nose into the nasopharynx.
- Once in the nasopharynx, ask the patient to swallow. Unless contra-indicated, the patient may take a small sip of water.
- While the patient swallows, advance the tube through the pharynx.
- Continue advancing the tube until the noted distance has been inserted.
- Remove the guide wire by gentle traction.
- Occlude the end of the nasogastric tube with a clean spigot.
- Secure the tube using hypoallergenic tape.

- Mark the tube at the exit point, from the nostrils check the tube position using the National Patient Safety Agency (NPSA) approved techniques p. 422-6, and measure the distance of the protruding tube.
- Discard the equipment using clinical waste disposal.
- Decontaminate your hands.
- Document the episode of care.

Practice tips

- Ask the patient to take sips of water once the tube is in the pharynx. This can facilitate passage of the tube.

Pitfall

- Administering feeds or drugs through a nasogastric tube before checking the tube position (📖 on p. 440).

Checking the fine-bore nasogastric tube position by X-ray

Background

Confirmation that the tip of a nasogastric tube is situated in the stomach is essential before initiating a feed or administering medication. Incorrect positioning in the bronchial tract could have fatal consequences. The National Patient Safety Agency has produced guidelines indicating the safest methods for checking correct positioning of nasogastric tubes.[1]

X-ray

An X-ray is the most accurate method of confirming the position of a nasogastric tube. However, radiological confirmation of nasogastric position is not routine and its need should be assessed by the health care professional team.

Common pitfalls

The following limitations of X-ray confirmation must be considered:
- X-rays can be misinterpreted.
- X-rays only confirm the position of the nasogastric tube at the time of X-ray.
- Cost of X-rays.
- Loss of feeding time.
- Patient exposure to X-rays.
- Difficulty with community patients accessing radiology services.

1. National Patient Safety Agency (2005). *Advice to the NHS on reducing harm caused by the mis-placement of nasogastric feeding tubes.* NPSA: London. http://www.mpsa.nhs.uk/health.alerts

Checking nasogastric tube position via gastric aspirate

Background
Testing the pH of gastric aspirate can be used as a method of checking the position of nasogastric tubes. The position should always be checked prior to administration of any feed or medication; after initial insertion; during episodes of vomiting, retching or coughing; following evidence of misplacement, and at least once daily during continuous feeds.

Equipment
- Non-sterile gloves.
- Disposable apron.
- Disposable receiver.
- pH indicator paper.
- 50mL syringe.
- Clean spigot.

Procedure
- Explain the procedure and gain consent.
- Decontaminate your hands.
- Put on a pair of gloves and an apron.
- Place a pH indicator strip into a clean disposable receiver.
- Attach a 50mL syringe to the end of the nasogastric tube.
- Gently withdraw the syringe plunger, aspirating 0.5–1mL of gastric aspirate.
- Occlude the end of the nasogastric tube with a clean spigot.
- Visually inspect the aspirate, noting its colour and consistency.
- Place a small quantity of aspirate onto the pH indicator strip, according to the manufacturer's guidelines.
- Wait the amount of time specified by the pH indicator strip manufacturer.
- Compare the colour of the indicator strip to the manufacturer's specified colour code.
- Read the pH measurement.
- The pH of the aspirate should be <4.0 to confirm gastric placement. A pH of >5.5 might indicate bronchial or intestinal placement.
- If bronchial placement is suspected, immediately remove the nasogastric tube.
- Discard the equipment using clinical waste disposal.
- Decontaminate your hands.
- Document the episode of care.

Practice tips
- Syringes of >30mL only should be used because the smaller syringes might generate excessive pressure on the nasogastric tube, increasing the risk of fractures occurring in the tube.
- If there is any query about position and/or the clarity of the colour change on the pH strip, particularly between ranges 5 and 6, do not commence feeding.

- Use pH indicator paper/strips with wide ranges of gradients, so the resulting colour change is easily distinguishable.
- If you have difficulty aspirating, then turn the patient on their side.
- Advance the tube 10–20cm for the adult patient if difficulty in obtaining aspirate persists.

Pitfalls

- Proton-pump inhibitors might ↑ the pH of the gastric aspirate.
- A stomach full of food might alter the pH of the gastric aspirate. Aspirate might be difficult to obtain owing to the positioning of the tip of the tube against the gastric mucosa.
- Using blue litmus paper to test the aspirate. This contravenes the National Patient Safety Agency recommendations[1].
- Using a small syringe to aspirate. Syringes of > 30mL only should be used because smaller syringes might generate excessive pressure on the nasogastric tube, increasing the risk of fractures occuring in the tube.

1. National Patient Safety Agency (2005). *Advice to the NHS on reducing harm caused by the misplacement of nasogastric feeding tubes.* NPSA: London. http://www.mpsa.nhs.uk/health.alerts

Checking nasogastric tube position by visually recognizable gastric contents

Background

This method may only be used in patients who have a sufficient swallow and can take oral fluids.

Equipment

- Non-sterile gloves.
- Disposable apron.
- Two 50mL syringes.
- Glass of easily identifiable liquid, e.g. blackcurrant cordial.
- Disposable receiver.

Procedure

- Explain the procedure and gain consent.
- Decontaminate your hands.
- Put on a pair of gloves and an apron.
- Position the patient in a semi-recumbent position.
- Ask the patient to swallow a small sip of the easily identifiable liquid, e.g. blackcurrant cordial.
- Attach a 50mL syringe to the end of the nasogastric tube.
- Gently withdraw the plunger of the syringe, aspirating a small amount of the gastric contents.
- Place the gastric aspirate into the disposable receiver.
- Compare the aspirate with the swallowed liquid; if similar, this might indicate that the nasogastric tube is situated in the stomach.
- Ensure the patient is comfortable.
- Discard the equipment using clinical waste disposal.
- Decontaminate your hands.
- Document the episode of care.

Practice tips

- No method of checking the nasogastric tube position is fail-safe; if there is any doubt about the correct positioning, expert help and advice should be sought.

Pitfall

- Using small syringes to aspirate. This might generate excessive pressure on the nasogastric tube, ↑ the risk of fractures occurring in the tube. Syringe of >30mL only should be used.

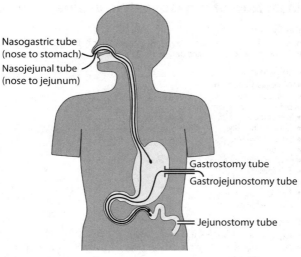

Nasogastric tube
(nose to stomach)
Nasojejunal tube
(nose to jejunum)

Gastrostomy tube
Gastrojejunostomy tube

Jejunostomy tube

Fig. 12.4   Nasogastric tube position. © Burdeff Institute, 2008.

Insertion of a nasogastric drainage tube

Background

Nasogastric drainage tubes can be inserted to empty the gastric contents. Indications for insertion are detailed in Table 12.6.

Equipment

- Nasogastric tube (Ryles).
- 50mL syringe.
- pH indicator paper.
- Receptacle.
- Lubricating jelly.
- Glass of water.
- Tissues.
- Hypoallergenic tape.
- Scissors.
- Water for flushing.
- Non-sterile gloves.
- Disposable apron.

Procedure

- Explain the procedure and gain consent.
- Agree a signal by which the patient can communicate if they want the procedure to stop.
- Stop the procedure immediately if the patient shows signs of distress, respiratory difficulties, coughing, or pain.
- Decontaminate your hands.
- Put on a pair of gloves and an apron.
- Assist the patient to sit in an upright position, with their head supported in the neutral position.
- Assess the patency of each of the patient's nostrils in turn by asking them to sniff with the other nostril closed. Choose the nostril that sounds the clearest.
- Measure the distance on the tube from the patient's earlobe to the bridge of the nose and add this to the distance from the bridge of the nose to the base of the xiphisternum. Make a note of the total distance.
- Lubricate the proximal end of the fine-bore nasogastric tube.
- Insert the rounded end of the tube into the chosen nostril and slide it along floor of the nose into the nasopharynx.
- Once in the nasopharynx, ask the patient to swallow. Unless contra-indicated, the patient may then take a small sip of water.
- While the patient swallows, advance the tube through the pharynx.
- Continue advancing the tube until the noted distance has been inserted.
- Secure the tube using hypoallergenic tape.
- Mark the tube at the exit point from the nostrils and measure the distance of the protruding tube.
- Check the tube position using the National Patient Safety Agency (NPSA)-approved techniques 📖 p. 432–436.[1]
- Attach a drainage bag.
- Ensure the patient is comfortable.

- Discard the equipment using clinical waste disposal.
- Decontaminate your hands.
- Document the episode of care.

Table 12.6 Indications for inserting a nasogastric tubes

Bowel obstruction
Gastrointestinal surgery
Excessive vomiting
Gastric dilatation
Pancreatitis
Endotracheal intubation
Positive pressure ventilation

Pitfall

- Inserting the nasogastric tube into bronchus, withdraw the tube immediately if the patient starts to cough or show signs of respiratory distress.

1. National Patient Safety Agency (2005). *Advice to the NHS on reducing harm caused by the misplacement of nasogastric feeding tubes.* NPSA: London. http://www.mpsa.nhs.uk/health.alerts

Parenteral feeding

Background

Parenteral nutrition (PN) is the aseptic delivery of nutritional substrates directly into the circulatory system. It should be used to prevent or treat malnutrition only in the event of the gastrointestinal tract being unusable or its function inadequate. Indications for PN are detailed in Table 12.7. Parenteral feeds are administered most commonly through central venous access, because they enable solutions of high osmolality and nutritional density to be infused. Occasionally, PN might be delivered through a peripheral venous line for short-term (<14 days) delivery only. PN must always be delivered through a volumetric infusion pump. The bag must be compounded under sterile conditions. Correct storage of PN bags is essential; bags of PN must be refrigerated before use. Patients receiving PN need careful monitoring to recognize and treat complications (Table 12.8).

Procedure: underlying principles

- Line insertion and any subsequent intervention should be carried out under strict aseptic conditions.
- PN bags and administration sets must be changed every 24 hours under strict aseptic conditions.
- There should be a designated lumen used solely for PN administration—PN should never mix with other drugs or infusions.
- A sterile transparent dressing should cover the central venous catheter insertion site.

Monitoring

- Monitor the patient's temperature, pulse, respiration, and blood pressure every 4–6 hours.
- Monitor the patient's body weight daily.
- Take accurate and comprehensive fluid balance measurements for the duration of PN administration.
- Urea and electrolytes, and full blood count—initially and then on alternate days.
- Blood glucose: every 4 hours initially; if stable, a minimum of twice daily.
- Serum phosphate: 48 hours after initiation of PN; twice a week thereafter.
- Serum magnesium: twice a week.
- Trace elements—monthly.
- Liver function tests—initially and then twice a week.
- Examine the venous catheter insertion site daily for signs of infection.

Table 12.7 Indications for PN

Following major intestinal surgery
Severe pancreatitis
Prolonged ileus
Severe mucositis
High-output intestinal fistulae
High-output stomas
Severe inflammatory bowel disorders
Severe intestinal insufficiency

Table 12.8 Complications of PN

Fluid overload
Dehydration
Hyperglycaemia
Hypoglycaemia
Azotaemia
Hypophosphataemia
Infection or catheter-related sepsis
Venous catheter leakage, cracking, or fracture
Venous catheter blockage
Phlebitis

Insertion of subcutaneous cannula

Background

Subcutaneous fluid administration (hypodermoclysis) is a valuable means of replacing fluids and maintaining hydration. It is a safe, minimally invasive method of delivering fluids. It should not be used for emergency fluid administration or to correct severe dehydration. A potential complication of hypodermoclysis is local oedema at the infusion site.

Equipment

- Subcutaneous cannula (butterfly).
- Sterile, transparent, occlusive dressing.
- Sterile gauze.
- 2% chlorhexidine gluconate in 70% isopropyl alcohol application.
- Sterile gloves.
- Disposable apron.

Procedure

- Explain the procedure and gain consent.
- Wash and dry hands.
- Check the expiry date and that packaging is intact on sterile equipment.
- Put on a pair of sterile gloves, ensuring they are put on by only touching the wrist end.
- Cleanse the chosen infusion site (Table 12.9) using 2% chlorhexidine gluconate in 70% isopropyl alcohol application.
- Allow to dry passively for 30 seconds.
- Gently secure the subcutaneous tissue between two gloved fingers.
- Insert the subcutaneous cannula into the subcutaneous tissue at a 30° angle.
- Secure the cannula in place using the sterile, transparent, occlusive dressing.
- Ensure the patient is comfortable.
- Discard the equipment using clinical waste disposal.
- Decontaminate your hands.
- Document the episode of care.

Practice tips

- The cannula should be changed every 48 hours.
- The type of infusion fluid depends on the patient's individual requirements. Electrolyte solutions (e.g. physiological saline and dextrose saline) are commonly used owing to their ability to correct intracellular deficits.
- The infusion site should be monitored for evidence of infection, inflammation, and oedema.

Table 12.9 Subcutaneous infusion sites

Inner thigh
Chest wall
Infrascapular (below the shoulder bone)
Infraclavicular (below the collar bone)
Lateral aspect of the upper arm
Abdomen

Stoma care

Background

A stoma is an artificial, surgical opening of the bowel or urinary system onto the abdomen. Types of stoma, their indications, and their outputs are detailed in Table 12.10.

The purpose of stoma care is to collect urine or faeces within a stoma appliance and ensure good skin and stoma hygiene. The choice of appliance depends on the type of stoma, effluent, siting of the stoma, condition of the peristomal skin, and individual patient considerations, e.g. preference, lifestyle, mental capacity, and disability.

Equipment

- Disposable kidney bowl.
- Tissues.
- Clean stoma appliance.
- Clinical waste bag.
- Tap water.
- Disposable wipes.
- Disposable measuring jug.
- Non-sterile gloves.
- Disposable aprons.
- Disposable protective pad.

Procedure

- Explain the procedure and gain consent.
- Decontaminate your hands.
- Assist the patient to sit in a comfortable position.
- Put on an apron and a pair of gloves.
- Place a clean protective pad underneath the stoma site.
- Drain the contents of the stoma bag into the measuring jug.
- Remove the existing stoma appliance and discard into the clinical waste bag.
- Remove effluent from the stoma and peristomal area using a damp disposable wipe.
- Examine the peristomal skin for:
  • Redness
  • Soreness
  • Inflammation
  • Infection
  • Excoriation
  • Herniation
  • Mucocutaneous separation
  • Ischaemia
  • Bleeding
  • Oedema.
- Examine the stoma for:
  • Inflammation
  • Infection
  • Oedema
  • Ischaemia

- Retraction
- Bleeding.
- Observe the colour, size, and extent of the protrusion.
- Wash and dry the stoma and peristomal site thoroughly using disposable wipes.
- Apply a clean stoma appliance.
- Ensure the patient is comfortable.
- Discard the equipment using clinical waste disposal.
- Decontaminate your hands.
- Document the episode of care.

Table 12.10 Types of stoma

Stoma	Indications	Output
Ascending/transverse colostomy Formed from a piece of colon	Trauma or perforation Obstruction Diverticulitis Crohn's disease Ulcerative colitis Fistula	Semi-fluid to mushy Foul odour
Descending/sigmoid colostomy Formed from a piece of colon	Trauma or perforation Obstruction Rectal cancer Diverticulitis Incontinence Fistula	Semi-formed to solid Minimal odour
Ileostomy Formed from a piece of ileum	Crohn's disease Ulcerative colitis Familial adenomatous polyposis Obstruction	Liquid to pasty High volumes Enzymatic and salty
Urostomy/ileo conduit Formed in the urinary tract using a section of ileum	Bladder cancer Bladder trauma Spinal cord injury Congenital anomaly	Liquid urine with mucus shreds

Management of constipation

Background

Constipation is the infrequent passage of stool: less than one bowel motion every 3 days. Effective management of constipation is essential because it can cause abdominal distension, halitosis, loss of appetite, urinary retention or incontinence, agitation and confusion, nausea and vomiting, faecal overflow, and haemorrhoids. If constipation and faecal impaction are left untreated, they may lead to cardiac or respiratory failure in susceptible individuals.

A constipation risk assessment tool (Table 12.11) predicts risk by taking into account the following factors:
- Patient knowledge and attitudes.
- Toileting activities and habits.
- Toilet position.
- Toilet facilities.
- Lifestyle factors.
- Dietary habits.
- Dietary fibre.
- Fluids.
- Exercise and activity.

Non Pharmacological treatment
- Increase daily intake of fibre. High fibre foods include fruit, vegetables, and cereals.
- Add bulking agents, such as wheat bran to the diet.
- Increase fluid intake—at least 1–2 litres of water a day.
- Foods with laxative properties include prunes, dried apricots, avocados, pineapples, and rhubarb.
- Exercise, e.g. a daily walk or run.

Pharmacological treatment

Once constipation has been diagnosed or a patient has been identified as high risk, a laxative agent might be necessary, in addition to dietary alterations to include higher fibre intake.

Laxatives

Bulk-forming laxatives

Bulk-forming laxatives imitate the natural action of fibre by increasing faecal mass, which stimulates peristalsis. An example is ispaghula husk.

Osmotic laxatives

Osmotic laxatives soften and lubricate faeces by retaining fluid in the bowel by osmosis. Examples include lactulose, a phosphate enema, and a micro-enema.

Faecal softener

Faecal softeners directly lubricate and soften the stool to enable ease of passage. An example is arachis oil.

Stimulant laxatives
Stimulant laxatives increase intestinal motility, which both softens the faeces and encourages bowel movements. Examples include bisacodyl, co-danthramer docusate, senna, sodium picosulphate, and glycerin suppositories.

Iso-osmotic laxatives
Iso-osmotic laxatives encourage water retention within the bowel, which in turn softens faeces by the iso-osmotic agent polyethyleneglycol. This type of laxative is mostly used for bowel preparation before investigations or surgical procedures. An example is Movicol®.

The treatment plan should be evaluated and reviewed regularly and additional laxative agents, enemas, and/or suppositories added, as necessary.

Table 12.11 Constipation risk assessment tool

Fluids	Mobility	Diet	Mental state	Predisposition	Score
Drinks 1500–2000mL/day 1	Fully mobile + active 1	Full diet 1	Normal and appropriate 1	Predisposing medication 3 Taking opioids 4	
Drinks <1000mL/day 2	Mobile but sedentary Use of aids 2	Small, unvaried diet 2	Confused, memory impairment 2	History of constipation 3	
Drinks <700mL/day 3	Immobile 4	Poor diet 3	Very confused 3	Predisposing medical condition 3	
Total					
Score of 5 or less	Minimal risk No immediate action required Patient should be encouraged to report any changes in bowel habit				
Score of 5–7	Medium risk Perform bowel assessment Encourage mobility Increase fluid intake, if possible Encourage fibre-rich food				
Score of 8+	High risk Intervention as for medium risk+ Maintain a bowel chart Consider an appropriate laxative Consider rectal and abdominal investigations				

Administration of suppositories

Background

A suppository is a medicated solid substance prepared for insertion into the rectum. Medications given by this route includes analgesics, e.g. paracetamol, non-steroidal anti-inflammatory drugs, e.g. diclofenac and epileptic medication, e.g. lorazepam. Rectal medications avoid liver metabolism and can have a predictable greater and faster effect that oral medications. Administration of a suppository might precipitate a vasovagal attack. If the vagus nerve is stimulated, a ↓ in heart rate and blood pressure, leading to collapse or faint, could ensue. Patients should be observed and monitored for signs of vagal stimulation throughout the procedure.

Equipment

- Prescribed suppository.
- Lubricating gel.
- Non-sterile gloves.
- Disposable apron.
- Tissues.

Procedure

- Check the suppository against the prescription chart.
- Check the expiry date of the suppository.
- Check the patient's case notes for any anal or rectal surgery or abnormalities—if present, seek medical advice before continuing.
- Explain the procedure and gain consent.
- Encourage the patient to urinate before the procedure.
- Decontaminate your hands.
- Put on a pair of gloves and an apron.
- Position the patient on their left side, with knees flexed.
- Place a disposable protective pad underneath the patient's hip and bottom.
- Examine the peri-anal area, noting any abnormalities—if necessary, seek medical advice before continuing.
- Lubricate the suppository with lubricating gel.
- Insert the blunt end foremost into the patient's anal canal.
- Clean the patient's peri-anal area using tissues.
- Ensure the patient is comfortable.
- Discard the equipment using clinical waste disposal.
- Decontaminate your hands.
- Document the episode of care.

Practice tip
- Explain to the patient that they may feel the need to defacate. They should try and avoid this to retain the medication.

Administration of enemas

Background

An enema is the procedure of introducing liquids into the rectum and colon through the anus. Indications and contraindications are listed in Table 12.12.

Administration of an enema might precipitate a vasovagal attack. If the vagus nerve is stimulated, a ↓ in heart rate and blood pressure, leading to collapse or faint, could ensue. Patients should be observed and monitored for signs of vagal stimulation throughout the procedure.

Equipment

- Non-sterile gloves.
- Disposable apron.
- Prescribed enema.
- Tissues.
- Disposable protective pad.

Procedure

- Check the enema against the prescription chart.
- Check the expiry date of the enema.
- Check the patient's case notes for any anal or rectal surgery or abnormalities—if present, seek medical advice before continuing.
- Explain the procedure and gain consent.
- Encourage patient to urinate before the procedure.
- Decontaminate your hands.
- Put on a pair of gloves and an apron.
- Position the patient on their left side, with knees flexed.
- Place a disposable protective pad underneath the patient's hip and bottom.
- Examine the peri-anal area, noting any abnormalities—if necessary, seek medical advice before continuing.
- Lubricate the nozzle of the enema with lubricating gel.
- Insert the entire length of the nozzle into the patient's anal canal.
- Gently squeeze the contents of the enema into the patient's rectum.
- Ask the patient to retain the contents in their rectum for as long as possible.
- Slowly withdraw the nozzle.
- Clean the patient's peri-anal area using tissues.
- Ensure the patient is comfortable.
- Discard the equipment using clinical waste disposal.
- Decontaminate your hands.
- Document the episode of care.

Practice tip
- Ensure a commode is nearby to avoid the embarrassment of the patient calling for help or trying to reach the toilet precipitously.

Table 12.12 Indications and contraindications for enemas

Indications for enemas
To clean the lower bowel before surgery or investigations
To introduce medications
To treat irritated bowel mucosa
To ↓ hyperkalaemia
To relieve constipation

Contraindications for enemas
Low platelet count
Malignancy of the peri-anal region
Recent lower gastrointestinal or gynaecological surgery
Allergies, e.g. latex, phosphate, or peanut oil
Neutropaenia

Manual removal of faeces

Background

The manual removal of faeces is occasionally required to empty the patient's rectum of faeces. It is an invasive procedure and should only be performed as a last resort, when other constipation management treatments have failed. A thorough physical assessment is necessary before the procedure. Manual removal of faeces should only be performed by a health care worker competent to do so, usually an advanced practitioner. Manual evacuation of faeces should be a multidisciplinary team decision, involving both medical and nursing staff.

Equipment

- Prescribed stool softener.
- Disposable bedpan.
- Mild sedative, if prescribed.
- Thermometer.
- Non-sterile gloves.
- Sphygmomanometer.
- Disposable apron.
- Disposable protective pad.
- Lubricating gel.
- Tissues.

Procedure

- Explain the procedure and gain consent.
- Take the patient's temperature, pulse, respiration, and blood pressure—if outside the patient's normal limits, seek medical advice before continuing.
- Check the prescribed sedative and stool softener against the prescription chart.
- Check the expiry dates of the sedative and stool softener.
- Administer the prescribed sedative and stool softener.
- Wait an appropriate amount of time, as guided by the drug manufacturers, until the patient is adequately sedated and the stool has adequately softened.
- Encourage the patient to urinate.
- Decontaminate your hands.
- Put on a pair of gloves and an apron.
- Position the patient in the left lateral position, with knees flexed.
- Place a protective pad underneath the patient.
- Inspect the patient's peri-anal area and observe for the following:
  - Fissures
  - Lesions
  - Scars
  - Inflammation
  - Discharge
  - Prolapse
  - Haemorrhoids
  - Polyps.

- Lubricate your gloved index finger with lubricating gel.
- Slowly insert your gloved finger into the patient's rectum.
- Advise the patient to take slow, deep breaths.
- Remove smaller particles of stool and break larger pieces up by inserting your finger into the stool.
- Collect the stool in the disposable bedpan.
- On completion of stool removal, wash the patient's peri-anal area using a disposable wipe.
- Replace the patient's clothing and ensure the patient is comfortable.
- Discard the equipment using clinical waste disposal.
- Decontaminate your hands.
- Take the patient's temperature, pulse, respiration, and blood pressure—seek medical advice if the measurements are outside the patient's normal limits.
- Decontaminate your hands.
- Document the episode of care.
- Observe the patient for abnormal signs—rectal bleeding, dizziness, chest pains, cramps, or pain.

Practice tips

- Continually inform the patient of your actions and describe to the patient what to expect.
- Where possible, advise the patient to bear down on exhalation.
- If necessary, monitor the patient's temperature, blood pressure, and respiration rate throughout the procedure.
- Two pairs of gloves are sometimes worn.

Genito-urinary system

Louise Stayt
Senior Lecturer in Professional Practice Skills, School of Health
& Social Care, Oxford Brookes University, Oxford, UK

Jacqueline Randle
Associate Professor, Clinical Skills Lead for Masters of Nursing
Science, School of Nursing, Midwifery & Physiotherapy,
University of Nottingham, UK

History-taking

Background

The genito-urinary system comprises the urinary tract and reproductive organs and structures. A full history of genito-urinary symptoms is essential in the assessment process. Some aspects of history-taking differ between ♂ and ♀.

Urinary system

Past medical history

Check for:
- Urinary tract infection.
- Kidney trauma.
- Kidney stones.
- Bladder disease.
- Kidney disease.
- Diabetes.
- Hypertension.
- Cardiovascular disease.

Current health

- Assess general health state.
- Check for allergies.
- Assess for specific symptoms, including details of onset and duration of symptoms:
  - Pain or burning on micturition (dysuria).
  - Altered urine colour.
  - Blood in the urine (haematuria).
  - Incontinence.
  - Frequency of voiding.
  - Retention.

Family health

Check for the following:
- Kidney disease.
- Cardiovascular disease.
- Diabetes.
- Bladder disease.
- Genito-urinary cancers.

Drug history

A full drug history of current and past medications must be obtained because many drugs are nephrotoxic, can alter the colour and appearance of urine, and can alter genito-urinary function, e.g. non-steroidal anti-inflammatory drugs, aminoglycosides, cisplatin, and lithium carbonate.

♀ genital health history

- Assess whether there is any possibility that the patient could be pregnant.
- Gain information about the patient's menstrual cycle, including:
  - Age of onset.
  - Duration of menses.

- Frequency of menses.
- Dysmenorrhoea (painful period/cramps).
- Metrorrhagia (mid-cycle spotting.
- Menorraghia (heavy bleeding).
- Onset of menopause (if appropriate).
- Obtain details of any pregnancies, including:
  - Number of pregnancies.
  - Whether deliveries were vaginal or Caesarian.
  - Any abortions.
  - Any miscarriages.
- Ask about the method of birth control.
- Assess sexual health by asking about:
  - Details of sexual practices.
  - Risk-taking behaviour.
  - Number of sexual partners.
  - Human immunodeficiency virus (HIV) status.
  - History of dyspareunia (pain during intercourse).
  - History of sexually transmitted diseases.
  - History of vaginal discharge.
  - Last cervical smear.
  - Papanicolaou (pap) test results.
  - Concerns or worries.

♂ genital health history

Ask about:
- Whether the patient has been circumcised, and, if so, the reasons for this and date of the procedure.
- Ease of foreskin retraction and replacement.
- Presence of peneal sores, lumps, or ulceration.
- Scrotal swelling.
- Penile discharge or bleeding.
- Trauma to the scrotum or penis.
- Undescended testicles.
- Details of sexual practices and preferences.
- Risk-taking behaviour.
- Number of sexual partners.
- HIV status.
- History of sexually transmitted diseases.
- Contraception.
- Pain on intercourse.
- Concern or worries.

Practice tip

- Sensitivity is required when gaining a patient's history.

Examination of the urinary system

Background

Examination of the ♀ and ♂ urinary systems is similar. Assessment of the patient's urinary system should be preceded by general observation of vital signs, weight, and mental status. Such parameters could provide an indication of renal impairment or failure.

Observe the patient's skin for:
- Pallor—anaemia is common in renal dysfunction.
- Uraemic frost—crystal formation from metabolic waste is common in renal impairment and failure.
- Signs of fluid imbalance—oedema, ascites, and dry mucous membranes.

Percussion of the kidneys

Background

Inflammation of the kidneys leads to costovertebral angle tenderness, which might be detected on percussion of the kidneys.

Procedure

- Explain the procedure and gain consent.
- Decontaminate your hands.
- Assist the patient into an upright sitting position, leaning forwards.
- Warn the patient that you will be hitting them gently and request that they try to relax.
- Using the ulnar aspect of your hand, carefully strike the patient, using small 'karate-chops'. Do this several times from the 10th rib to just below the renal angle in a linear fashion (Fig. 13.1).
- Pain experienced only when striking over the renal angle is indicative of renal tenderness on that side.
- Repeat on the opposite side.
- Ensure the patient is comfortable.
- Decontaminate your hands.
- Document the episode of care.

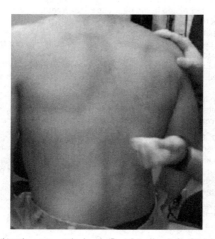

Fig. 13.1 Striking the costavertebral angle. From http://medinfo.ufl.edu/year1/bcs/slides/abdomen/slide29.html. With permission from Richard Rathe, MD, University of Florida.

Palpation of the kidneys

Background
The kidneys are palpated as part of a full abdominal examination. They are not usually palpable unless they are enlarged. You may however be able to palpate them in thinner patients. Both kidneys descend during inspiration. The right kidney is usually easier to palpate than the left because it is positioned lower. Normal kidneys feel smooth and rubbery. Causes of kidney enlargement include tumours, cysts and hydronephrosis. Bilateral enlargement occurs in polycystic disease.

Procedure
- Explain the procedure and gain consent.
- Decontaminate your hands.
- Lie the patient supine on the bed or examination couch.
- Ask the patient to inform you if they experience pain during the examination.

Palpation of the Right Kidney
- Stand on the right-hand side of the patient.
- Place your left hand behind the patient just below and parallel to the 12th rib.
- Lift your left hand up trying to displace the kidney anteriorly.
- Place your right hand in the right upper quadrant lateral and parallel to the rectus muscle (see fig. 13.2a).
- Ask the patient to take a deep breath.
- At the peak of inspiration press your right hand firmly into the right upper quadrant.
- Try to "capture" the kidney between your two hands.
- If palpable, note the size and shape of the kidney and any tenderness elicited.
- Ask the patient to breathe out.
- Slowly release the pressure from your left hand and feel for the kidney's return to its expiratory position.

Palpation of the Left Kidney
- Reach over and place your left hand behind the patient just below and parallel to the left 12th rib.
- Place your right hand in the left upper quadrant lateral and parallel to the rectus muscle (see fig. 13.2b).
- Repeat the procedure as for the right kidney.
- Ensure that the patient is comfortable.
- Decontaminate your hands.
- Document the episode of care.

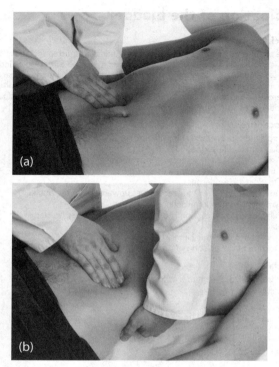

Fig. 13.2 (a) Palpation of the right kidney; (b) palpation of the left kidney. Reproduced with permission from Thomas and Monaghan (2007) *The Oxford handbook of clinical examination and practical skills.* With permission from Oxford University Press and the authors.

Palpation of the bladder

Background

The bladder normally cannot be palpated unless it is distended above the pubic symphysis. Causes of bladder distension include outlet obstruction due to an enlarged prostate or urethral structure, medications (in particular anticholinergics) and neurological disorders such as stroke or multiple sclerosis. A distended bladder is uncomfortable and tender to palpate. Bladder infectious cause more profound suprapubic tenderness.

Procedure

- Explain the procedure and gain consent.
- Decontaminate your hands.
- Assist the patient into the supine position.
- Palpate the lower abdomen using a light, passing motion (📖 on p. 394).
- Observe for tenderness.
- Percuss (📖 on p. 292 for technique) upwards from the public symphysis to check for dullness.
- Palpation and percussion should delineate the upper border of the bladder.
- Decontaminate your hands.
- Document the episode of care.

Pitfall

- Mistaking a pregnant uterus for a bladder. Consider in women of childbearing age.

Examination of the ♀ external genitalia

Background

Assessment of these organs is essential in the detection of reproductive organ disorders because signs and symptoms associated with reproductive disorders might be mild.

Equipment

- Non-sterile gloves.
- Disposable apron.

Procedure

- Explain the procedure and gain consent.
- Ask the patient if they require a chaperone. A chaperone should always be present when doing an intimate examination on the opposite sex.
- Ensure the patient has an empty bladder.
- Decontaminate your hands.
- Put on a pair of non-sterile gloves and an apron.
- Help the patient into the dorsolithotomy position (laid supine or semi-supine, with legs parted).
- Observe the pubic hair for the level of sexual maturity.
- Observe the labia for:
  - Colour
  - Signs of inflammation
  - Infection
  - Discharge (colour and odour)
  - Lesions.
- Observe the urethral meatus for:
  - Colour
  - Discharge
  - Ulceration
  - Infection
  - Inflammation.
- Observe the vestibule for:
  - Inflammation
  - Colour
  - Lesions
  - Discharge
  - Odour.
- Observe the vaginal opening for:
  - Colour
  - Discharge
  - Odour
  - Lesions.
- Ensure the patient is comfortable.
- Discard the equipment using waste disposal.
- Decontaminate your hands.
- Document the episode of care.

Practice tips

- The labia are normally pink in colour; the urethral meatus, vestibule, and vaginal opening are normally pink and moist in appearance.
- It is normal to see some vaginal discharge, which is usually clear and odourless. Abnormal vaginal discharge might be creamy or brown–green in colour and usually has an offensive odour.
- Respect the wishes of the patient at all times during the examination.

Pitfall

- Not having a chaperone present when doing an intimate examination, particularly on the opposite sex.

Examining the vagina and cervix

Background

Examination of the vagina and cervix is a specialist procedure and additional training and assessment are required before performing this skill.

Equipment

- Cuscoe speculum.
- Non-sterile gloves.
- Disposable apron.
- Wipes.

Procedure

- Explain the procedure and gain consent.
- Ask the patient if they require a chaperone. A chapter should always be present when doing an intimate examination on the opposite sex.
- Decontaminate your hands.
- Put on a pair of non-sterile gloves and an apron.
- Position the patient in a semi-recumbent position.
- Reveal the patient's genitalia, ensuring privacy and dignity.
- Warm the speculum by running it under a hot tap.
- Encourage the patient to take deep breaths.
- Insert the speculum obliquely (45° angle) while maintaining a posterior direction toward the rectum.
- Always apply pressure downward during insertion and never upwards.
- Rotate the speculum to a horizontal position and grasp handle with non-dominant hand.
- Continue to insert speculum until flush against the perineum.
- Open and position speculum by depressing the thumb rest slowly approximately 2–3cms or until the cervix is visible between the blades.
- Inspect the vaginal lining, cervix, and cervical os.
- Take swabs for microbiology culture and sensitivity screening, if required prepare beforehand.
- To remove speculum, rotate clockwise, applying posterior pressure on the pelvic floor.
- Remove the blades at an oblique angle and avoid pulling pubic hair or pinching labia.
- Replace the patient's clothing and ensure the patient is comfortable.
- Discard the equipment using clinical waste disposal.
- Decontaminate your hands.
- Document the episode of care.

Practice tips

- Speculums should only be lubricated with water because many commercial lubricants contain a bacteriostatic agent that could affect the microbiology culture results.
- The patient should be encouraged to take deep breaths while the speculum is inserted, to relax the abdominal muscles and ease insertion.
- Respect the wishes of the patient at all times during the examination.

Pitfall

• Not having a chaperone present when doing an intimate examination, particularly on the opposite sex.

Examination of the ♂ external genitalia

Background
Examination of the ♂ external genitalia is essential to detect both urinary and reproductive disorders.

Equipment
- Non-sterile gloves.
- Disposable apron.

Procedure
- Explain the procedure and gain consent.
- Ask the patient if they require a chaperone. A chaperone should always be present when doing an intimate examination on the opposite sex.
- Decontaminate your hands.
- Put on a pair of non-sterile gloves and an apron.
- Position the patient in a comfortable semi-supine position.
- Reveal the patient's genitalia, ensuring privacy and dignity.
- Fully retract the foreskin (if patient has one).
- Observe the penis for:
  - Lesions
  - Inflammation
  - Discharge
- Take swabs for microbiology culture and sensitivity screening, if required.
- Replace the foreskin.
- Observe the scrotum for:
  - Size.
  - Appearance.
  - Inflammation.
  - Redness.
  - Presence of nodules.
  - Ulceration.
  - Lesions.
  - Cysts.
  - Oedema.
  - Parasites.
- Ask the patient to stand and bear down.
- Observe for bulges (hernias) in the inguinal (groin) and femoral (thigh) areas.
- Replace the patient's clothing and ensure the patient is comfortable.
- Discard the equipment using clinical waste disposal.
- Decontaminate your hands.
- Document the episode of care.

Palpation of the testicles

Palpation of the testicles might detect abnormal masses, tenderness, or swelling.

Equipment

- Non-sterile gloves.
- Disposable apron.

Procedure

- Explain the procedure and gain consent.
- Ask patient if they require a chaperone. A chaperone should always be present when doing an intimate examination on the opposite sex.
- Decontaminate your hands.
- Put on a pair of non-sterile gloves and an apron.
- Position the patient in a comfortable semi-supine position.
- Reveal the patient's genitalia, ensuring privacy and dignity.
- Palpate the testicles using your thumb and first two fingers.
- Observe for:
  - Size
  - Shape
  - Tenderness
  - Irregular areas
  - Lumps.
- Replace the patient's clothing and ensure the patient is comfortable.
- Discard the equipment using clinical waste disposal.
- Decontaminate your hands.
- Document the episode of care.

Practice tips

- Transillumination (examination of the testicles) can be performed by holding the head of a torch against the scrotum and helps distinguish a mass from fluid. The testicle, lumps, warts, and blood vessels appear as opaque shapes. Examine both testicles using this method and compare the findings.
- Respect the wishes of the patient at all times during the examination.

Palpation of the prostate gland

Background

Palpation of the prostate is required to detect enlargement. If the prostate gland protrudes into the rectal lumen, it is probably enlarged. Additional training and assessment are required before performing this skill.

Equipment

- Non-sterile gloves.
- Disposable apron.
- Lubricant gel.
- Disposable protective pad.
- Disposable wipes.

Procedure

- Explain the procedure and gain consent.
- Ask the patient if they require a chaperone. A chaperone should always be present when doing an intimate examination on the opposite sex.
- Decontaminate your hands.
- Put on an apron and a pair of gloves.
- Position the patient in the left lateral position, with knees flexed.
- Place a protective pad underneath the patient.
- Lubricate your gloved index finger with lubricating gel.
- Slowly insert your gloved finger into the patient's rectum.
- Palpate the prostate gland through the anterior rectal wall.
- Sweep your gloved finger from side to side across the posterior surface of the gland.
  - The prostate should feel smooth and be the size of a walnut.
  - Its consistency is rubbery, firm but not hard.
  - It is moderately mobile.
- Determine shape and size, consistency, surface texture, presence of nodules or tenderness and mobility.
- Wipe the patient's peri-anal area.
- Discard the equipment using clinical waste disposal.
- Ensure the patient is comfortable.
- Decontaminate your hands.
- Document the episode of care.

Practice tips

- Palpation of the gland may cause discomfort but should not cause pain.
- Keep fingernails short.
- Check your gloved finger for stool, mucus, malaena, pus or pale stool.

♀ urethral catheterization

Background

Urethral catheterization is commonly carried out to relieve anatomical obstruction of the urinary tract, postoperatively, and to measure and monitor urine output. Urethral catheterization can be used to manage urinary incontinence, but only if all other management techniques have been explored. There is no legal position on ♂ professionals catheterizing ♀ patients or vice versa; however, the patient's wishes should be respected at all times.

Equipment

- Procedure pack.
- Sterile gauze swabs.
- Two pairs of sterile gloves.
- Disposable protective pad.
- Sterile syringe (check catheter manufacturer's guidelines for size—usually 10mL).
- Sterile urinary drainage bag.
- Alcohol hand rub.
- 6mL local anaesthetic gel.
- Two ♀-length catheters of appropriate size and material (see below).
- Disposable apron.
- 0.9% saline solution for irrigation.
- Sterile water for injection.
- Catheter fixator.
- 50mL bladder syringe.
- 2% chlorhexidine gluconate in 70% isopropyl alcohol application.

Procedure

- Explain the procedure and gain consent.
- Ask the patient if they require a chaperone. A chaperone should always be present when doing an intimate procedure on the opposite sex.
- Decontaminate your hands.
- Ensure the dressing trolley is clean. If visibly dirty, clean it using detergent and water.
- Assemble the equipment and put it on the bottom shelf of the trolley.
- Put on a clean disposable apron.
- Decontaminate your hands.
- Position the patient in either the supine position, with knees bent and hips flexed, or the lateral fetal position, with knees slightly parted by a pillow.
- Place the disposable protective pad underneath the patient's hips and bottom.
- Wash and dry your hands.
- Commence aseptic non-touch technique ⊞ on p. 80.
- Draw up the required amount of water to inflate the balloon in accordance with manufacturer's guidelines.
- Position the sterile dressing towel over the disposable pad.
- Cleanse the vulval area from the pubic bone towards the perineum using gauze soaked in 0.9% saline solution.

- Use a new piece of gauze for each cleansing action.
- Remove the sterile gloves and wash and dry your hands or use an alcohol hand rub.
- Apply a new pair of sterile gloves.
- Insert local anaesthetic gel into the urethra and wait for 2min.
- Place the catheter in the sterile receiver and position it on the sterile dressing towel.
- Separate the labia using one hand and identify the urethral orifice.
- Insert the catheter until urine drains.
- Insert the catheter a further 5cm.
- If no urine drains, the catheter might have been inserted in the vagina; leave the catheter in and attempt insertion up the urethra using a clean catheter.
- Once the catheter is in position, inflate the catheter balloon using the required amount of sterile water for injection.
- Gently withdraw the catheter until resistance is felt.
- Attach the catheter to the drainage bag.
- Anchor the catheter to the thigh using a catheter-fixator device.
- Measure and record the amount of residual urine drained.
- Discard the equipment using clinical waste disposal.
- Ensure the patient is comfortable.
- Decontaminate your hands.
- Document the episode of care and size of catheter used.

Practice tips

- Choose the smallest urinary catheter size possible. Larger urethral catheters might lead to bladder irritation, pain, spasms, and leakage. Usually ♀ will require a 10–12-ch urethral catheter.
- While cleansing the vulval area, ensure you cleanse the labia majora, labia minor and urethral meatus. Areas should be cleaned from the clitoral area towards the peri-anal region using a new swab for each cleansing action.
- If resistance is felt or the patient complains of pain or discomfort during insertion of the catheter, stop the procedure immediately and report to the appropriate medical staff.
- Always support the weight of the catheter bag; catheter tubing must be secured using a catheter fixator. The weight of the catheter bag and continual drag of the tubing might result in pressure necrosis.
- Some dressing packs include foam swabs.

♂ urethral catheterization

Background

Urethral catheterization is commonly carried out to relieve anatomical obstruction of the urinary tract, postoperatively, and to measure and monitor urine output. Urethral catheterization can be used to manage urinary incontinence, but only if all other management techniques have been explored. Owing to the potential complications and difficulties associated with ♂ urethral catheterization (e.g. urethral strictures, stenosis, and prostate enlargement), additional training and assessment is required. There is no legal position on ♀ health care workers (HCWS) catheterizing ♂ patients or vice versa; however, the patient's wishes should be respected at all times.

Equipment

- Sterile procedure pack.
- Sterile gauze swabs.
- Two pairs of sterile gloves.
- Apron.
- Disposable protective pad.
- 0.9% saline solution for irrigation.
- Sterile syringe (check catheter manufacturer's guidelines for size— usually 10mL).
- Sterile water for injection.
- Sterile drainage bag.
- Catheter fixator.
- Alcohol hand rub.
- 50mL bladder syringe.
- 11mL local anaesthetic gel.
- Two ♂-length catheters of appropriate size and material.
- 2% chlorhexidine gluconate in 70% isopropyl alcohol application.

Procedure

- Explain the procedure and gain consent.
- Ask the patient if they require a chaperone. A chaperone should always be present when doing an intimate examination on the opposite sex.
- Decontaminate your hands.
- Ensure the dressing trolley is clean. If visibly dirty, clean it using detergent and water.
- Assemble the equipment and put it on the bottom shelf of the trolley.
- Put on a clean disposable apron.
- Decontaminate your hands.
- Position the patient in the supine position, with legs extended.
- Place the disposable protective pad underneath the patient's hips and bottom.
- Wash and dry your hands.
- Commence aseptic non-touch technique 🕮 on p. 80.
- Draw up the required amount of water to inflate the balloon, as per the manufacturer's guidelines.
- Position the sterile dressing towel across the patient's thighs and suprapubic area.

- Cleanse the glans penis and underneath the prepuce (foreskin) if present.
- Use a new piece of gauze for each cleansing action.
- Remove the sterile gloves and wash your hands or use alcohol hand rub.
- Apply a new pair of sterile gloves.
- Holding the penis upright, retract foreskin if necessary and insert local anaesthetic gel into the urethra and wait for 5min.
- Place the catheter in the sterile receiver and position it on the sterile dressing towel.
- Hold the shaft of the penis firmly at an angle of 60–90° to the body.
- Gently insert the catheter into the urethra until urine drains and then advance the catheter to the bifurcation of the catheter tube.
- Once the catheter is in position, inflate the catheter balloon using the required amount of sterile water for injection.
- Ask the patient to tell you of any discomfort and observe them for manifestations of discomfort or pain.
- Gently withdraw the catheter until resistance is felt.
- Attach the catheter to the drainage bag.
- Return the prepuce over the glans penis.
- Anchor the catheter to the thigh using a catheter-fixator device.
- Measure and record the amount of residual urine drained.
- Discard the equipment using clinical waste disposal.
- Ensure the patient is comfortable.
- Decontaminate your hands.
- Document the episode of care and size of catheter.

Practice tips

- If continued resistance is felt or the patient complains of pain or discomfort while the catheter is inserted, stop the procedure immediately and report to the appropriate medical staff.
- Choose the smallest urinary catheter size possible; larger urethral catheter sizes might lead to bladder irritation, pain, spasms, and leakage. Usually ♂ require a 12–14-ch urethral catheter.
- Always support the weight of the catheter bag; catheter tubing must be secured using a catheter fixator. The weight of the catheter bag and the continual drag of the tubing might result in pressure necrosis.

Pitfall

- Failing to return the foreskin to its correct position after the procedure.

Urethral catheter care

Background
Owing to the potential risk of infection, it is essential that urethral catheters are cleansed daily. The cleansing procedure can be carried out by the health care worker (HCW) or patient, if able.

Equipment
- Non-sterile gloves.
- Disposable apron.
- Soap.
- Warm water.
- Disposable wipes.

Procedure
- Explain the procedure and gain consent.
- Position the patient so they are in a comfortable position, with the catheter exposed.
- Decontaminate your hands.
- Put on a pair of gloves and an apron.
- Clean the protruding length of catheter tubing using disposable wipes, soap, and warm water. Wipe the catheter tubing in the direction away from the patient.
- For ♀ patients, gently cleanse the meatus and surrounding area using wipes, soap, and water. For ♂ patients, gently retract the prepuce (foreskin) and cleanse the glans penis using wipes, soap, and water. Return the prepuce once finished.
- Observe the area for inflammation, infection, discharge, or bleeding.
- Dry the area thoroughly.
- Discard the equipment using clinical waste disposal.
- Ensure the patient is comfortable.
- Decontaminate your hands.
- Document the episode of care.

Practice tips
- Ordinary soap is adequate for daily cleansing. The use of antiseptic preparations does not help prevent infection and might interfere with the body's natural flora; ∴ it is not recommended for use in daily catheter cleansing.
- Encourage the patient to carry out their daily catheter cleansing themselves.
- Ensure the catheter is placed below the level of the bladder to ensure good drainage and prevent backflow of urine.
- Avoid breaking the sealed system between the catheter tube and the drainage bag.
- Do not allow bags to touch floor as this a point of entry for infection.

Emptying a catheter drainage bag

Background
Catheters should only be emptied when they are three-quarters full. Minimal disturbance to the closed catheter circuit helps prevent the entrance of infection.

Equipment
- Clean disposable measuring jug.
- Non-sterile gloves.
- Disposable apron.
- 2% chlorhexidine gluconate in 70% isopropyl alcohol application.
- Disposable protective pad.

Procedure
- Explain the procedure and gain consent.
- Decontaminate your hands.
- Put on a pair of gloves and an apron.
- Place a disposable protective pad on the floor beneath the drainage bag.
- Place a disposable measuring jug underneath the drainage bag tap.
- Open the tap and drain the urine into the jug.
- Close the tap.
- Wipe the tap and rim using a clean tissue.
- Clean the tap and rim using 2% chlorhexidine gluconate in 70% isopropyl alcohol application and allow to dry.
- Measure the amount of urine collected in the jug.
- Discard the equipment using clinical waste disposal.
- Ensure the patient is comfortable.
- Decontaminate your hands.
- Document the episode of care and record the urine output.

Practice tips
- Gloves are single-use only and a new pair should be worn for the emptying of each catheter.
- The patient should be informed of the signs of urinary tract infection.

Removal of a urethral catheter

Background
A urethral catheter might need to be removed if no longer needed, occluded, or expired and needs changing.

Equipment
- Non-sterile gloves.
- Disposable apron.
- Sterile syringe (check catheter manufacturer's guidelines for size—usually 10mL).
- Clean receiver.
- 2mL of sterile water.

Procedure
- Explain the procedure and gain consent.
- Refer to the catheter manufacturer's guidelines or patient's case notes to ascertain how much water was used to inflate the catheter balloon.
- Decontaminate your hands.
- Put on an apron and a pair of gloves.
- Attach the syringe to the valve and allow the pressure of the water to push the plunger back to the appropriate level (usually 10mL).
- If the water does not drain, insert 2mL of sterile water for injection and withdraw back immediately.
- If the water still does not drain and the balloon remains inflated, seek appropriate medical advice.
- Otherwise, withdraw the catheter slowly until fully removed.
- Place the catheter in the receiver.
- Ensure the removed catheter is intact.
- Ensure the patient is comfortable.
- Discard the equipment using clinical waste disposal.
- Decontaminate your hands.
- Document the episode of care.

Practice tip
- Try to remove the urethral catheter in the evening or at bedtime. The bladder might then fill while the patient is relaxed and their natural diuresis pattern will promote urination in the morning.

Pitfall
- Not checking the amount of sterile water used to inflate the baloon and attempting removal when it is still partially inflated.

Intermittent self-catheterization: patient education

Background

Clean intermittent self-catheterization (ISC) is an accepted form of treatment for neuropathic bladder dysfunction and other causes of incomplete bladder emptying. It can ↓ the incidence of urinary tract infection and renal disease and lead to fewer complications than other management options, e.g. indwelling suprapubic or urethral catheters.

Procedure: underlying principles

Patients might be taught ISC in the hospital, clinic, or home setting. Success depends on:

- Motivation—the indications for ISC should be fully explained to the patient and potential benefits highlighted. However, other management options should also be discussed. Patients should then be allowed to choose their preferred option.
- Facilities and resources—the teaching location and resources might greatly affect the speed at which the patient learns the technique. The patient's usual routine and home facilities must be considered.
- Preparation—patients must be advised to observe good hand hygiene and use alcohol hand wipes or wet wipes if hand-washing facilities are unavailable. It is suggested that the genital area is cleaned once daily using mild soap and water.
- Position—patients might be taught to perform ISC in several different positions, e.g. lying in bed, sitting on a toilet, or standing over a toilet. Patient preference, mobility, home facilities, and disabilities must be considered when choosing an appropriate position for ISC.
- Technique—there are two techniques used to perform ISC. The first technique involves directing the catheter into the urethra using a mirror for visualization (see p. 486). The second technique involves directing the catheter into the urethra by touch. The choice of technique depends on the patient's eyesight, finger sensation, dexterity, and disabilities.
- Constipation—constipation can effect catheter placement and subsequent drainage. Therefore patients need advice regarding the management of their bowels, including dietary advice.
- Catheter choice—there are a wide range of products available (e.g. uncoated or coated PVC nelaton and rigid or flexible), which come in a variety of sizes. The choice of catheter depends on the patient's preference, comfort, lubrication, and frequency.
- Frequency—the frequency with which a patient is required to perform ISC depends on the underlying aetiology. Catheterization must be frequent enough to prevent bladder distention and also keep the patient dry. Some patients, who cannot empty their bladder at all, might have to perform ISC four to six times daily. Patients who can pass some urine only need to perform ISC once daily to once weekly, just to prevent the build up of urine.

- Ongoing support—a good support network is necessary for ISC to succeed. Support from health care professionals is required to monitor progress and troubleshoot problems and complications. Patient organizations (e.g. Incontact) and local self-help groups might also be of assistance. Good communication between the different support services is paramount for ongoing patient care.

Intermittent self-catheterization

Background

Intermitted self catheterisation can be taught to patients so that they can perform it independently. The principles underpinning patient education for this procedure are outlined on page 484.

Equipment

- Urinary catheters.
- Tissues.
- Clean jug or bowl.
- Mirror.
- Protective pad.
- Lubricant gel.

Procedure

- Explain the procedure and gain consent.
- Arrange the equipment on a clean surface.
- Ask the patient to remove any inhibiting clothing.
- Ensure the patient thoroughly washes and dries their hands.
- Decontaminate your hands.
- Help the patient to position themselves in a comfortable position, either lying on a bed on a protective pad or sitting on or standing over a toilet.
- Teach the patient to identify the urethra using a mirror.
- Ask the patient to open the chosen catheter packet. If it is an unlubricated variety, ensure the patient lubricates the tube with water or lubricant gel.
- Ensure the funnel end of the catheter tube is in a receiver or clean jug or bowl if the procedure is undertaken in bed or over the toilet bowl, respectively.
- Encourage the patient to insert the catheter tip into the urethral opening and continue until urine drains.
- Tell the patient to insert the catheter a further 4–6cm to ↓ the risk of contamination.
- Once the urine flow has stopped and bladder is empty, ask the patient to gently remove the catheter from the urethra using a rotating action.
- Ask the patient to rinse the used catheter using warm water and dry it using a clean tissue.
- Discard the equipment using clinical waste disposal.
- Encourage the patient to wash and dry their hands thoroughly.
- Decontaminate your hands.
- Answer any concerns or worries.
- Document the episode of care.

Bladder washout

Background

A bladder washout is the lavage of the bladder using sterile fluid. A bladder washout can be carried out under the following circumstances:

- To clear an obstructed catheter.
- To remove blood clots.
- To remove sediment.

Equipment

- Sterile dressing pack.
- 60mL bladder syringe.
- Alcohol hand rub.
- Disposable protective pad.
- Sterile jug.
- Sterile 0.9% saline solution for irrigation.
- Sterile receiver.
- Sterile gloves.
- Disposable apron.
- Clamp.
- Clean dressing trolley.
- Sterile catheter drainage bag.
- Sterile gauze.
- 2% chlorhexidine gluconate in 70% isopropyl alcohol application.

Procedure

- Explain the procedure and gain consent.
- Decontaminate your hands.
- Ensure the dressing trolley is clean. If visibly dirty, clean it using detergent and water.
- Assemble the equipment and put it on the bottom shelf of the trolley.
- Put on a clean disposable apron.
- Decontaminate hands.
- Place the disposable protective pad underneath the catheter join.
- Clamp the catheter tubing.
- Wash and dry your hands.
- Commence aseptic non-touch technique 📖 on p. 80.
- Draw up 0.9% saline solution for irrigation into the 60mL bladder syringe.
- Place a sterile towel underneath the catheter join, on top of the disposable protective pad.
- Disconnect the catheter tube from the catheter drainage bag and place the end on the sterile towel.
- Apply alcohol hand rub.
- Clean the end of the catheter tubing using sterile gauze and 2% chlorhexidine gluconate in 70% isopropyl alcohol application.
- Insert the filled 60mL bladder syringe into the end of the catheter tubing, release the clamp, and gently inject the fluid into the bladder.
- Remove the syringe and allow the bladder contents to drain into the sterile receiver, noting how much fluid is injected and how much is returned.

- Continue to inject and drain fluid until the contents run clear.
- If the fluid does not drain, gently aspirate using the 60mL bladder syringe.
- Once washout is complete, clean the end of the catheter tubing using gauze and 2% chlorhexidine gluconate in 70% isopropyl alcohol application.
- Attach a new sterile catheter drainage bag to the catheter tubing.
- Ensure the patient is comfortable.
- Discard the equipment using clinical waste disposal.
- Decontaminate your hands.
- Document the episode of care.

Practice tips

- Use isotonic solutions because they are less likely to alter the patient's fluid and electrolyte balance.
- Never use sterile water because it is readily absorbed by the bladder and could ∴ alter the patient's fluid and electrolyte balance.
- Solutions, such as 0.02% chlorhexidine and 1% mandelic acid, can be prescribed to prevent or ↓ bacterial growth.
- Citric acid preparations can be prescribed to prevent and dissolve crystallization in the catheter and bladder.

Continuous bladder irrigation

Background

Continuous bladder irrigation is the continuous washout of the bladder using sterile fluid. Bladder irrigation might be indicated to prevent the formation of blood clots following prostatic surgery or during severe bladder infection. Patients requiring continuous bladder irrigation will need a three-way urinary catheter. Usually a large gauge catheter is selected to facilitate the removal of blood clots and debris.

Equipment

- Sterile dressing pack.
- Alcohol hand rub.
- 2% chlorhexidine gluconate in 70% isopropyl alcohol application.
- Clamp.
- Prescribed sterile irrigation fluid (usually saline).
- Irrigation giving set.
- Drip stand.
- Sterile jug.
- Disposable protective pad.
- Sterile gloves.
- Disposable apron.
- Dressing trolley.

Procedure

- Explain the procedure and gain consent.
- Wash and dry your hands.
- Ensure the dressing trolley is clean. If visibly dirty, clean it using detergent and water.
- Assemble the equipment and put it on the bottom shelf of the trolley.
- Put on a clean disposable apron.
- Decontaminate your hands.
- Place the disposable protective pad underneath the catheter join.
- Clamp the catheter tubing.
- Decontaminate your hands.
- Commence ANTT 📖 on p. 80.
- Place a sterile towel under the catheter join on top of the disposable protective pad.
- Remove the spigot from the irrigation arm of the three-way catheter.
- Discard the spigot and gloves and put on a new pair of sterile gloves.
- Clean the irrigation arm using gauze and 2% chlorhexidine gluconate in 70% isopropyl alcohol application.
- Attach the irrigation giving set to the irrigation arm of the catheter.
- Release the clamp on the catheter and empty the urine from the drainage bag.
- Discard the equipment using clinical waste disposal.
- Decontaminate your hands.
- Set the irrigation fluid at the required rate by adjusting the roller clamp on the giving set.
- Ensure the fluid is draining into the catheter bag.
- Ensure the patient is comfortable.

- Decontaminate your hands.
- Document the episode of care.
- Maintain an accurate fluid-balance chart.

Practice tips

- Accurate fluid-balance monitoring has to be maintained during continuous bladder irrigation to monitor urine output and ensure the early detection of complications, e.g. renal dysfunction, or a blocked catheter. ▶ Document how much irrigation is going in and the total amount of fluid draining out of the catheter. The difference between these two values is the patient's urine output:
  - Input: irrigation fluid infused (IFI).
  - Output: total drainage from catheter (TD).
  - Urine output $\approx$ TD – IF.
- Monitor the colour of the drainage from the catheter and alter the irrigation infusion rate accordingly. If the drainage in the catheter is dark red and blood-stained, the irrigation fluid infusion rate must be increased. If the drainage in the catheter is pale and clear, the irrigation infusion rate can be slowed down slightly. The ideal colour of the drainage is pale rose.

Urinanalysis

Background

Urinanalysis tests the characteristics and composition of freshly voided urine. Reagent strips typically test for the presence of glucose, blood, white blood cells, proteins, ketones, nitrites, urobilinogen, bilirubin, and pH of the urine. Urinanalysis might be performed on admission, daily, or in response to the presence of any urinary symptoms.

Equipment

- Reagent sticks.
- Disposable bedpan.
- Non-sterile gloves.
- Disposable apron.
- Tissues.

Procedure

- Explain the procedure and gain consent.
- Decontaminate your hands.
- Put on a pair of gloves and an apron.
- Ask the patient to urinate in the disposable bedpan, ensuring a clean and fresh specimen.
- Dip the reagent strip fully, but briefly, into the urine sample.
- Tap excess urine back into the disposable bedpan.
- Wait the required time interval, according to reagent stick manufacturer's guidelines.
- Compare the reading on the reagent stick with the manufacturer's colour charts.
- Ensure the patient is comfortable.
- Discard the equipment using clinical waste disposal.
- Decontaminate your hands.
- Document the episode of care.

Musculoskeletal system

Alison Whitfield
Emergency Nurse Practitioner, Clinical Educator in Emergency
Medicine, Trauma and Orthapaedics Emergency Department,
Nottingham University Hospitals NHS Trust, UK

Musculoskeletal history taking: non-trauma

Background

The musculoskeletal system provides form, stability, protection and movement to the body. It is made up of bones, muscles, tendons, ligaments, joints, cartilage and other connective tissue. Patients may present with an injury or non-traumatic symptoms relating to one or more joints or body regions. The depth and focus of the history will depend on the circumstances and the training and experience of the health care worker (HCW). It will also be influenced by whether the presentation is traumatic (📖 on p. 498) or non-traumatic and whether it is acute or chronic. Musculoskeletal problems may be part of multisystem disorders, such as systemic lupus erythematosus or inflammatory bowel disease, and can be associated with blood dyscrasias. Musculoskeletal diseases can also affect other systems, e.g. lung involvement in rheumatoid arthritis.

Presenting complaint (PC)

- Non-traumatic conditions present with some or all of the following: *pain, swelling, stiffness, redness, weakness* and *limitation of movement or activity*.
- The problem may be located to one area or joint or more than one area or joint. Involvement of one joint is termed monoarticular and more than one polyarticular.

History of the PC

Ask the following questions about the PC:
- Location of the affected joint or area.
- Time of onset of symptoms.
- Mode of onset—sudden or gradual?
- Duration of symptoms. Acute onset of knee swelling suggests monoarthritis, whereas bony knee swelling due to osteoarthritis may have been present for years.
- Progression of symptoms: whether persistent or waxing or waning.
- Aggravating and relieving factors, such as rest or medications. Ankylosing spondylitis for example often improves after exercise.
- Whether symptoms are worse in the morning or evening—does the pain waken the patient at night?
- Pattern of involvement and whether in polyarthropathy, the symptoms are symmetrical or asymmetrical—are they migratory (moving from joint to joint)? Different diseases have characteristic distribution of joint involvement, e.g. rheumatoid arthritis tends to be symmetrical with early involvement of the small joints of the hands and feet (usually sparing the distal interphalangeal joints of the hand, which are affected in osteoarthritis).
- Ask about pain in the usual manner (📖 on p. 105). The main questions to ask about pain in addition to the above relate to *radiation* (e.g. hip pain can radiate to the knee and vice versa) and *severity* which can be rated on a scale of 0–10.

- Ask about loss of function and effect on activities of daily living (ADL)—e.g. eating, dressing, and hygiene.
- Enquire about associated symptoms:
  - general malaise, fever, chills, sweating, nausea, vomiting, anorexia, weight loss, backache, eye symptoms, rashes, inflammatory bowel symptoms of diarrhoea, bleeding per rectum (PR), mucus PR and genito-urinary symptoms (e.g. urethral or vaginal discharge, particularly in young, sexually active patients).
- Ask whether the patient has had previous similar episodes.

Past history

Enquire about:
- Similar problems in the past or any history of musculoskeletal disease.
- Previous injury or operations to the affected part.
- Recent illness or infection.
- Chronic medical conditions—musculoskeletal pain might be associated with a wide range of diseases. A patient with psoriasis might have developed a spondyloarthopathy. Other conditions might impact on management or on the choice or medication. An intensive physiotherapy regime may not be appropriate for a patient with severe ischaemic heart disease. Patients with peptic ulcer disease should not be prescribed non-steroidal anti-inflammatory drugs (NSAIDs).
- Significant conditions in the past, e.g. a history of breast cancer would raise the possibility of metastases in a patient with back pain.
- A history of tuberculosis or exposure to it. Tuberculosis arthritis (particularly of the spine) is on the increase.

Medications/allergies

- Ascertain what medications and doses the patient is on.
- The patient might already be taking analgesics or other medications that will impact on further prescribing decisions e.g. NSAIDS should not be prescribed to patients on warfarin.
- A large number of medications can cause joint or muscle pain as a side-effect—e.g. omeprazole, phenytoin, salmeterol, atorvastatin, and montelukast.
- Corticosteroids cause thinning of bones (osteoporosis), making the patient more susceptible to fractures as well as the rarer avascular necrosis.
- Diuretics cause a rise in serum uric acid predisposing to gout.
- Enquire about over-the-counter, herbal or alternative therapies. Patients often forget these or discount them as medications. Some herbs (e.g. garlic or ginkgo biloba) may make bleeding worse.
- Enquire about allergies to drugs and materials.

Habits

- Enquire about smoking and alcohol. Smoking is a risk factor for osteoporosis and for cancers that may present with bony secondaries.
- Alcohol is a risk factor for gout and its abuse contributes to musculoskeletal injuries.

Sexual history

- Gonococcal arthritis is the commonest cause of septic arthritis in young adults. Enquire about sexual activity, safe sex precautions and genito-urinary symptoms such as penile or vaginal discharge.

Family history

- Enquire about musculoskeletal disease in the family. Some musculoskeletal conditions are hereditary or have a familial link— e.g. ankylosing spondylitis and systemic lupus erythematosus.
- It is important to bear in mind that patients who develop musculoskeletal symptoms and have close relatives with severe joint disease are likely to be particularly concerned.

Social history

- The impact of musculoskeletal disease on a patient's lifestyle and psychological welfare can range from mild to very severe. Detailed enquiry should be made about their work, living conditions, the effect of their symptoms on their ADL, and hobbies, in addition to the social support mechanisms available to them.

Systems review

- A thorough review of systems is important in a patient presenting with joint or muscle pain or weakness. It might provide clues to aid diagnosis of systemic diseases with musculoskeletal manifestations and can highlight the effects of musculoskeletal diseases on other systems.

Practice tips

- See p. 26–41 for general tips relating to history-taking.
- Pain disturbing sleep is a priority for treatment.
- Active involvement of only one joint suggests trauma, septic arthritis, or gout/pseudogout.
- Redness over a joint almost always indicates infection, trauma, or gout/pseudogout.
- Consider gonorrhoea infection in sexually active patients who have joint pain.

Pitfalls

- Missing vital diagnostic clues in the history or failing to ask about appropriate systemic symptoms.
- Failing to ask about previous injuries or operations and disability or deformity resulting from them—the patient does not always volunteer this information.

Musculoskeletal history taking: trauma

Background

In a mechanical injury caused by a known insult, the history will focus on the details of the injury and the components of the history relevant to management and treatment. The family history and systems review are not as important as they are in non-traumatic presentations. Multiply injured patients need assessment by a team of highly experienced and skilled health care workers (HCWs). Management of the airway, breathing and circulation is the priority in these patients (□ on p. 500).

Presenting complaint (PC)

- Traumatic conditions usually present with *pain, swelling, limitation of movement* or *symptoms of instability*.

History of the PC

Enquire about:

- Time, place, and mechanism of injury.
- Magnitude, direction, and duration of force.
- First aid measures.
- Whether played on after the injury—if it occurred in sport.
- Symptoms and progression of symptoms, e.g. very rapid swelling in a joint following injury indicates a haemarthrosis (blood in the joint) whereas swelling taking 12–24 hours to develop is more likely to be due to a reactive effusion of synovial fluid.
- Special points relating to the anatomical region—e.g. 'locking' of the knee which may point to a meniscal injury or 'giving way' which may result from instability due to ligamentous disruption.
- Enquire about 'pins and needles' and numbness which may give clues to neurovascular damage.
- Tetanus status—if there is a wound.

Past history

Enquire about:

- Previous injury or operations to the affected part and prior disability.
- Previous or current medical problems, in particular conditions that are likely to make the patient more susceptible to fractures, e.g. osteoporosis, increase bleeding, e.g. blood dyscrasias or impact on soft-tissue healing, e.g. diabetes mellitus.
- Peptic ulcer disease, renal failure, asthma if planning to prescribe or recommend NSAIDS as they are either contraindicated or to be used with caution in these conditions.

Medications/allergies

- Ascertain what medications and doses the patient is on
- Corticosteroids cause thinning of bones (osteoporosis), making the patient more susceptible to fractures
- ► Know whether a patient who has sustained trauma is on anticoagulant therapy. This will make them more susceptible to external and internal bleeding. Also patients on warfarin should not be

prescribed NSAIDS as they can cause a potentially fatal increase in the INR (International Normalised Ratio).
- Enquire about over-the-counter remedies, herbal or alternative therapies. Patients often forget these or don't view them as medications. Some (e.g. garlic, ginkgo biloba) may make bleeding worse.
- Enquire about allergies to drugs and materials such as latex or elastoplast.

Social history
- The impact of an injury on a patient's lifestyle and psychological welfare can range from mild to very severe. Elderly patients can be severely debilitated by apparently minor injuries. A relatively trivial finger injury could threaten the livelihood of a professional violinist. If appropriate, detailed enquiry should be made about the patient's work, living conditions, the effect of their symptoms on their ADL (Activites of Daily Living) and hobbies, in addition to the social support mechanisms available to them.

Practice tips
- Take a detailed history of the mechanism of injury in trauma.
- Patients often complain of an injured limb feeling cold. This is usually due to it not being used. Vascular damage however should always be considered and ruled out.
- 'Pins and needles' or numbness can have a variety of causes in trauma. It is important to rule out serious neurological or vascular causes. These symptoms may also result from swelling, mild neuropraxia (nerve bruising) or due to lack of use of a painful limb.

Pitfalls
- Attributing non-traumatic pain to coincidental trauma (often minor)— ensure the symptoms are consistent with the trauma sustained and temporally linked as expected.
- Failing to take an accurate history.
- Failing to ask about previous injuries or operations and disability or deformity resulting from them—the patient does not always volunteer this information.
- Not seeking expert haematological advice in patients with blood dyscrasias, e.g. haemophilia presenting with injury.

Physical assessment: musculoskeletal system

Background

Examination of the musculoskeletal system should be systematic and thorough. Use the 'look–feel–move' system of examination, which involves inspection, palpation of bony landmarks, joints, and soft tissue structures, assessment of range of movement, and special manoeuvres to test specific functions. The examination might be localized to one body part (e.g. in minor trauma) or be more comprehensive.

Procedure

- Explain the procedure and gain consent.
- Assess the patient's general appearance, body proportions, and ease of movement.
- Obtain vital signs if appropriate, e.g. patient unwell or presenting with hot swollen joint.
- Expose the area involved adequately—compare with the opposite limb.
- 'Look' for bruising, swelling, deformity, erythema, muscle wasting, scars and obvious foreign bodies.
- 'Feel' for tenderness, swelling, warmth and crepitus.
- 'Move'—active joint movement, passive joint movement and resisted movements checking muscles and tendons.
- 'Stress test' ligaments—test the stability of the joint in all directions.
- 'Special' tests relevant to the area being examined, e.g. the Thomas test for fixed flexion of the hip or the impingement test for the shoulder.
- Test function, e.g. ability to button clothes in hand arthritis.
- Check distal neurovascular function—power, sensation, skin colour changes, skin temperature, pulses and capillary refill beyond the affected area.
- Complete the assessment by examining the joints above and below.

Practice tips

- Know your anatomy and keep a mental picture of the structures under your fingertips.
- Many patients will be anxious and difficult to examine—distract the patient while you are palpating. Watch for facial expressions of pain rather than continually asking 'does it hurt?'
- Offer analgesia if the patient is in pain. This will not mask any injury and will make examination easier to perform.
- Observe the patient's gait and mobility unobtrusively as they enter the examination room and sit on the chair or couch. This will often provide more accurate information than formal observation.
- Sensation may be a more reliable indicator of nerve injury, particularly if there is a fracture where power may be limited by pain and mechanical dysfunction.

Pitfalls

- Not measuring the temperature in patients with non-traumatic musculoskeletal pain.
- Not exposing the affected part adequately and comparing with the contralateral side.
- Not exerting firm enough pressure to elicit tenderness.
- Putting pressure on two points simultaneously when examining for tenderness, e.g. pressing on a tender distal ulna when examining for anatomical snuff box (ASB) tenderness and assuming the reaction to pain is owing to ASB tenderness.
- Failing to test tendons against resistance. This may result in partial tears or tendon inflammation (tendonitis) being missed.
- Failing to examine the joint above and below.
- Failing to examine for neurovascular deficit distal to the injury.
- Missing a more serious injury in a patient presenting with a 'minor injury', e.g. a splenic rupture in a patient presenting with wrist pain following a pedal cycle collision. Always perform vital signs and examine the head, chest, and abdomen if the patient looks or feels unwell, e.g. complaining of dizziness or looking pale. Seek senior help early.

Initial assessment of a multiply injured patient

Background

Multiply injured patients should be assessed by a multidisciplinary team of highly experienced and skilled health care workers (HCWs). Management follows ATLS (acute trauma life support) principles. An initial 'primary survey' to detect and treat life-threatening injuries is followed by a 'secondary (head to toe) survey' when the patient has been stabilized. If the patient deteriorates at any stage they must be reassessed beginning again with the airway.

Procedure

Before the patient's arrival
- The leader of the resuscitation should be identified and team roles defined.
- The bay should be prepared and equipment set out and checked.
- The team should put on protective clothing.
- Relevant specialties and departments, e.g. CT, blood bank, and theatre, should be alerted. On arrival in hospital, the priority is to detect and treat life-threatening problems beginning with the airway.
- Essential pre-hospital information to be sought is outlined in Box 14.1.

History

- Critical questions to ask in the history are illustrated in Box 14.2 using the mnemonic AMPLE.
- The history is taken from the patient if they are conscious, pre-hospital personnel, witnesses, relatives or friends.
- A detailed history of the mechanism of injury is vital, e.g. the distance in falls from a height, the type of weapon in penetrating trauma etc.
- In a road traffic collision (RTC) enquire about the speed of impact, intrusion into the vehicle, wearing of seat belt, airbag deployment, position of patient in car, ejection from the vehicle and fatalities in the accident.

Examination

Primary survey
- **A – Airway with cervical spine control.** Assess and secure the airway as outlined 📖 p. 202–208. Endotracheal intubation (📖 on p. 220) will be necessary in unconscious patients. Rarely cricothyroidotomy will be indicated if the airway cannot be secured by any other methods (e.g. in severe facial trauma). The cervical spine should be immobilized 📖 on p. 528 and maintained in a neutral position with manual immobilization when establishing an airway. When the airway has been secured the patient should receive 100% oxygen at 15 L/minute.
- **B – Breathing control.** Assess breathing as outlined on p. 210. Do a thorough examination of the neck and chest looking for signs of trauma. Life-threatening chest injuries, amenable to immediate treatment, include tension and open pneumothoraces.
- **C – Circulatory and haemorrhage control.** Control any major external haemorrhage by direct pressure. Assess the circulation as

outlined on ☐ p. 239. If the patient has signs of hypovolaemic shock, insert 2 wide-bore peripheral cannulae. Take blood for haematological and biochemical analyses and group and cross match. Commence fluid resuscitation. Ascertain in which of the 5 likely locations blood loss is occurring – i.e. into the chest, abdomen or pelvis, from multiple long bone fractures or 'onto the floor' from external bleeding. This is done during the primary survey by means of physical examination, X-rays of the chest and pelvis or ultrasound or CT. Unstable patients not responding to fluid resuscitation usually need an immediate operation and should not be sent to CT.

- **D – Disability.** Assess the level of consciousness (GCS Score) ☐ on p. 582. Look at the size, equality and reaction of the pupils. Assess limb power and symmetry of limb movements.
- **E – Exposure.** Completely undress the patient, covering them with a warm blanket as soon as they have been examined to avoid hypothermia. Log roll the patient and perform a rectal examination if indicated.
- **'Adjuncts' to the primary survey** include urinary and gastric catheters and ECG recording.

Pitfalls

- Being distracted by the most obvious or gruesome injury, e.g. a badly crushed limb, and attending to that before assessing ABC.
- Not having an identified team leader and a clear allocation of roles amongst HCWs managing the trauma.
- Not involving senior personnel early.
- Not being systematic and thorough in the examination, e.g. not palpating or auscultating the axillae and missing decreased breath sounds, wounds, rib fractures or subcutaneous emphysema.
- Not examining the front and back of the body and missing injuries.
- Failing to identify early signs of hypovolaemic shock (e.g. tachycardia) and not realizing that hypotension is a late sign.
- Delaying transfer of the patient to theatre when urgent surgery is required.

Box 14.1 Essential pre-hospital information

- Location time and nature of the incident
- Number, age and sex of the casualties
- The patient's injuries
- Airway, breathing and circulatory status
- GCS
- Any treatment to date and its effect
- Estimated time of arrival

Box 14.2 AMPLE – critical questions in the history

A – Allergies
M – Medications
P – Past medical history
L – Last meal
E – Events/environment related to the injury

Applying a broad arm sling

Background
A broad arm sling is used for limb injuries that require support rather than elevation, e.g. a fractured clavicle.

Equipment
- Sling.
- Safety pin or elastic adhesive tape.

Procedure
- Explain the procedure and gain consent.
- Remove all jewellery from the patient's neck and injured arm.
- Flex the elbow of the injured arm to ~100° with the forearm across chest. Ask the patient to use their opposite hand to support the arm at the wrist.
- Slide the sling between the patient's chest and forearm, with the point behind the elbow of the injured limb and the long straight side parallel to the sternum (Fig. 14.1a).
- Lay a corner of the sling across the opposite shoulder and then around the back of the neck.
- Bring the lower end of the sling upwards and over the shoulder of the injured arm, enfolding the forearm (Fig. 14.1b).
- Tie the ends over the hollow of the clavicle on the injured side using a reef knot (i.e. take the ends right over left and then back again, left over right) (Fig. 14.1c).
- Fold the remaining corner neatly around the elbow and secure it with a safety pin or elastic adhesive tape.
- Ensure the fingertips are visible to check circulation.
- Check distal neurovascular status after application of the sling.
- Give the patient advice about removing the sling at regular intervals and performing exercises on the uninjured joints of the affected limb to avoid stiffness.
- Document the episode of care.

Practice tip
- For added comfort and to relieve pressure on the patient's neck, insert a piece of sponge, measuring ~8 × 2cm—make two holes at intervals of one-third of the length of the sponge and insert the ends of the sling through it before tying them around the patient's neck.

Pitfalls
- Tying the sling incorrectly either at the back of the patient's neck or on the uninjured side, causing discomfort or injury.
- Failing to remove jewellery around the patient's neck or rings on the injured limb.

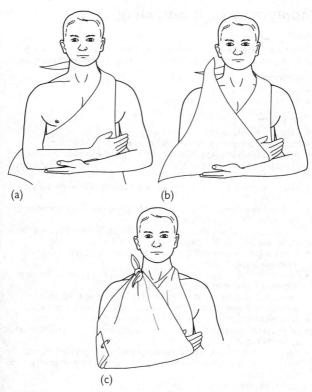

Fig. 14.1 (a) Slide the sling between the arm and chest. (b) Enfold the forearm. (c) Tie on the injured side.

Applying a high arm sling

Background

A high arm sling is used if swelling of the hand, wrist, or forearm is probable (e.g. a fractured wrist). It provides elevation in addition to support.

Equipment

- Sling.
- Safety pin or elastic adhesive tape.

Procedure

- Explain the procedure and gain consent.
- Remove all jewellery from the patient's neck and injured arm.
- Ask the patient to place the hand of the injured arm onto the shoulder of the uninjured side, bringing their elbow to the midpoint of the ribs on the affected side (Fig. 14.2a).
- The patient might support the injured arm on the elbow with their other hand.
- Hold the two corners of the short edge of the sling, with the point to the elbow of the injured side (Fig. 14.2b).
- Lay the sling over the arm, with a short overlap at the elbow, and the other end over the shoulder, dangling down the patient's back.
- Tuck the long edge under the arm, starting at the hand and working downwards (Fig. 14.2c).
- The free corner is then taken around the back and upwards, to meet the other free corner lying over the shoulder.
- Tie both ends in the centre of the patient's back, using a reef knot i.e. take the ends right over left and then back again, left over right (Fig. 14.2d).
- Fold over the corner at the elbow and secure it with a safety pin.
- Check distal neurovascular status (sensation and capillary refill) after application of the sling.
- Give the patient advice about removing the sling at regular intervals and performing exercises on the uninjured joints of the affected limb to avoid stiffness.
- Document the episode of care.

Practice tips

- Ask the patient to hold the edge of the sling on their shoulder with their thumb to hold the sling in place until it is secured.
- After securing the sling, ask the patient to relax into it and ensure the arm doesn't slip downwards.
- Consider how the patient will cope at home. It might be worth placing the sling under their clothing, so that they can undress without having to undo the sling first.

Pitfalls

- Placing the patient's arm across their chest without sufficient elevation of the hand.
- Not securing the sling at the elbow resulting in the arm slipping downwards.
- Tying the knot too high, putting pressure on the patient's neck.

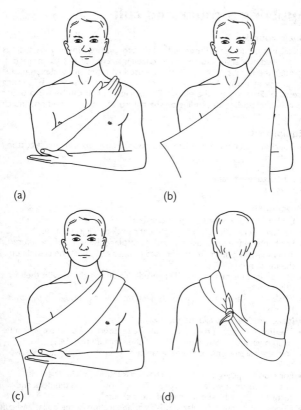

Fig. 14.2 (a) Support the arm; (b) position the sling; (c) tuck under the arm; (d) tie in the centre of the patient's back.

Applying a collar and cuff

Background

A collar and cuff can be used with the hand elevated for injuries such as a fractured humeral head and neck, enabling gravity to put some traction through the fracture site. It can also be used with the elbow flexed to 90° for elbow injuries, where a broad arm sling might cause pain by putting pressure directly onto the elbow. The collar and cuff can be worn under or over the clothes, depending on the nature of the injury and how much mobility is to be encouraged.

Equipment

- Collar and cuff material: ~4cm-wide sponge covered with a soft cotton material.
- Tie wrap.
- Elastic adhesive tape
- Scissors.

Procedure

- Explain the procedure and gain consent.
- Remove all jewellery from the patient's neck and injured arm.
- For humeral fractures, ask the patient to place the wrist of the injured arm against the sternum; the fingertips will rest against the clavicle on the uninjured side.
- The patient might support the injured arm on the elbow with their other hand.
- Make a loop around the patient's neck that is long enough to slip over their head.
- Make another loop around their wrist.
- The figure of eight produced should be secured in the centre with a tie wrap over the proximal one-third of the sternum (Fig. 14.3).
- Snip the surplus end of the tie wrap and cover it with elastic adhesive tape.
- For elbow injuries, the above technique is followed with the wrist at the xiphisternum level, making a larger loop around the neck and securing at the distal one-third of the sternum.
- Check distal neurovascular status after application of the collar and cuff.
- Give the patient advice about removing the collar and cuff at intervals and performing exercises on the uninjured joints of the affected limb to avoid joint stiffness.
- Document the episode of care.

Practice tips

- Consider how the patient will cope at home. It might be worth placing the collar and cuff under their clothing, so that they can undress without having to undo it first.

Pitfall

- Using a collar and cuff for injuries such as clavicular fractures, where the weight of the arm should be supported.

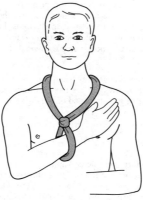

Fig. 14.3 A collar and cuff.

Applying a mallet splint

Background

A mallet splint is the mainstay of treatment for a mallet digit caused by the common Type 1 mallet injuries, which are closed injuries involving rupture of the terminal extensor tendon or avulsion of a fragment of its bony insertion. The patient cannot actively extend the distal interphalangeal joint (DIPJ) (Fig. 14.4a). The mallet splint holds the end of the digit in extension, to enable healing. Mallet splints may also be used with other modes of treatment for the more complex Type 2, 3 and 4 mallet injuries.

Equipment

- A mallet splint. Splints range in size and are made of rigid moulded plastic. There is a window over the nail on the dorsal aspect which enables the colour of the distal end of the digit and capillary refill to be checked.
- Elastic adhesive tape.
- Scissors.

Procedure

- Explain the procedure and gain consent.
- Remove any jewellery from the patient's affected digit.
- Ensure that there are no external injuries to the skin.
- Use the equivalent digit on the other hand (allowing for swelling) to choose an appropriately sized splint.
- Angle the splint slightly so that the long edge is at ~20° to the dorsum of the finger. Slide the splint onto the finger until the pulp fits snugly into the tip of the splint and the nail is visible through the cut-out section (Fig. 14.4b).
- The DIPJ should be straight—neither hyperextended nor flexed.
- The splint should reach the proximal interphalangeal joint (PIPJ) but still allow the joint to flex fully. If the splint is longer and covers the joint, mark the length required and trim the splint using scissors. Ensure the edges of the splint are smooth before reapplying it.
- Secure the splint at the PIPJ using elastic adhesive tape (Fig. 14.4c).
- Less commonly, a mallet deformity can affect the thumb. In this case, apply the splint up to the first metacarpophalangeal joint (MCPJ) but still allowing movement at that joint.
- Continuous splinting of the finger for 6 weeks is recommended followed by 2 weeks of night splinting.
- Advice should be given to the patient about how to remove the splint at home to clean the finger. The patient should be told to place their hand, with the palm downwards, on a flat surface and slide out of the splint. They should keep the finger flat and not allow the DIPJ to bend before reapplying the splint, by sliding it back on.
- The DIPJ should not be allowed to flex at any point after the initial fitting of the splint, until the splint is no longer required.
- Document the episode of care.

Pitfalls
- Not trimming the splint to the correct length, preventing flexion at the PIPJ.
- Failing to emphasize to the patient the importance of not allowing the DIPJ to bend if the splint is removed for examination or cleaning.

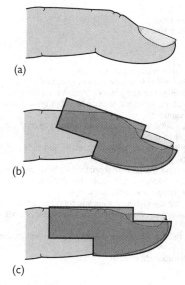

(a)

(b)

(c)

Fig. 14.4 Application of a mallet splint.

Applying neighbour strapping

Background
Neighbour (or buddy) strapping is used for digit fractures or ligamentous injuries. The injured digit is strapped to the adjacent digit which provides support, pain relief and encourages early mobilization.

Equipment
- Elastic adhesive tape.
- Cotton tubular bandage.
- Scissors.

Procedure
- Explain the procedure and gain consent.
- Remove any jewellery from the patient's digits.
- Decide which finger or toe you will strap to the affected digit. If the injury is a collateral ligament, choose the digit on the side that will provide best support.
- Ensure that no skin injuries will come in the way of the strapping.
- Ask the patient to fully extend both digits.
- Cut two lengths of cotton tubular bandage and slide them over the selected digits.
- Apply tape around the proximal phalanx of both digits, ensuring the proximal joint is free—do not apply any tension.
- Repeat at the middle and distal phalanges.
- If the injury is new, a high arm sling will be required to ↓ swelling.
- Advise the patient to remove the tape if they experience any parasthesiae.
- They should also be advised to exercise the fingers or toes within the strapping.
- Document the episode of care.

Practice tip
- A Bedford splint is a double layer of elasticated tubular bandage material sewn down the centre to make two tubes to slide over the two digits—this is more comfortable than tape and is easier to apply.

Pitfalls
- Applying tape over joints, preventing movement.
- Applying tape too tightly or loosely.
- Not applying tubular bandage or soft strapping material between digits may lead to skin damage due to rubbing of bony prominences.

Applying a futura splint

Background

Futura splints are used to provide support for patients with wrist sprains or tendonitis. They can be used for suspected fractures if a back slab is not indicated and for buckle fractures in children. The splints come in small, medium, large, and extra large sizes for both adults and children, with left or right fittings.

Equipment

* Futura splint.

Procedure

* Explain the procedure and gain consent.
* Select the correct size and left or right fitting—the metal bar fits against the palm and the velcro fastens on the dorsal aspect of the hand and forearm.
* Undo the velcro straps.
* Ask patient to hold out the hand on the affected side, with their palm facing downwards and the thumb extended.
* Place the rigid bar against the palm and palmar aspect of the wrist. The fingers should be free and the cut-out section should fit around the thumb.
* The velcro straps should attach across the dorsal aspect of the wrist and through the first webspace. Apply light tension.
* The splint should fit with a small gap between the edges under the velcro. Do not allow the edges to overlap because this will cut into the patient's skin.
* Check capillary refill after application.
* Advise the patient to loosen the straps if they have any parasthesiae in the limb.
* Advise the patient to move their fingers frequently to avoid stiffness. They should also be told to seek medical advice if they experience continuing symptoms and follow-up has not been arranged.
* Document the episode of care.

Practice tips

* Encourage the patient to do frequent finger movements to avoid stiffness.
* Advise the patient to seek further medical advice if they continue to experience symptoms. The splint should not be worn long term without further medical input.

Pitfalls

* Applying the splint too tightly or loosely.
* Applying right splint to left hand or vice versa and strapping on palmar aspect of the wrist.

Applying an elasticated tubular support bandage

Background
An elasticated tubular bandage is applied to limbs to give support and ↓ swelling after sprains and strains. It is sized alphabetically from A to H in ascending widths.

Equipment
- Elasticated tubular bandage of appropriate size.
- Measuring tape.
- A metal cage applicator.

Procedure
- Explain the procedure and gain consent.
- Ensure the patient is not allergic to latex.
- Expose the area to which the tubular bandage is to be applied.
- Treat and dress any skin wounds as appropriate.
- Remember that the tubular bandage should be applied from the joint above to the joint below the injury site, e.g. for an ankle sprain, it should be applied from the knee to the toes.
- Measure the circumference of the limb at the widest point to be covered.
- Lay the tubular bandage along the limb to measure the required length.
- Make a small pen mark onto the material, as a guide, and then double the length of the tubular bandage before cutting.
- Stretch one open end of the tubular material over the end of the metal cage applicator and then concertina the remaining material onto it.
- Hold the applicator with your thumbs inside and fingers outside, supporting the material to stop it slipping off.
- Pass the limb through the centre of the applicator up to the joint above the affected one.
- Pull a little of the material over the end of the applicator onto the skin, and then, after returning your hands to the position described in the last step, move down the limb, allowing the material to flow out.
- Use your fingers to alter the tension as the material feeds out—to stop wrinkles developing.
- On reaching the joint below the injury, stop and move back up the limb, still feeding out the material. This will give you a double layer of material, with the fold at the distal joint.
- Trim any excess material—the second layer should be ~1–2cm shorter than the bottom layer, to prevent a tourniquet-type effect.
- Do not fold over any excess material because this will ↑ pressure.
- Check capillary refill time and distal sensation after the procedure.
- Give the patient advice on after care—the patient should be advised to remove the tubular bandage at night to prevent constriction. If they develop 'pins and needles' the tubular bandage should be removed and medical advice sought if the symptoms persist after removal. The tubular bandage should not be used for >1 week, and the same tubular

bandage should not be re-used on another limb injury because it has been specifically measured for this injury.
- Document the episode of care.

Practice tips

- Place the applicator on a solid surface at about hip height, stretch one end over the cage, and use your thumbs to pull the remaining material on—this technique leaves your fingers free to stop the material slipping back upwards.
- Ask the patient to hold the top of the tubular bandage while you apply it to stop slippage.

Pitfall

- Cutting the length too short or long.
- Applying a single layer. The tubular bandage is designed to create the correct tension with a double layer.
- Inaccurate measurement of limb diameter resulting in the tubular bandage being too tight or loose.

Applying a Richard splint

Background

A Richard splint is used to immobilize the knee following soft-tissue injuries, such as meniscal tears or collateral ligament sprains. The splint is lighter than a plaster of Paris cast and can be removed to wash. It is available in sizes of 20 and 24 inches (length).

Equipment

- Richard splint.
- Rayon stockinette e.g. Tubinette®

Procedure

- Explain the procedure and obtain consent.
- Choose the correct size of splint for the patient—it should fit from mid-thigh when the cut-out section is aligned with the patella.
- Ensure the patient's leg is exposed to the point of application.
- Apply a layer of stockinette underneath the splint for added comfort. This should be slightly longer than the Richard splint.
- Remove the side panels that are attached by velcro.
- Place the large section underneath the leg, with the widest part underneath the thigh, and fasten the velcro straps to secure the splint.
- Attach the sides so that the panels meet and the patella is visible through the cut-out section.
- The straps are then passed across the front of the leg, through the buckles on the opposite side, and back to the velcro on the side the strap originated from.
- Advise the patient not to remove the sections at home and only to open the velcro straps.
- Document the episode of care.

Practice tip

- Lay side panels beside the patient when arranging the splint before fitting to ensure no mix up between the sides.

Pitfalls

- Applying the Richard splint over clothing causes discomfort and can cause pressure sores.
- Inappropriate selection of a splint that is too small causing pressure sores due to pressure from the side panels.
- Applying elastic tubular bandage instead of rayon stockinette under the splint.

Applying a cast

Background

Casts are applied to treat fractures and soft-tissue and tendon injuries; they provide immobilization, support, and pain relief. Plaster of Paris is the favoured material for casts for all new fractures or if swelling or bleeding might occur, but synthetic resin-based materials are preferable if a lighter cast is required.

Equipment

- Plaster of Paris bandage.
- Bucket of warm water.
- Non-sterile gloves.

Procedure

- Explain the procedure and gain consent.
- Ideally two members of staff should carry out the procedure—one person holds the limb in the correct position and the other person applies the cast.
- Prepare all the equipment before starting the application.
- The limb positioning will be determined by the injury—maintain the chosen position throughout the procedure until the cast is completely set; movement could cause ridges that might cause pressure sores.
- Stockinette should be applied 1 inch longer than the required plaster length.
- Any prominent bony areas, such as the ulna styloid or malleoli, should be protected by a small square of orthopaedic felt.
- A layer of undercast padding should be applied in a smooth and even spiral with an overlap of one-third—do not apply tension.
- Plaster of Paris or resin bandages should be immersed in warm water, according to the manufacturer's instructions.
- Squeeze gently to remove excess water.
- Bandages should be rolled on, starting from the distal end of the limb covering ~one-third of the previous turn smoothly, without tension.
- The remainder of the Plaster of Paris/resin bandages should be applied quickly, before the previously applied bandage has set.
- Before the last roll is applied, the stockinette can be turned back to provide a soft edge.
- Constant smoothing and moulding of the wet plaster is necessary to facilitate adherence of the layers and to avoid formation of ridges.
- Trim the cast with strong scissors while it is drying, to enable full movement of the joints not held by the cast.
- Check the distal pulses and sensation once the cast is dry.
- Cut a window in the plaster over skin wounds to enable observation and dressing changes
- Instruct the patient on aftercare of the cast.
- Document the episode of care.

Practice tips

- Split the plaster if the limb is likely to swell, e.g. with a new injury.

- Ensure all materials are at hand before beginning procedure—plaster sets quickly.
- Wear a plastic apron to protect your clothing.
- Drape an apron over the patient to protect their clothing.
- The water temperature should comply with the manufacturer's instructions—this is generally lukewarm, because cold water slows the setting process and hot water quickens it.
- Warn the patient that they will feel a warm sensation during the setting process. Plaster of Paris setting is an exothermic reaction.
- Use your palms to mould the cast and give a smoother finish.
- Damp undercast padding cleans plaster off the skin and shoes.

Pitfalls

- Using your fingers, rather than the palms of your hands, to mould the cast can cause dents in the cast.
- Allowing movement during application.
- Restriction of movement of other joints because the cast is too long.
- Extremes of water temperature are uncomfortable for the patient and interfere with the plaster setting times.
- Applying the cast too tightly or not splitting it in situations where swelling might occur.
- Using too much plaster.

Assisting with the removal of skeletal pins/wires

Background
The removal of skeletal pins or wires can be carried out within the clinical setting or under general anaesthetic in the theatre. A medical practitioner generally carries out the procedure.

Equipment
- Pliers.
- Chuck and chuck key.
- Wound toilet supplies.
- Entonox for pain management, if required.
- Gloves.
- Antiseptic solution.
- Wound dressings.

Procedure
- Ensure the patient understands the procedure and that consent has been obtained.
- Prepare the materials and equipment required on a dressing trolley.
- All metal equipment should be cleaned with soapy water before the procedure.
- Position the patient and pin site.
- The area around the pin site should be cleansed using antiseptic solution. If the pins pass through the limb, both sides must be cleansed to prevent the possibility of infection being pulled through the bone.
- A health care worker (HCW) should support the limb while another HCW (usually a doctor) removes the pins/wires.
- Metalwork should be disposed of appropriately.
- Normal wound care protocols apply.
- Advise the patient to leave the dressing *in situ* until the area around the pin site has healed over. Explain to the patient that there may be some localized swelling after pin or wire removal and that this is normal. Advise them to seek medical advice if they have symptoms or signs of infection which should be explained to them.
- If the patient is to be supported by a plaster cast, a non-adhesive dressing should be applied and the limb prepared for casting. For wrist injuries, a futura splint might be used.
- Document the episode of care.

Practice tip
- Use mouthwash sponges to clean around pin sites.

Care of the residual limb postoperatively

Background

The most common reasons for limb amputation are poor circulation and infection secondary to diabetes. Care of the residual limb wound in the early postoperative period is crucial and involves care of the wound and positioning of the residual limb to ↓ oedema. Encouraging early mobilization and exercise helps to prevent contractures and promote independence. The patient might need psychological support for acceptance of the loss of their limb.

Equipment

- Limb board.
- Dressings.

Procedure

- Explain the procedure and gain consent.
- The residual limb might be bandaged or have a light dressing, depending on the preference of the surgeon—this should be kept intact, but observe for leakage.
- Normal wound care protocols apply.
- The wound can be left exposed after 72 hours, providing there are no signs or symptoms of infection.
- The residual limb should be kept elevated, except during exercise, to prevent oedema.
- A limb board can be placed under the residual limb of a below-knee amputation—to enable extension of the knee while elevating.
- Encourage the patient to touch the residual limb, handling and massaging helps to desensitize the area and aids proprioception.
- Massaging the residual limb after wound healing helps prevent adhesions and keeps the flesh mobile and supple.
- Exercises should be performed at least twice daily—extension of the hip by lying prone and pushing the residual limb down into the mattress for a count of five. If the patient can tolerate it, they should also lie supine and extend the thigh off the bed.
- Use of a compression sock aids circulation and might ↓ pain 📖 on p. 524.
- Daily checks of the stump for sores should be initially carried out, with education of the patient to do this independently as soon as possible.

Practice tips

- Avoid the use of the term 'stump' to describe the residual limb because the patient might find it offensive.
- The patient might find it comfortable to sit or kneel on a stool to shower.
- Always rule out deep venous thrombosis (DVT) as a cause of oedema of the limb during the postoperative period following amputation.

Pitfalls

- Allowing the patient to sit for long periods without performing exercises can cause contractures.
- Inexperienced staff should not carry out bandaging of the stump because, if it is not performed correctly, it can cause circulatory problems and an irregular residual limb shape.

Applying a compression garment to a residual limb

Background

A compression garment, often referred to as a 'stump shrinker', is applied to help control swelling, promote healing and shape the residual limb. It is applied ~7–10 days postoperatively, before fitting of a prosthesis (📖 on p. 525). After the prosthesis is fitted, it is still worn at night for up to 1 year and might be worn indefinitely if a prosthesis is not fitted. It can be worn while there is a wound, providing there is no sign of infection.

Equipment

• Compression garment.
• Possibly, an applicator.

Procedure

• Explain the procedure and gain consent.
• Measure for the correct size of garment, according to the manufacturer's instructions.
• Stand next to the patient on the same side as the residual limb.
• Face the area the compression garment will be applied to. Observe from the same angle as the patient, this aids their learning because most will be expected to perform this skill for themselves in time.
• Gather the garment like a sock, holding it with both hands and gently pulling it over the residual limb.
• Smooth any wrinkles by stroking upwards with the palms of your hands.
• A tube applicator made of plastic material can be used to ease application—the sock is threaded onto the tube and the residual limb is then passed into the tube to lie against the end of the garment. Slide tube upwards until the garment slides off onto the thigh and then pass the tubing off the limb.

Practice tips

• Inspect the pressure garment for foreign bodies prior to application.
• If the stump is still sensitive and no applicator is available, rather than pulling the garment on like a sock, turn the garment inside out, except the part at the distal end. Place the residual limb into the garment and fold back the material along the leg.
• Women might find suspenders keep the compression garment in place overnight.

Pitfalls

• Fitting the garment incorrectly—it should be removed if the patient complains of pain.
• Using a compression garment with staples still *in situ*—the staples might catch on the material.

Care of a residual limb and prosthesis

Background

In general, the earlier a prosthesis is fitted, the better. A general assessment is made of the suitability for prosthesis within 3 months of amputation.
► Teach the patient a good routine for stump care because sores prevent them wearing their prosthesis and limit their mobility.

Procedure

- Explain the procedure and gain consent.
- Check the residual limb for infection, allergy, ulceration or swelling.
- Wash the residual limb at least once daily using unperfumed soap. Pat it dry with a soft towel; do not rub the skin.
- Wash the prosthesis socket daily using mild soap and water. Rinse thoroughly because residual soap might cause irritation of the skin.
- Carefully apply a clean prosthetic sock, ensuring there are no wrinkles.
- Socks should never be worn for >1 day and should be changed more often in hot weather.
- Remove the prosthesis if the patient feels uncomfortable on standing. Reapply, but if discomfort persists, seek advice from the prosthetic department.

Practice tips

- Preparation of the patient before surgery aids their recovery.
- Suggest using a mirror to see areas that are difficult to get at.
- A hairdryer is useful for drying the residual limb after washing and avoids the pain caused by friction of a towel on sensitive skin. Caution must be exercised to avoid burns if the patient has altered levels of sensation.
- Wash in the evening if the prosthesis will be left off for the night.
- In hot weather, wash the residual limb more regularly to prevent soreness and rashes.
- Prosthetic socks are available in 3, 5, and 6 ply—a mix of these produces a greater choice of thickness (e.g. 3 ply + 5 ply = 8 ply). This is commonly known as 'sock juggling'.

Pitfalls

- Applying perfumed moisturiser or lotions to the skin of the residual limb, which might cause irritation or sores.
- Using tape, which can cause breakdown of thin skin.
- Using crutches initially—the patient is likely to fall until the body has adjusted to loss of the limb.

Assessing the need for immobilization of the cervical spine in alert and stable patients

Background

The decision to immobilize a cervical spine (with collar, sandbags, and tape—i.e. 'triple immobilization') or remove immobilization depends on several factors elicited from the history and examination. The Canadian cervical spine rule (Table 14.1) is a validated clinical decision-making tool that can be used in *alert and stable* patients with recent trauma (<48 hours). All patients with altered consciousness levels and potential neck injuries should be immobilized.

Procedure

- History—an accurate history must be obtained from the patient, including:
  - Demographics, including age.
  - Circumstances and mechanism of injury.
  - Time of onset and site of pain.
  - The presence or absence of neurological symptoms—paraesthesia/ loss of power.
- If any of the following **high-risk** *factors* are present, immobilize the cervical spine:
  - Age >65 years.
  - Presence of previous spinal disease, e.g. ankylosing spondylitis or rheumatoid arthritis.
  - Any high-risk mechanism—see Table 14.1.
  - Neurological symptoms at any time since the injury.
  - The presence of a severe distracting injury, e.g. rib, sternal or femoral fractures.
- If the patient has no high-risk factors, determine whether any one of the following five low-risk factors is present:
  - Delayed onset of pain.
  - Walking following the injury.
  - Sitting up for examination.
  - A simple rear-end collision.
  - No midline cervical spine tenderness—palpate for midline tenderness without moving the neck.
- If **no** low-risk factors are present, immobilize the cervical spine.
- If any **one** of the above low-risk factors (and no high-risk factors) is present, ask the patient to actively rotate their neck as far as they can to each side.
- Stop the patient actively rotating if they complain of paraesthesia or loss of power while they do so.
- If the patient cannot rotate their neck to 45° on both sides, immobilize the cervical spine.
- Immobilization is not required if the patient has no high-risk factors, at least one low-risk factor, and can rotate their neck to 45° to each side.

Practice tip

- Even if an alert patient has some pain on rotation, as long as they have no high-risk factors and one low-risk factor, it is safe to allow them to actively rotate their neck.

Pitfalls

- Failing to take an accurate history of the mechanism of injury and missing a high-risk mechanism.
- Failing to take a previous medical history, including previous spinal disease or injury.
- Not appreciating the significance of pre-existing vertebral disease predisposing a patient to spinal injury from apparently trivial mechanisms.

Table 14.1 Adaptation of the Canadian C-Spine Rule[1,2] as a decision tool for spinal immobilisation (for alert and stable trauma patients > 16 years where neck injury is a concern).

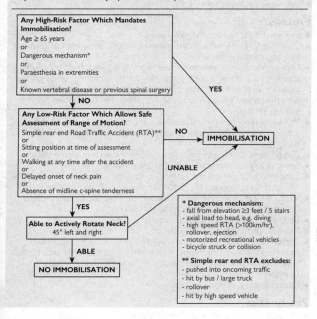

. Stiell IS, Well GA et al. (2001) The Canadian Cervical Spine Rule for radiology in alert stable trauma patients. *JAMA* **286**:1841–8.

. Miller P, Coffey F et al. (2006 Jul) Can emergency nurses use the Canadian Cervical Spine Rule to reduce unnecessary patient immobilisation? *Accid Emerg Nurs* **14(3)**:133–40.

Immobilizing the cervical spine

Background

Triple immobilization with a collar, sandbags, and tape is required to safely immobilize the cervical spine. Ideally, two people perform the procedure—one person maintaining inline immobilization, while the other person applies the collar. The manufacturer's guidelines should be followed to select the correct size of collar for a patient.

Equipment

- Cervical collar.
- Sandbags.
- 5cm-wide elastic adhesive tape.

Procedure

- Explain the procedure and gain consent.
- Continue to converse with the patient because being immobilized can be a frightening experience.
- One person should immobilize the head throughout the procedure—standing behind the patient, place your hands with the thumbs on the patient's forehead and fingers splayed to obtain the greatest contact with the patient's head. Lean your elbows on the trolley/bed/floor to provide stability.
- The second person should remove the clothing from around the patient's neck—observe for any swelling, bruising, or wounds while doing this.
- Cut off tight clothing to prevent excessive movement of the spine.
- Remove any jewellery, which will interfere with X-ray.
- Slide the collar behind the patient's head until it sits centrally, hold the velcro strap to prevent the collar slipping while fitting the front part.
- Wrap the collar around the patient's neck, ensuring the chin support fits snugly and the base is centrally located on the sternum.
- Secure the collar with the velcro strap.
- Place sandbags against both sides of the patient's head.
- Attach one end of the tape to a solid section of the trolley/bed. Pass the tape over the forehead and attach it to the other side of the trolley/bed. Ensure the tape tension is the same on both sides, to prevent head rotation.
- Document the episode of care.

Practice tips

- 1L bags of saline can be used as an alternative to sandbags.
- Fold the edge of the elastic adhesive tape. to prevent it sticking to the patient's eyebrows.

Pitfalls

- Releasing inline immobilization before the patient is fully immobilized.
- Attaching the tape to the mattress or other moveable points.
- Leaving patients unsupervised when they are immobilized. Their airway could be compromised if they vomit

- Attempting to manipulate the neck to neutral in a patient with pre-existing fixed flexion of the cervical spine. Extreme caution should be exercised in these patients and a senior medical opinion should be obtained. It might be appropriate to omit the collar component of triple immobilization in such patients.
- Not obtaining a history of allergy to elastic adhesive tape.

Performing a log roll

Background

A log roll is used to turn a patient onto their side while maintaining their spine in a neutral alignment. It is used if there is a suspected or actual spinal injury. It requires four people to complete the procedure safely.

Procedure

- Explain the procedure and gain consent. It is vital that the patient understands they must not move during the procedure. If a rectal examination is to be performed during the log roll obtain consent from a conscious patient and explain the rationale for doing it.
- Gather and brief all personnel before performing the procedure.
- Ensure that there is enough slack on all lines, tubes and monitor wires so that they are not displaced during the procedure.
- Person one maintains manual inline immobilization of the patient's head and neck—this person should ideally be a senior clinician because they will lead the procedure.
- The other three people should arrange themselves alongside the patient, with the tallest person at the shoulders (person two), the mid-height person at the waist (person three), and the shortest person at the legs (person four).
- Person one slides their hands onto the patient's shoulders, palms upwards. Their thumbs should anchor against the patient's clavicles and fingers splay behind the neck and shoulders. Their forearms should rest against the side of the patient's head.
- Once the head and neck are manually immobilized, person one instructs person four to remove the sandbags and tape. Person four then returns to their allocated place at the lower legs.
- Person two holds the shoulders and waist.
- Person three holds the pelvis with the hand closest to the patient's head and supports the patient underneath the thigh with the other hand.
- Person four supports the patient underneath the knee and calf.
- Person one checks everyone is in position and gives clear instructions as to when to move the patient—e.g. 'I will say one, two, three, and roll.'
- On command, all members of the team simultaneously roll the patient towards themselves maintaining the neutral alignment.
- After the examination and any interventions are complete, person one gives clear commands to return the patient to a supine position.
- Person four returns to the head to replace triple immobilization before person one releases their manual hold.
- Document the episode of care.

Practice tips

- Person one should avoid covering the patient's ears; they must be able to hear any instructions or questions.
- Reassure the patient before, during and after the procedure.
- Clear debris from the trolley before returning the patient to the supine position.

Pitfalls

- Members of the team taking instructions from anyone other than person one leading the log roll.
- Not achieving triple immobilization before person one releases manual immobilization.
- Not standing close enough to the edge of the bed or trolley to prevent patient falling off if rolled near edge.
- Displacing lines, tubes or monitor wires during the log roll.

Wound care

Pat Frakes
Emergency Nurse Practitioner, Emergency Department,
Nottingham University Hospitals NHS Trust, UK

History-taking

Background
A wound is a break in the skin or body tissue caused by injury or surgical incision. Wounds can be classified as:
- Acute (owing to injury or surgery) or chronic (failure to heal within an expected timeframe)—chronic wounds usually have an underlying problem, such as poor circulation or diabetes.
- By depth of tissue involvement.
- By closure—primary intention (wound edges apposed and held in place by mechanical means, e.g. sutures or steristrips) or secondary intention (wound left open to heal).

Successful management of wounds demands treatment of the whole person, meticulous wound care, an understanding of wound healing and dressings, and management of the patient's underlying condition.
▶ Take an accurate history before assessing a wound.

Presenting complaint/current health
Enquire about:
- Hand dominance, if an upper limb injury.
- Location, cause, timing, and progression of the wound.
- Exact mechanism, if an injury.
- First aid treatment.
- The possibility of a foreign body in the wound.
- Pain, bleeding, or discharge from the wound.
- Tetanus immunization status (see Table 15.1 for the most recent tetanus guidelines.)

Past history
Enquire about:
- Processes and diseases likely to adversely affect wound healing, e.g. poor circulation, diabetes, cancer, human immunodeficiency virus (HIV), or sickle cell disease.
- Previous wound healing.

Medications/allergies
Enquire about:
- The patient's medications, specifically asking about drugs likely to impede wound healing, e.g. steroids and chemotherapeutic agents.
- Over-the-counter and alternative medications and herbal remedies.
- Allergies to medications.
- Allergies to latex, dressings or adhesive plasters.

Social history/habits
Enquire about:
- Social circumstances and support, nutrition, occupation, hobbies, and cigarette and alcohol history. All of these factors impact on or are affected by wound healing.

Family history
Enquire about:
• Illnesses in the family, specifically noting familial or hereditary
  conditions that affect healing and predispose to chronic wounds.

Systems review
A full review of systems should be performed in patients with chronic
wounds.

Practice tips
• Generic practice tips for history-taking are on 📖 p. 26–41.
• Use a pain assessment tool to determine the type of pain and its
  severity.

Pitfalls
• Failing to elicit a history of factors and diseases impacting on wound
  healing.
• Failing to identify the tetanus immunization status, especially in burn
  wounds.
• Failing to identify non-accidental injury or domestic violence. Ensure
  the wound is consistent with the mechanism of injury and look for
  other clues, e.g. unusual sites and delayed presentation.

Physical assessment

Background

The assessment of a patient presenting with a wound might require a full top-to-toe physical examination. Particular attention should be paid to evidence of systemic disease that might impact on wound healing, nutritional status, and factors local to the wound, e.g. ischaemia, venous insufficiency, and neuropathy. Accurate assessment of the wound itself is crucial for appropriate wound care and for monitoring progress. Examination of the wound involves assessment of its overall appearance, size, depth, edges, floor and the surrounding skin. Table 15.2 shows the acronym 'COMPLETE', which is a useful aide memoire for wound assessment.

Equipment

- Non-sterile gloves.
- Disposable apron.

Procedure

- Explain the procedure and gain consent.
- Put on a pair of non-sterile gloves and an apron.
- Inspect the wound for its general appearance:
  - size, depth, tissue type(s)
  - exposed underlying structures (e.g. bone, joint, tendon, or nerve)
  - curling or rolling of the wound edges
  - presence of granulation tissue, slough or exudate (amount, colour, and odour), necrosis, or underlying haematoma
  - Look also for bruising, erythema, dessication, and signs of poor vascularization.
- Palpate the skin and assess for turgor and local temperature. To assess turgor, rub a finger across the patient's skin, looking for any sliding of the epidermis from the dermis.
- Measure the surface area, depth, and volume of the wound 📖 on p. 538.
- Assess for undermining/tunnelling—📖 on p. 538.
- Assess the local neurovascular status:
  - temperature
  - hair growth
  - skin quality
  - oedema
  - varicosities
  - haemosiderin deposition, which results from venous stasis and causes hyperpigmentation (usually a brown/orange colour) of the skin
  - sensation, pulses, and capillary refill.
- Document the findings accurately. Wounds healing by 2° intention (📖 on p. 534) might be categorized as hypergranulating, granulating, epithelializing, necrotic, infected, or sloughy or a combination of these categories.

Practice tip

- Digital photographs can help to support, but should not replace, the practitioner's description of the wound. The patient's consent must be obtained for photography of the wound.

Pitfalls

- Mistaking erythema limited to the wound edges as a sign of infection—it is usually present in normal healing.
- Failing to identify or treat underlying factors affecting wound healing.
- Being unaware that the presence of pain in the chronic inflammatory phase of wound healing (2–5 days) or delayed bleeding might be indicative of infection.
- Being unaware that the absence of pain might be indicative of an underlying neuropathic disorder or a full-thickness burn.

Table 15.1 Tetanus Immunisation Recommendations[1]

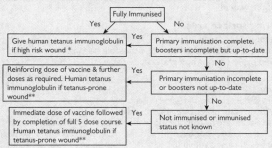

* wound heavily contaminated with material likely to contain tetanus spores and/or extensive devitalised tissue

** compound fractures; systemic sepsis present; puncture wound; significant degree of devitalised tissue; delay of surgical intervention > 6hrs

Table 15.2 The 'COMPLETE' acronym for wound assessment

C	Clinical assessment of the patient	Vital signs and general appearance
O	Overall appearance of the wound	Tissue type, wound edges, and surrounding skin
M	Measure wound	Length, width, depth, area, and volume
P	Pain assessment	Presence or absence, type, and severity
L	Location of the wound	Site of wound, and high or low tension
E	Exudate	Quantity, quality, and odour
T	Tunnelling/undermining	Presence or absence
E	Evaluate/re-evaluate	Monitor the wound regularly

Adapted from Department of Health (2006) tetanus immunisation recommendations - Immunisation against Infections Disease, The Green Book, Crown Publications.

Measuring wounds

Background

Wounds are measured so that wound healing can be monitored. At the same time, impediments to healing (e.g. tunnelling, undermining, or sinus tracts) are sought. Acute wounds should be measured at each dressing change and chronic wounds should be measured every 2–4 weeks. A ↓ in the surface area and depth of a wound indicates that wound healing has taken place. Probing under the wound edges with a swab or probe will detect any tunnelling, undermining, or sinus tracts invisible from the external surface, and enable accurate measurement of the length and width of the wound.

Measuring surface area

Equipment
- Lesion measure acetate paper, with disposable backing.
- Squared paper (if using non-grid acetate paper).
- Pen.

Procedure
- Explain the procedure and gain consent.
- Place the acetate paper over the wound.
- Create a template by marking the wound edges on the acetate paper.
- Place the acetate paper over the squared paper and record the number of squares enclosed within the template. Each square measures 1cm^2.

Measuring depth

Equipment
- Wound swab or probe.
- 0.9% saline.
- Marker pen.

Procedure
- Explain the procedure and gain consent.
- Dip the wound swab into the normal saline.
- Insert the moistened wound swab or a probe into the deepest part of the wound.
- Mark the swab or probe at the level of the wound edges.
- Measure the distance from the tip of the swab or probe to the marker.

Measuring and mapping, tunnelling and undermining

Equipment
- Probe or cotton-tipped wound swab.
- 0.9% saline solution.
- Marker pen.

Procedure
- Explain the procedure and gain consent.
- If using a cotton-tipped swab dip it into the 0.9% saline solution.
- Insert the swab or probe into the length of the undermined space.
- At the end point, gently push upwards to produce a bulge in the skin.
- Mark the bulging skin with a pen.

- Repeat this process at regular intervals around the perimeter of the wound.
- Connect the marked points on the skin using the marker pen.
- Measure the length and width of the tunnelling/undermining.
- Multiply the length of tunnelling/undermining by the width of tunnelling/undermining to obtain an overall tunnelled/undermined estimate.

Practice tips

- Record the amount of dressing used for cavity wounds at each dressing. A ↓ is indicative of wound healing.
- Take care not to force the swab/probe when detecting and mapping any tunnelling/undermining.
- It is preferable to have the same practitioner doing sequential measurements of wound parameters.
- A crude measurement of wound area can be obtained by multiplying the greatest length by the greatest breadth.

Pitfalls

- Being unaware that, if there is slough present in a wound, there might be an initial ↑ in the size of the wound as it de-sloughs.
- Failing to remove loose debris, resulting in an inaccurate measurement.

Wound cleaning

Background

Wounds must be cleaned thoroughly if they contain contaminants, debris, or residual dressing parts. The majority of acute traumatic wounds require cleaning; uncontaminated surgical wounds and clean chronic wounds do not. High-pressure wound irrigation (>7 per square inch) is the preferred method for cleaning wounds. It is usually performed with a syringe and narrow-bore needle. Sterile plastic containers (steripods) containing 0.9% saline solution or spray cleaners might also be used.

Equipment

- Sterile dressing pack.
- Gallipot.
- Sterile 0.9% saline solution.
- Dressing trolley or suitable working surface.
- Sterile gloves.
- Alcohol hand rub.
- Isopropyl alcohol-impregnated swabs.
- Disposable apron.
- Protective eyewear
- 35mL or 65mL syringe.
- 19G needle.

Procedure

- Explain the procedure and gain consent.
- Wash and dry your hands.
- Prepare the trolley or working surface and the dressing pack and equipment 📖 on p. 80.
- Decontaminate your hands.
- Put on protective eyewear (goggles/glasses)
- Put on sterile gloves.

Irrigating a wound

- Draw up warmed 0.9% saline using a 35mL or 65mL syringe.
- Attach a 19G needle to the syringe.
- Irrigate the wound using the needle and syringe until the wound is clean.
- Use copious amounts of 0.9% saline, particularly in areas of poor vascularity.
- Dry the skin surrounding the wound.

Cleaning a contaminated wound with residual debris after irrigation

- Dip a folded piece of gauze into warmed 0.9% saline and perform a single swab of the wound.
- Swab from the least contaminated area of the wound towards the highest contaminated area.
- Discard the gauze.

- Repeat the process until the wound is clean.
- Dry the skin surrounding the wound.

Scrubbing a wound
- The wound might require scrubbing with a surgical scrub if there are deeply embedded contaminants, e.g. road grit. Scrubbing can damage healthy tissue and should only be performed if irrigation and swabbing have failed. The decision to scrub a wound should be discussed with a senior clinician.

After the procedure
- Discard the equipment using clinical waste disposal.
- Decontaminate your hands.
- Clean the trolley.
- Document the episode of care.

Practice tips
- Use entonox or a local anaesthetic agent if cleaning is painful for the patient.
- Ensure that you have containers and absorbent sheets to collect the overflow of irrigating fluid.

Pitfalls
- Failing to remove contaminants for fear of hurting the patient, potentially leading to wound infection or 'tattooing' of the skin.
- Omitting to wear the correct protective clothing. Splash-back from the wound during irrigation can put the practitioner at risk of cross-infection.

Wound debridement using larval therapy

Background

Larval therapy is used to treat ischaemic and diabetic ulcers, infected wounds, and sloughy/necrotic wounds. The enzymes secreted by the sterile maggots of the fly *Lucilia sericata* break down necrotic tissue into a semi-liquid form, which the maggots then ingest. Larval therapy is used after autolysis has commenced in the wound. A successful outcome is usually achievable after a single application. Larval therapy is contra-indicated in dry necrotic wounds, malignant fungating wounds and in wounds that contain fistulae or connect to vital organs. It should not be used in areas of poor blood supply and should be used with caution near exposed blood vessels. Patients on warfarin need to be closely observed.

Equipment

- Dressing trolley or suitable working surface.
- Sterile dressing pack/gallipot.
- Sterile 0.9% saline solution.
- 35mL or 65 ml sterile syringe/19G needle (for wound irrigation)
- Sterile gloves/alcohol hand rub.
- Isopropyl alcohol-impregnated swabs.
- Disposable apron/protective eyewear.
- Sheet of acetate.
- Hydrocolloid dressing/sterile scissors.
- Loose larvae or bio-bags (larvae-filled bags)—maximum of 10 larvae/cm^2, depending on the amount of necrotic tissue.
- Sterile fine nylon mesh (supplied with larval pack).
- Roll of sleek. (supplied with larval pack)
- Non-adherent dressing.
- An absorbent dressing pad or gauze.
- Tape or bandage.

Procedure

- Explain the procedure and gain consent.
- Wash and dry your hands.
- Prepare the trolley or working surface and the dressing pack and equipment 📖 on p. 80.
- Decontaminate your hands
- Put on sterile gloves.
- Clean the wound 📖 on p. 540.
- Make a template of the wound by tracing the wound edges onto a sheet of acetate.
- Place the template over the hydrocolloid dressing and cut out the shape of the wound. Discard the piece cut out.
- Apply the remainder of the hydrocolloid dressing to the patient, aligning the edges of the hole with the wound edges.
- Loosen the larvae from their container with 0.9% saline and place them into the wound.
- Cover the larvae with the fine-bore nylon net, supplied with the larvae

- Secure the edges of the net with waterproof tape (sleek) over the hydrocolloid dressing.
- Place moistened gauze over the net to prevent the larvae from drying out and cover with a non-adherent dressing.
- Cover with an absorbent pad or gauze/secure with tape or a bandage.
- Advise the patient not to sit or lie close to heating appliances, which can cause the larvae to dry out.

After the procedure
- Discard the equipment using clinical waste disposal.
- Decontaminate your hands.
- Clean the trolley.
- Document the episode of care.
- After 3 days, remove the larvae with gloved fingers or forceps, or rinse them from the wound with 0.9% saline.
- Dispose of the larvae as clinical waste.

Practice tips

- Larvae find it hard to penetrate hard necrotic tissue. The use of a hydrocolloid dressing or hydrogel before larval therapy helps to soften or rehydrate the dead tissue. Hydrogels containing propylene glycol should not be used because larvae react adversely to this substance.
- For heavily exuding wounds, light padding should be applied over the net and secured round the edges.
- Net sleeves and boots are available for hand and foot wounds. The outer dressing might need to be watered in dry atmospheres.
- For non-compliant patients, the use of a biobag is preferable. The larvae are contained in a bag that is simply placed in the wound. This method is not as effective as wound debridement using free-range larvae.
- In the case of death of the patient, cover the wound with an occlusive dressing to suffocate the larvae or insert nugel into the wound to kill the larvae.

Pitfalls

- Occluding the area with heavy padding. This suffocates the larvae.
- Using normal saline instead of water to maintain a moist wound environment. This kills the larvae.
- Using an excessive volume of water to maintain a moist wound environment might drown the larvae.
- Being unaware that the powerful enzymes produced by the larvae have the potential to cause irritation of healthy tissue if excessive numbers of larvae are used or they are left in place too long after debridement has been completed.
- Mistaking the expected ↑ in the amount of exudates for infection. This exudate might be discoloured and malodorous.
- Mistakenly thinking that some of the larvae must have escaped from the wound if there are fewer larvae on removal of dressing. The larvae have a tendency to eat each other.

Applying and removing a wound dressing

Background

Dressings are applied to wounds to protect them from further contamination and to promote wound healing. They should be removed only to perform assessment of the wound or to undertake a specific treatment. In uninfected wounds, it is preferable to leave the dressing in place for several days, to minimize the disturbance to wound healing. Any decision on the length of application should however be in accordance with manufacturer's guidelines.

Equipment

- Sterile dressing pack.
- Sterile 0.9% saline solution contained in 35mL or 65mL syringe and 19G needle or plastic tubing or aerosol can.
- Dressing trolley or suitable surface.
- Sterile gloves.
- Alcohol hand rub.
- Disposable apron.
- Protective goggles where appropriate.
- Suitable dressing.

Procedure

- Explain the procedure and gain consent.
- Check the patient's allergies and potential contraindications to dressings, e.g. povidone iodine in patients with thyroid disorders.
- If a dressing is *in situ* carefully remove it taking note of any blood, exudate or smell. If the dressing does not come off easily it may need to be soaked to prevent disturbance of the new granulation.
- Clean the wound 📖 on p. 540.
- Dry the skin surrounding the wound.
- Assess the wound and choose an appropriate dressing 📖 on p. 546.
- Apply the dressing according to the manufacturer's instructions.

After the procedure

- Discard the equipment using clinical waste disposal.
- Decontaminate your hands.
- Clean the trolley.
- Document the episode of care.
- For large cavity wounds, record the number of dressings required to fill the cavity.

Practice tips

- Warming a hydrocolloid dressing between the palms of the hands before applying it to a wound enables malleability on application.
- When packing small cavity wounds with an alginate dressing, do not pack too tightly because the formation of a plug of hard alginate might prevent efficient drainage of exudates.
- When applying film dressings to awkward areas, e.g. elbows and heels, apply them in overlapping strips.
- To remove a film dressing, gently lift one corner of the dressing from the surrounding skin and then gently stretch horizontally away from the skin in the direction of hair growth. This releases the adhesive and enables the dressing to be removed without damaging fragile skin or body hair.
- Soak dressings that have become adhered to the wound to prevent damage to the new granulation.
- Use nitrous oxide gas or a local anaesthetic agent if removal is painful for the patient.

Pitfalls

- Applying a hydrogel dressing to a wound with a compromised blood flow, or copious exudate, leading to maceration of the wound edges.
- Overapplication of hydrogel dressings, leading to maceration of the healthy tissue surrounding the wound.
- ↓ the efficacy of a film dressing by covering it with a 2° dressing and/or clothing, This might affect the control of the passage of water vapour from beneath the dressing.
- Not taking sufficient care to avoid creases when applying a film dressing over vulnerable skin, which puts the skin at risk of pressure damage.
- Failing to ensure that, when removing alginate dressings from a wound, no residue remains. Retained fibres might stimulate an inflammatory response.
- Moistening an alginate dressing before application. This affects the gelling process and might limit the capacity of the dressing to absorb exudate. Rarely should the dressing be moistened before application.
- Failing to change povidone–iodine dressings daily for wounds with copious exudates. The exudates ↓ the efficacy of the povidone–iodine dressing.
- Removal of both primary and secondary dressings for exudate if replacement of the secondary dressing would have sufficed.

Choosing a wound dressing

Background

Dressings should provide and maintain an environment in which wound healing can take place at the maximum rate. Dressings can also be used in the absence of a wound to protect fragile skin. This will depend on the site and nature of the wound. It is also important to consider patient preference, social circumstances and frequency of bathing, when deciding upon the suitability of a dressing, and how it will be secured.

Procedure

- Assess the patient and their wound 📖 on p. 536–538.
- Choose the wound dressing depending on the type of wound (Table 15.3), the wound site, known sensitivity and the fragility of the skin.
- Document the choice of wound dressing including the rationale for its selection. This enables continuity of care by other health care workers.
- Apply the wound dressing 📖 on p. 544.

Practice tips

- The choice of hydrogel should depend on the state of wound hydration because different hydrogels have different fluid-handling capacities.
- If a wound is malodorous owing to proteolytic organisms, e.g. a fungating tumour, a hydrogel with a ready-mixed preparation of metronidazole to combat the odour can be used.

Pitfalls

- Incorrect choice of dressing owing to inaccurate assessment of the wound or inadequate knowledge of the various dressings.
- Routinely using film dressings with hydrogels, which could lead to excessive maceration of the wound tissue. They should only be used if there is hard black eschar.

Table 15.3 Choice of wound dressing according to wound type

Type of wound	1° dressing	2° dressing	Action
Necrotic	Hydrogel	Film, hydrocolloid, or foam	Rehydrates/ debrides
Sloughy	Hydrofibre or alginate	Occlusive or Semi-occlusive	De-sloughs/ debrides
Granulating cavity with medium to high exudates	Alginate, hydrofibre, or foam	N/A	Absorbs exudate
Granulating flat with minimal exudate	Hydrocolloid wafer, flat foam adhesive, or nonadhesive	N/A	Protects
Epithelializing	Hydrocolloid, semi-permeable film, silicone, or wound contact layers	N/A	Protects and ↓ potential for infection
Infected	Povidone–iodine-impregnated dressing Silver dressing Honey dressing	Low-adherent face dressing	Treats cause of local infection

Applying a wound drainage bag

Background

Wound drainage bags are used to drain liquid or semi-solid matter from wounds or open drains inserted perioperatively. The indications for wound drainage include postoperative open drainage, heavily infected wounds, dehisced wounds, sinuses and fistulae.

Equipment

- Sheet of acetate.
- Pen.
- Gloves.
- Wound drainage bag.
- Filler paste.
- Hydrocolloid dressing.
- Dressing trolley.

Procedure

- Explain the procedure and gain consent.
- Prepare the trolley and the equipment.
- Place the acetate paper over the wound.
- Create a template by marking the wound edges on the acetate paper.
- Make the template slightly larger than the wound.
- Apply the template to a wound drainage bag and cut a hole in it.
- Put on gloves.
- Clean and thoroughly dry the skin surrounding the wound.
- Fill any crevices with paste or cover the area surrounding wound with a thin hydrocolloid.
- Apply the bag by pressing down carefully to ensure a good seal.
- Use a bag with a porthole if the wound requires dressing, irrigation, or regular inspection.
- Leave the bag in place for 4–7 days because frequent removal can cause skin irritation.

After the procedure

- Discard the equipment using clinical waste disposal.
- Decontaminate your hands.
- Clean the trolley.
- Document the episode of care.

Practice tips

- Ensure the patient is lying flat, to ensure accurate wound measurement.
- Stoma paste can be applied to the wound edges to aid adherence of the drainage bag.
- If the surrounding skin is broken, consider using an alcohol-free stoma paste, e.g. Pelican® paste.
- Apply a barrier cream to the skin underneath the hydrocolloid dressing for added protection and to ↓ the risk of non-adherence caused by perspiration.
- Position the drainage port/tap strategically to enable easier emptying of the drainage bag.

Pitfalls

- Ill-fitting or poorly applied drainage bags will put the surrounding skin at risk of corrosion by the wound effluent.
- Applying alcohol-based stoma paste to broken skin, causing discomfort to the patient.

Infiltration of local anaesthetic for wounds

Background

The action of local anaesthesia is limited to the discrete area of the body to which it is applied. It can be used to anaesthetize wounds that require suturing, exploration, or thorough cleaning. The commonest local anaesthetic agent used is lidocaine. The maximum dose for an average adult is 3mg/kg body weight or ~20mL of 1% lidocaine solution.

Equipment

- Sterile dressing or toilet and suture pack.
- Sterile 0.9% saline solution.
- Dressing trolley.
- Sterile gloves.
- Disposable apron.
- Alcohol hand rub.
- Isopropyl alcohol-impregnated swabs.
- Protective eyewear.
- 5mL or 10mL luer-lock syringe.
- 23G and 27G needles.
- Anaesthetic agent.
- 35mL or 65mL syringe.
- 19G needle.

Procedure

- Explain the procedure and gain consent.
- Ensure that the patient is not allergic to the anaesthetic agent.
- Wash and dry your hands.
- Prepare the trolley or working surface and the dressing pack and equipment 🕮 on p. 80.
- Decontaminate your hands.
- Put on sterile gloves.
- Check the name, dose, and expiry date of the anaesthetic agent.
- Use either a 5mL or a 10mL syringe and a 23G needle to draw up the anaesthetic agent and then change to a 27G needle.
- Dip a folded piece of gauze into the 0.9% saline solution and, starting at one end of the wound, wipe along one edge, finishing at the opposite end of the wound. Discard the gauze.
- Repeat the process along the opposing edge of the wound.
- Insert the needle, with its bevelled side facing upwards, subcutaneously into one end of the wound, and then push the needle horizontally as far as possible towards the opposite end of the wound.
- Aspirate, to ensure that the tip of the needle is not in a vascular structure, and then inject into the wound while simultaneously drawing the needle back through the wound.
- If the wound is large, repeat the process at intervals until you reach the opposite end.
- If the wound is highly contaminated or infected, the needle should be inserted intradermally ~3mm from the wound edge.

- Repeat the process on the opposing wound edge.
- Check the wound is anaesthetized before performing the intervention.

Practice tips

- Lie the patient on a couch or trolley when giving local anaesthetic because the procedure can induce vasovagal episodes.
- Be aware of where the resuscitation equipment is in case the patient has an adverse reaction to the anaesthetic agent.
- Be aware where to access in the event of cardiac arrest due to local anaesthetic toxicity.
- Consider using distraction therapy and entonox for children.
- Consider using entonox for patients who have a needle phobia or for wounds in sensitive areas, e.g. the plantar aspect of the foot.

Pitfall

- Not aspirating before infiltration, with the risk of injecting a bolus of anaesthetic agent into a vascular structure.

Performing a digital nerve block

Background

A digital nerve block (ring block) involves injecting a local anaesthetic agent into the base of a digit to anaesthetize it. This numbs the digit and enables minor surgical procedures to be performed without pain. The common digital nerves run with the digital vessels on the palmar (hand) or plantar (foot) aspect of a digit; there are smaller nerves on the dorsal aspect. A lidocaine block will numb a digit for 1–2 hours. A bupivcaine block will last for ~6–8 hours.

Equipment

- Sterile dressing or toilet and suture pack.
- Sterile 0.9% saline solution.
- Dressing trolley.
- Sterile gloves.
- Alcohol hand rub.
- Isopropyl alcohol-impregnated swabs.
- Disposable apron.
- Protective eyewear.
- 5mL or 10mL luer-lock syringe.
- 23G and 27G needles.
- Local anaesthetic.

Procedure

- Explain the procedure and gain consent.
- Ensure that the patient is not allergic to the anaesthetic agent.
- Wash and dry your hands.
- Prepare the trolley or working surface and the dressing pack and equipment 📖 on p. 80.
- Decontaminate your hands.
- Put on sterile gloves.
- Check the name, dose, and expiry date of the anaesthetic agent.
- Use either a 5mL or a 10mL syringe and a 23G needle to draw up the anaesthetic agent and then change to a 27G needle.
- Dip a piece of folded gauze into the 0.9% saline solution and clean the base of the digit.
- Rest the palmar/plantar aspect of the digit on a flat, sterile field.
- Hold the syringe like a dart and insert the needle at an angle of 45° into one side, at the base of the digit, just proximal to where the webspace begins.
- Aim for the centre of the dorsal aspect, until the tip of the needle touches the proximal phalanx.
- Pull back slightly to release the tip of the needle from the bone.
- Straighten the needle to a 90° angle and gently push the needle downwards through the soft tissue until the tip of the needle meets resistance from the skin on the palmar/plantar aspect.
- Aspirate to ensure that the tip of the needle is not in a blood vessel.
- Inject ~1mL of the anaesthetic agent into the digit while drawing the needle slowly back out of the digit.
- Repeat the process on the other side of the digit.

- To block the dorsal nerve, insert the needle horizontally from one side, at the base of the dorsal aspect of the digit, with the bevelled side facing upwards.
- Push the needle across the dorsal aspect, until the tip of it meets resistance from the skin on the other side of the digit. Take care not to pierce through the skin.
- Aspirate and then proceed to inject ~1mL of the anaesthetic agent into the digit while simultaneously drawing the needle back through the digit.
- Check the digit is anaesthetized before performing the procedure.

After the procedure
- Inform the patient of the potential problems associated with ↓ of sensation for the period that the digit remains numb.
- Discard the equipment using clinical waste disposal.
- Decontaminate your hands.
- Clean the trolley.
- Document the episode of care.

Practice tips
- Lie the patient on a couch or trolley because the procedure can induce a vasovagal episode.
- Consider using entonox because patients often find this a very painful procedure.
- For children, use distraction therapy and consider entonox.
- If ring blocking a thumb, ask the patient to place the thumb on top of the hand dressing trolley and the remaining digits under the trolley to obtain optimal access to the radial aspect of the thumb.

Pitfalls
- Piercing the skin on the palmar/plantar surface, causing ↑ pain for the patient.
- Placing your finger underneath the patient's digit—there is a high risk of needlestick injury and cross-contamination if the palmar/plantar skin is accidentally pierced.
- Not aspirating before infiltration, with the risk of injecting a bolus of anaesthetic agent into a vascular structure.
- Failing to administer sufficient anaesthetic agent. ~1mL should be injected into each side of the finger and a further 1mL should be injected across the dorsal aspect, enough to see visible soft-tissue swelling. Occasionally higher doses are required.
- Administering too much local anaesthetic agent (>8mL) can cause vascular compromise and ischaemia.

Vacuum-assisted wound closure

Background

The application of controlled levels of negative pressure has been shown to accelerate wound debridement and promote healing. Vacuum-assisted closure can accelerate healing in chronic wounds, e.g. pressure ulcers, and is used for venous, arterial, and diabetic ulcers. It can be used for traumatic wounds, flaps, grafts, burns and for infected and dehisced surgical wounds. The technique is contraindicated in malignancy and in the presence of active bleeding. It should not be used for wounds opening into body cavities or near vulnerable body organs. Other contraindications include fistulae of unknown origin, untreated osteomyelitis, and the presence of dry necrotic tissue. Caution should be exercised when treating patients on anticoagulant therapy.

Equipment

- Sterile dressing pack.
- Sterile 0.9% saline solution.
- Dressing trolley.
- Sterile gloves.
- Alcohol hand rub.
- Isopropyl alcohol-impregnated swabs.
- Disposable apron.
- Black open-cell foam for cavity wounds or white, flat, small-cell foam for flat wounds.
- Therapeutic regulated accurate care (TRAC™) pad.
- Film dressing.
- VAC (vacuum-assisted closure) therapy machine—either an ATS mains/4 hour battery back-up with a 500mL canister or a portable freedom system with a 300mL canister, depending on the amount of exudate and mobility of the patient.

Procedure

- Explain the procedure and gain consent.
- Ensure the patient is in a comfortable position, with optimal access to the wound.
- Wash and dry your hands.
- Prepare the trolley or working surface and the dressing pack and equipment 📖 on p. 80.
- Decontaminate your hands.
- Put on sterile gloves.
- Remove the existing dressing.
- Clean the wound 📖 on p. 540.
- Dry the skin surrounding the wound.
- Cut and tailor the foam to the shape of the wound, ensuring a snug contact with the edges and surfaces of the wound.
- Seal the area with an airtight film dressing.
- Cut a 1cm² hole in the film membrane over the centre of the wound.
- Attach the TRAC™ pad over the hole.
- Connect the tubing to the machine canister.

- Set the control to the optimal setting for the wound, following local guidelines (125mmHg is recommended for most wounds, but ↓ the pressure for skin grafts and leg ulcers).
- Switch the machine on.
- Leave the machine on a continuous vacuum for 48 hours or set it to intermittent vacuum pressure (e.g. 5 minutes on and 2 minutes off).

After the procedure
- Discard the equipment using clinical waste disposal.
- Decontaminate your hands.
- Clean the trolley.
- Document the episode of care.
- Dressings should be changed every 48 hours.
- Change the canister when it is full or every fourth day.

Practice tips
- The placement of a hydrocolloid dressing over the surrounding skin can aid adherence of the film dressing if difficulty is experienced in obtaining an airtight seal owing to the location of the wound or excessive moisture.
- Instead of discarding the transparent side of the dressing package, use it as a wound template by placing the sterile side on the wound and trace the outline with a pen. Then transfer the template to the foam and cut it out using a scalpel.
- To avoid pressure damage to the surrounding skin of wounds smaller than the TRAC™ pad, apply another piece of foam, cut to the size of the TRAC™ pad and with a 1cm^2 hole in its centre aligned with the hole in the film membrane, before applying the TRAC™ pad.
- Become fully familiar with the functions of the therapy unit— i.e. pressure setting, therapy mode, and lock/unlock function.
- Take care to avoid trapping or kinking tubing.

Pitfalls
- Allowing the foam dressing to overlap the wound edges, with potential damage to the surrounding healthy tissue.
- Applying the TRAC™ pad to a wound smaller than the size of the pad, putting the surrounding healthy skin at risk of pressure damage.
- Setting the therapy unit at incorrect parameters, which might ↓ the efficacy of the treatment.

Wound closure using adhesive tape

Background

Adhesive tapes are suitable for closing dry, superficial wounds under minimal tension. They can be used for flap lacerations and wounds with friable edges that are unsuitable for suturing, e.g. pretibial lacerations. They are excellent for fingertip lacerations, particularly in children. Adhesive tapes should not be used if there is poor apposition of the wound edges or over joints or in areas of high tension. They are unsuitable for deep or bleeding wounds or wounds in moist areas. They cannot be used on mucous membranes.

Equipment

- Sterile dressing pack.
- Sterile 0.9% saline solution.
- Dressing trolley.
- Alcohol hand rub.
- Isopropyl alcohol-impregnated swabs.
- Disposable apron.
- Protective eyewear.
- Non-sterile and sterile gloves.
- 35mL or 65mL syringe.
- 19G needle.
- Adhesive tapes.
- Non-adherent dry dressing.

Procedure

- Explain the procedure and gain consent.
- Wash and dry your hands.
- Prepare the trolley or working surface and the dressing pack and equipment 📖 on p. 80.
- Decontaminate your hands.
- Put on the sterile gloves.
- Draw up warmed 0.9 % saline solution using a 35mL or 65mL syringe.
- Attach a 19G needle to the syringe.
- Irrigate the wound using the needle and syringe, until the wound is clean.
- Use copious amounts of 0.9% saline solution, particularly in areas of poor vascularity.
- The wound might require scrubbing with a surgical scrub if there are deeply embedded contaminants, e.g. road grit. Scrubbing can damage healthy tissue and should only be performed if irrigation and swabbing have failed.
- Explore the wound for damage to underlying structures, e.g. tendons.
- Dry the skin surrounding the wound.
- Tear along the perforated card, holding the tapes to expose their ends.
- Peel off a single tape using either forceps or your fingertips.
- Place one half of the tape onto the skin adjacent to the centre of the wound, up to the wound edge, ensuring that the tape adheres to the skin.

- Push the opposing wound edge with the index finger of your non-dominant hand, to appose the wound edges.
- Bring the tape straight across the apposed wound edges and press down onto the skin of the opposing wound edge, ensuring that the tape adheres well.
- Repeat the procedure, leaving a space of ~5mm between each tape.
- Cover with a dry dressing.
- Advise the patient to keep the wound clean and dry until removal of tapes in 5–7 days, depending on the expected rate of wound healing. The patient could soak the tapes to aid removal.

After the procedure
- Discard the equipment using clinical waste disposal.
- Decontaminate your hands.
- Clean the trolley.
- Document the episode of care.

Practice tips
- When peeling the tape off the card, use the index finger of the nondominant hand to catch the other end of the tape, to prevent it from curling up and adhering to itself.
- To improve adhesiveness, prepare the skin with compound benzoin tincture before application of the tapes. Take care not to get any of the agent into the wound because this causes pain.
- Lie another tape across the ends of the tapes, to anchor them into position and prevent them from curling up.

Pitfalls
- Applying steristrips to deep or high tension wounds where tissue adhesive or sutures might be more appropriate e.g. wounds over joints or deep forearm wounds.
- Failing to clean the wound thoroughly before application of the tapes. An anaesthetic agent should be used if pain does not permit thorough cleaning of the wound.
- Apposing the wound edges by securing the tape to one side and then pulling the free end of the tape across to the other side of the wound, causing uneven tension on the wound edges.
- Failing to leave an adequate gap between tapes, this could impede the release of exudate/pus from the wound if it became infected.
- Failing to evaluate the wound adequately after the procedure, to ensure adequate closure has been achieved.

Wound closure using tissue adhesive

Background

Tissue adhesive ('glue') is used to close relatively dry wounds that are under minimal tension. It has the advantages of being quick to apply and relatively painless. It avoids the necessity for follow-up. Tissue adhesive is waterproof and provides antimicrobial protection. There are two types: butylcyanoacrylate and octylcyanoacrylate. Butylcyanoacrylate forms an opaque, brittle bond, whereas octylcyanoacrylate forms a transparent, flexible, and stronger bond, enabling it to be applied to non-uniform surfaces.

Equipment

- Sterile dressing pack.
- Sterile 0.9% saline solution.
- Dressing trolley.
- Sterile gloves.
- Alcohol hand rub.
- Isopropyl alcohol-impregnated swabs.
- Disposable apron.
- Protective eyewear.
- 35mL or 65mL syringe.
- 19G needle.
- Tissue adhesive.

Procedure

- Explain the procedure and gain consent.
- Wash and dry your hands.
- Prepare the trolley or working surface and the dressing pack and equipment 📖 on p. 80.
- Decontaminate your hands.
- Put on sterile gloves, ensuring they are put on by only touching the wrist end.
- Clean the wound 📖 on p. 540.
- Explore the wound for injury to the underlying structures (e.g. tendons).
- Dry the skin surrounding the wound.

Application of butylcyanoacrylate tissue adhesive

- Twist the end of the applicator to remove it. Invert the applicator and tap it to expel air from the nozzle.
- Apply the fine nozzle attachment, if included.
- Appose the wound edges with your fingers.
- Squeeze the applicator to expel a small spot of adhesive onto the apposed wound edges. Repeat the process, expelling several small spots along the full length of the wound, effectively spot-welding the wound together.
- Continue to appose the wound edges until the adhesive has dried.

Application of octylcyanoacrylate tissue adhesive
- Gently crush the vial to break the inner chamber.
- Invert the vial and squeeze it until the adhesive soaks through the tip of the applicator and forms a small drop at the tip.
- Appose the wound edges with your fingers.
- Apply the adhesive onto the apposed wound edges in a continuous sweeping movement.
- Continue to appose the wound edges until the adhesive has dried.
- Apply a second layer of adhesive.

After the procedure
- Provide the patient with advice on wound care.
- Discard the equipment using clinical waste disposal.
- Decontaminate your hands.
- Clean the trolley.
- Document the episode of care.

Practice tips
- For a simple non-jagged linear cut, placing your finger and thumb at either end of the wound and stretching it lengthways might achieve optimal apposition. Adhesive can then be applied without fear of it running onto your fingers.
- Alternatively, if wound apposition is difficult without placing your fingers close to the wound, the edges can be apposed using adhesive tape (steristrips). Tissue adhesive can then be applied over the tape. The tape stays *in situ* until the adhesive 'scab' naturally falls away from the wound.
  The ends of tape will require trimming if they curl up from the skin.
- Have a saline-soaked piece of gauze to hand to wipe away any run-off of adhesive.
- If using adhesive for wounds to the forehead, ensure that the patient is lying flat. A trolley that enables lowering of the patient's head is preferable, to prevent any run-off of adhesive from getting into the patient's eyes or ears.
- If there is a risk of adhesive getting in the patient's eyes or ears, cover them with gauze or surround the wound with petroleum jelly to function as a barrier. Eye goggles localized to the orbits might also be worn.

Pitfalls
- Failing to make an accurate wound assessment and, consequently, inappropriately choosing tissue adhesive as the method of closure.
- Failing to clean the wound thoroughly before applying the tissue adhesive, leaving the wound prone to infection.
- Squeezing too hard on the applicator/vial, causing an excess of adhesive to be expelled and leading to a run-off of adhesive.
- Attempting to apply adhesive to a wound that is actively bleeding, this clogs the end of the applicator and negates the ability of the adhesive to close the wound.
- Not achieving successful wound apposition, which allows the tissue adhesive to run inside the wound and function as a foreign body, preventing wound healing and ↑ the risk of infection.

Wound closure using hair ties

Background

Simple scalp lacerations can be closed using the patient's own hair. The wound edges can be apposed without the use of sutures or an adhesive. This procedure is ideal for use in children because it is less traumatic than suturing. However, it cannot be performed if the hair is very short.

Equipment

- Sterile dressing pack.
- Sterile 0.9% saline solution.
- Dressing trolley.
- Sterile gloves.
- Alcohol hand rub.
- Isopropyl alcohol-impregnated swabs.
- Disposable apron.
- Protective eyewear.
- 35mL or 65mL syringe.
- 19G needle.
- Tissue adhesive.

Procedure

- Explain the procedure and gain consent.
- Wash and dry your hands.
- Prepare the trolley or working surface and the dressing pack and equipment 📖 on p. 80.
- Decontaminate your hands.
- Put on sterile gloves, ensuring they are put on by only touching the wrist end.
- Draw up warmed 0.9% saline solution using a 35mL or 65mL syringe.
- Attach a 19G needle to the syringe.
- Irrigate the wound using the needle and syringe, until the wound is clean.
- Dry the skin surrounding the wound.
- Ensure that the hair is dry, if necessary blot with gauze.
- Grasp small locks of hair from each side of the wound.
- Pull the locks of hair together, criss-crossing them over the wound.
- Apply tissue adhesive to the hair knots to hold them in position.

After the procedure

- Advise the patient that the hair surrounding the wound cannot be washed, combed, or brushed for 5–7 days. They should also avoid contact sports for 5–7 days.
- Discard the equipment using clinical waste disposal.
- Decontaminate your hands.
- Clean the trolley.
- Document the episode of care.

Practice tip

- On occasions, an additional pair of hands is needed to secure the hair ties particularly in uncooperative patients or young children.
- If skin adhesive is not available long hair can be tied in a reef knot and compound benzoin tincture or plastic skin dropped on to prevent slippage.

Pitfalls

- Allowing hair to stray into the wound ↑ the risk of infection.
- Not cleaning the wound thoroughly, particularly when using hair ties as a less traumatic closure method to avoid inflicting pain.

Wound closure using staples or clips

Background

Staples or clips can be used for scalp lacerations and non-facial linear cuts. They are easy to use and ↓ the risk of needlestick injury. Staples or clips are contraindicated in high-tension wounds and wounds in which the bleeding has not been controlled. They should not be applied before CT scanning.

Equipment

- Sterile dressing pack.
- Sterile 0.9% saline solution.
- Dressing trolley.
- Sterile gloves.
- Alcohol hand rub.
- Isopropyl alcohol-impregnated swabs.
- Disposable apron.
- Protective eyewear.
- 35mL or 65mL syringe.
- 19G needle.
- Stapler and staples.

Procedure

- Explain the procedure and gain consent.
- Wash and dry your hands.
- Prepare the trolley or working surface and the dressing pack and equipment 📖 on p. 80.
- Decontaminate your hands.
- Put on sterile gloves, ensuring they are put on by only touching the wrist end.
- Draw up warmed 0.9% saline solution using a 35mL or 65mL syringe.
- Attach a 19G needle to the syringe.
- Irrigate the wound using the needle and syringe, until the wound is clean.
- Use copious amounts of saline, particularly in areas of poor vascularity.
- The wound might require scrubbing with a surgical scrub if there are deeply embedded contaminants, e.g. road grit. Scrubbing can damage healthy tissue and should only be performed, after discussion with a senior clinician, if irrigation and swabbing have failed.
- Dry the skin surrounding the wound.
- Explore the wound for injury to underlying structures (e.g. tendons).
- Line up the wound edges with the centre-line indicator on the head of the stapler.
- Squeeze the trigger of the stapler to insert the staple.
- Slightly pull backwards to disengage the stapler from the staple.
- Repeat the process, as required, ensuring even spacing between staples (~5mm apart).
- Apply a suitable dressing, if required.

After the procedure
- Provide the patient with advice on wound care.
- Discard the equipment using clinical waste disposal.
- Decontaminate your hands.
- Clean the trolley.
- Document the episode of care.

Practice tip
- To ensure even spacing, place the first staple at the centre of the wound and a staple at either end of the wound. Place the next two staples equidistantly between the centre staple and the end staples. Continue to divide the spaces between the staples evenly with further staples until successful wound apposition has been achieved.

Pitfalls
- Pressing too hard with the stapler, causing excessive depression of the skin.
- Failing to remove adequately any haematoma present in a scalp wound, leading to ↑ risk of infection.

Wound closure using simple interrupted sutures

Background

Simple interrupted sutures are used to close wounds that require high tensile strength (deep or high-tension wounds) or if there is difficulty achieving haemostasis. They are used for wounds overlying joints and indicated in wounds with inverted edges. In most cases, non-absorbable nylon is used to close the skin, and vicryl is used to close the subcutaneous layers of deep wounds requiring closure in layers. The disadvantages of suturing compared with other methods of wound closure include the risk of needlestick injury, the requirement for local anaesthesia in nearly all cases, and the fact that usually sutures must be removed. Suturing in children can be extremely difficult and a significant proportion of adults have needle phobias.

Equipment

- In-date sterile toilet and suture pack, including a pair of scissors, needle holder, toothed forceps, gauze, two galley pots, and one non-absorbent and two absorbent drapes.
- Sterile 0.9% saline solution.
- Dressing trolley.
- Sterile gloves.
- Alcohol hand rub.
- Isopropyl alcohol-impregnated swabs.
- Disposable apron.
- Protective eyewear.
- 35 or 65mL syringe.
- 19G needle.
- Suture.
- Dressing.

Procedure

- Explain the procedure and gain consent.
- Follow the procedure for infiltration of local anaesthetic (📖 on p. 550) or digital nerve block (📖 on p. 552).
- Draw up warmed 0.9% saline solution using a 35 or 65mL syringe.
- Attach a 19G needle to the syringe.
- Irrigate the wound using the needle and syringe, until the wound is clean.
- Use copious amounts of 0.9% saline, particularly in areas of poor vascularity.
- The wound might require scrubbing with a surgical scrub if there are deeply embedded contaminants, e.g. road grit. Scrubbing can damage healthy tissue and should only be performed, after discussion with a senior clinician, if irrigation and swabbing have failed.
- Dry the skin surrounding the wound.
- Explore the wound for injury to underlying structures (e.g. tendons).
- Open the suture by tearing along the arrow marked on the outside packaging.

- Pick up the needle holder, placing your thumb and ring fingers in the fingerholds, middle finger on top of the fingerhold, above the ring finger, and index finger on the downward curve of the needle holder.
- Partially supinate your hand to turn the needle holder onto its side.
- Place the part of the exposed suture needle nearest to the suture between the tips of the needle holder, with the point of the needle facing upwards at an angle of 90° from the packaging and pull the suture out from the internal packaging.
- Holding the toothed forceps in the opposite hand, with your fingers in an upward position, as if holding a pen, hook and secure the wound edge.
- Point the needle straight down by pronating the hand holding the needle holder and insert the needle into the skin, 3–4mm from the wound edge.
- Push the needle through the skin, at an angle of 90°, supinating the hand slowly to allow the needle to follow its natural curve until the tip of the needle has come up through the centre of the wound or in narrow wounds equidistant on the opposite side (📖 see fig 15.1).
- Secure the tip of the needle with the forceps before releasing the needle from the needle holder.
- Pull the full length of the needle through the skin with the toothed forceps and then reposition the needle holder, as before.
- Hook and raise the opposing wound edge with toothed forceps and, with the hand holding the needle holder in full pronation, slide the needle under the wound edge, inserting the point of the needle 3–4mm from the wound edge and ensuring that the point of insertion is equidistant on both wound edges.
- Push the needle through the skin, again allowing the needle to follow its curve, and secure the tip of the needle with the forceps.
- Release the needle holder and pull the full length of the needle through the skin with the forceps.
- Release the forceps and, using the needle holder to hold the needle, continue to pull the suture through until ~2.5cm of suture remains.
- Release the needle holder and drop the needle down onto the sterile field in an area that ensures safety from a sharps injury to both patient and practitioner.
- Holding the suture in one hand and the needle holder in the other hand, begin to throw the first knot by twice winding the suture around the tip of the needle holder in a forwards motion.
- Secure the end of the suture between the tips of the needle holder and slide the suture off the needle holder. Keeping the hand holding the needle holder still, use the other hand to continue to pull the suture until a knot has formed close to the skin.
- If the knot is lying between the wound edges, it will be necessary to gently pull the suture with both hands, to lift the knot up and over to one side of the wound to prevent interference with wound healing.
- Throw a second knot by repeating the above process but only winding the suture around the tip of the needle holder once and in the opposite (backward) direction.
  Throw a third and final knot by again repeating the above process, winding the suture around the tip of the needle holder once in a forward direction.

- Adopting the same finger positioning used for holding the needle holder, use the scissors to cut the suture ~4–5mm from the knot.
- Repeat the process, as required, ensuring even spacing between sutures.
- On closure of the wound, apply a suitable dressing.

Practice tips

- When first removed from its packaging, the suture is springy and has a tendency to fall forwards in front of the needle. To prevent this from happening, pull the suture taut and secure it under the index finger resting on the needle holder.
- Use gentle movements when throwing the second knot because pulling unduly hard on the suture might cause the first knot to loosen.
- When securing the end of the suture with the needle holder, place the tip of the needle holder at the end of the suture to prevent it from doubling over and getting caught in the knot.
- To ensure even spacing for linear wounds, place the first suture at the centre and work to one side, placing the second suture halfway between the centre suture and the end of the wound. Continue to evenly divide the wound with further sutures until successful wound apposition has been achieved.
- For uneven wound edges, whereby one edge is everted and the other edge inverted, it is necessary to use a deeper bite on the inverted edge to ensure even wound apposition.
- Consider using vertical or horizontal mattress sutures for inverted wound edges or wide wounds that are difficult to appose without placing extreme tension on the wound.

Pitfalls

- Failing to create a bloodless field and adequately explore the wound for injury to underlying structures.
- Failing to secure the needle with the toothed forceps, resulting in the needle being pulled back through the skin when the needle holder is released.
- Using figures rather than the forceps to reposition the needle in the needle holder. This can result in a needle stick injury.
- Holding the point of the needle with the needle holder causing blunting of the needle.
- Winding the suture around the needle holder close to the wound when throwing the knots can pull the end of the suture through the wound.
- Failing to remove and replace a suture that has poorly apposed the wound edges.

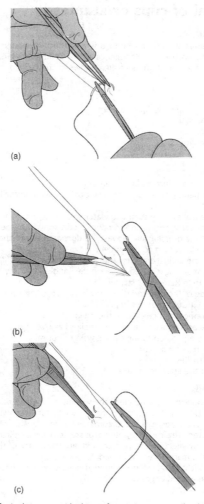

Fig. 15.1 (a) Begin the suture with plenty of pronation to enter the skin; (b) observe the needle tip in the wound to match up the depth of bite on the other side; (c) pushing down on the skin just beyond the emerging needle will help it to emerge perpendicular to the surface. Reproduced from Tulloch and Lee (2007) *Foundations of Operative Surgery*. With permission from Oxford University Press.

Removal of clips or staples

Background
Clips and staples should be removed when sufficient wound healing has taken place to ensure non-dehiscence of the wound margin. If they are not removed they function as foreign bodies in the wound, causing local inflammation.

Equipment
- Appropriate staple or clip removers.
- Sharps container.
- Sterile forceps.
- Non-sterile gloves.
- Gallipot.

Procedure
- Explain the procedure and gain consent.
- Ensure the patient is in a comfortable position, with optimal access to the wound.
- Clean your hands using soap and water and an alcohol hand rub.
- Put on non-sterile gloves and remove any dressing from the wound.
- Dispose of the dressing and gloves, and decontaminate hands.
- Place the gallipot next to the patient.
- Open the staple/clip removers and gently slide the lower 'lip' under the staple/clip at an angle of 90°. Squeeze the handles to lower the top 'lip', which will then flatten the staple/clip.
- Lift one side of the clip, and then the other side, using a rocking motion and gently lift out the staple/clip.
- Place the removed staple/clip in the gallipot.
- Repeat the procedure until all staples/clips have been removed.
- Discard the equipment using clinical waste disposal.
- Decontaminate your hands.
- Clean the trolley.
- Document the episode of care.

Practice tips
- If the wound is discharging, clean the wound using an aseptic technique 📖 on p. 540. Remove the staple/clip furthest away from the contaminated area first and continue to work towards the contaminated area, removing alternate staples/clips to minimize the spread of any infection and prevent sudden dehiscence of the whole wound if the margin has not healed.
- If there is slight gaping to the wound, use adhesive tape (steristrips) to appose the wound edges (📖 on p. 558).

Pitfall
- Failing to make an accurate re-assessment of the wound following removal of the staples/clips and thereby missing signs of potential wound dehiscence.

Removal of sutures

Background

Sutures should be removed when sufficient wound healing has taken place to ensure non-dehiscence of the wound margins. If non-absorbent sutures are left *in situ* too long they function as foreign bodies in the wound causing local inflammation and scarring.

Equipment

- Sterile dressing pack or suture-removal pack.
- Sterile stitch-cutter/scissors.
- Non-sterile gloves.

Procedure

- Explain the procedure to the patient and gain consent.
- Ensure the patient is in a comfortable position, with optimal access to the wound.
- Clean your hands using soap and water and an alcohol hand rub.
- Put on non-sterile gloves and remove any dressing from the wound.
- Dispose of the dressing and gloves, and decontaminate your hands.
- Place a piece of gauze next to the wound.
- Gently pull the knot of the suture upwards with a forceps and cut one side of the suture underneath the knot, as close to the skin as possible.
- Gently pull on the end of the suture containing the knot to remove the suture. Do not cut off the knot as it will leave the remaining suture under the skin.
- Place the suture on the gauze after removal.
- Repeat the procedure until all sutures have been removed.
- Reassess the wound and document the findings of the reassessment and the number of sutures removed.

After removal of sutures

- Discard the equipment using clinical waste disposal.
- Decontaminate your hands.
- Clean the trolley.
- Document the episode of care.

Practice tips

- If the wound is discharging, clean the wound using an aseptic technique 📖 on p. 540. Remove the suture furthest away from the contaminated area first and continue to work towards the contaminated area, removing alternate sutures (or the first 5cm of a continuous suture), to minimize the spread of infection and prevent sudden dehiscence of the whole wound if the margin has not healed.
- Before commencing suture removal, find out the number of sutures used to close the wound from the patient's notes or discharge advice and check this number against the number of sutures removed, to ensure that no sutures are left in the wound.

Pitfalls

Failing to remove sutures hidden under dried blood or wound exudate.
Failure to reassess the wound following removal of sutures, missing signs of potential wound dehiscence.

Assessing pressure areas

Background

Pressure areas are parts of the body that are more susceptible to formation of pressure sores. They are found over bony prominences, particularly if there is little subcutaneous tissue between skin and bone (e.g. the sacrum, greater trochanters of the hips, ischial tuberosities, and heels). Any area can become vulnerable if it is subjected to prolonged pressure (e.g. the nares from oxygen cannulae, the female labia or tip of the penis from urethral catheters, or the skin under tight casts or splints). Risk factors for the development of pressure sores include old age, immobility, paralysis, sensory loss, prolonged surgery, spinal boards, oedema, dehydration, circulatory disorders, anaemia, incontinence, and previous pressure sores. Risk-assessment tools quantify the risk. Appropriate assessment and preventive measures can minimize the risk of developing sores.

Equipment

- A risk-assessment tool, e.g. the Waterlow or Douglas scoring systems.

Procedure

- Explain the procedure and gain consent.
- Quantify the risk of development of pressure sores using a risk-assessment tool.
- Inspect the skin over areas of pressure (including under braces and casts).

  Look for:
  - Skin discolouration—redness is the first sign.
  - Blanching.
  - Taut shiny or oedematous skin.
  - Temperature changes—the temperature might initially be warmer than surrounding tissues and subsequently become cooler as the pressure sore develops.
- Re-evaluate the pressure sore risk score if a patient's condition alters and at least every 48 hours in acute care but more frequently in high-risk patients.
- Document the risk score and findings from inspection of the pressure areas.

Equipment issues

- All equipment used by patients at risk (e.g. wheelchairs, lounge chairs, cushions, mattresses, shower chairs, commodes, toilet seats, and car seats) should be evaluated for pressure risk.
- Equipment should be reviewed and maintained at regular intervals and if there is any change in the health or functional status of the patient.

Practice tips

- Observe the patient's preferred position in bed or on a chair. This might highlight areas in which pressure might be unexpectedly exerted especially if contractures are present.
- Assess pressure areas at every opportunity, e.g. when you are assisting patients to change position or with their hygiene needs.
- Remove trauma patients from spinal boards as soon as possible.

Pitfalls

- Not assessing pressure areas as thoroughly and/or as frequently as required.
- Not assessing risk factors adequately.
- Not maintaining clean and dry skin, particularly groin and skin folds.
- Not paying adequate attention to equipment, e.g. having the footplate too high in a wheelchair, which can ↑ pressure on the ischial tuberosity.

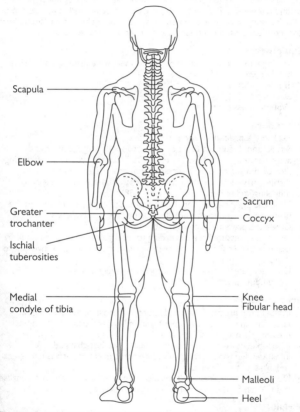

Scapula

Elbow

Greater trochanter

Ischial tuberosities

Medial condyle of tibia

Sacrum

Coccyx

Knee
Fibular head

Malleoli

Heel

Fig. 15.2 Bony prominences that are main sites of pressure sores. Reproduced from Castledine and Close (2007) *Oxford Handbook of General and Adult Nursing*. With permission from Oxford University Press.

Assessing pressure sores

Background

Pressure sores are areas of localized damage to the skin and underlying structures caused by pressure, shearing, or frictional forces. Most sores develop over bony prominences, e.g. the sacrum or heels. They can also develop in non-bony locations owing to pressure from equipment (e.g. the nares from oxygen cannulae or female labia or tip of the penis from urethral catheters). Risk factors for pressure sores include old age, immobility, sensory loss, prolonged surgery, oedema, dehydration, circulatory disorders, anaemia, incontinence, and previous pressure sores.

Equipment

- Tracing film, pen, and tape measure to measure existing areas of skin breakdown.
- Sterile cotton swab.
- Dressings.
- Wound assessment chart.

Procedure

- Explain the procedure and gain consent.
- Assess and document the location, size, depth, stage, colour, and appearance of the wound 📖 on p. 538. Trace the wound, using tracing film, or draw it on a wound-assessment chart. If appropriate, use a sterile cotton swab to measure the depth of the wound. Check for tunneling and undermining (📖 on p. 538).
- Note the presence of granulation tissue, drainage and odour, and the presence of any necrotic areas or particulate contamination.
- Grade the pressure sore as in Table 15.4.
- Dress the pressure sore, according to local guidance or as directed by tissue viability specialists, e.g. with alginate, hydrocolloid, or hydrofibre dressings, as appropriate.
- Consider referral to a plastic surgeon in severe cases.
- Document episode of care.

Practice tips

- Evaluate the pressure sore and appropriateness of the dressings at each dressing change: document the findings and date for the next dressing change.
- If possible, write on the dressing when it was last changed.
- In darker skin tones, grade I pressure sores might appear as persistent red, blue, or purple hues.
- Do not re-dress pressure sores more frequently than required because this will have a detrimental effect on the healing process.

Pitfall

- Inadequate assessment and documentation of pressure areas, resulting in development of a pressure sore owing to poor preventive management.

Table 15.4 Pressure sore grading

Grade	Appearance	Depth
Grade I	Redness of intact skin that does not blanch on pressure	Dermis remains intact
Grade II	Abrasion, blister or shallow crater	Damage to the epidermis extends into, but not through, the dermis
Grade III	Crater with or without undermining of adjacent tissue	Full-thickness skin loss may extend into the subcutaneous tissue, but not through the underlying fascia
Grade IV	Deep crater with or without undermining of adjacent tissue or sinus tracts	Full-thickness skin loss, with damage to the muscle, bone or tendon

Medication history

- What prescribed medications are being taken?
- Is the patient concordant?
- Is the patient taking any over-the-counter medication or homeopathic medicines?
- Is there any recreational drug use?

Social history

- Home circumstances
- Personal status, e.g. married, widowed
- Occupation
- Family/carer support
- Smoking
- Alcohol intake
- Diet
- Does patient have a driving license?

Family history

- Any history of neurological disease within the family? Some neurological conditions are genetic and/or have a familial link, e.g. Huntington's chorea, Alzheimer's disease.

Specific questioning

Ask the patient to describe their symptoms in the order in which they occurred. Specific signs and symptoms require further questioning and should include detail regarding:[1]

	Examples
Headache	Severity
	Character, for example throbbing, sharp, dull
	Any precipitating factors, e.g. coughing, straining at stool? Any relieving factors, e.g. analgesia, rest?
Any loss or alteration in conscious level	Head injury
	Tongue-biting
	Limb-twitching
	Urinary or faecal incontinence
	Alcohol or drug use
Visual disorder	Loss in one or both eyes, total or partial
	Diplopia
	Hallucinations
Sensory disorder	Site
	Type (pain, numbness, tingling)
	Any loss of sensation?
Motor disorder	Incoordination
	Loss of balance
	Weakness
	Involuntary movement

Speech disorder	Difficulty in articulation, expression or understanding
Mental disorder	Deterioration or change in: Memory Intelligence Personality Behaviour
Swallowing difficulties	Slow to swallow Dribbling Weight loss Chest infection
Lower cranial nerve disorder	Deafness/tinnitus Vertigo Balance problems Swallowing difficulties Voice change
Sphincter disorder	Incontinence Retention Difficulty in control

Practice tips

- Allow the patient time to speak, without interruption.
- In cases where the history is vague, or the patient is unable to give a detailed history, a witness account and/or a detailed history from family, friends or carers can be invaluable.
- Provide a brief summary of the essential points to the patient at the end to make sure you have correctly interpreted the patients account.
- Review the history and consider possible diagnoses prior to undertaking the full examination.

Pitfall

- Failing to ensure that there is a common understanding of the words used by you and the patient when describing signs and symptoms. For example dizziness might be interpreted as vertigo or light-headedness.

1. Lindsay K, Bone I, Callander R (2002) Neurology and Neurosurgery Illustrated (3rd Edition) Churchill Livingstone, Edinburgh.

Neurological assessment[1]

Background

If the history is suggestive of possible neurological disease, a full neurological assessment will be needed. This requires a systematic examination that assesses:

- Conscious level 📖 on p. 582
- Speech
- Higher cerebral function
- Cranial nerve function
- Examination of the upper limbs—motor and sensory function
- Examination of the lower limbs—motor and sensory function
- Tendon reflexes
- Coordination and gait

Practice tip

Depending on the presenting signs and symptoms it may be possible to exclude certain elements of the full neurological assessment and conduct a problem-focused assessment instead.

---

1 Full neurological examination and assessment is complex and beyond the scope of this book. As such, this text will limit itself to consideration of the neurological assessment using the Glasgow Coma Scale and associated neurological observations (see Fig. 16.1). For additional information on neurological examination, the reader should refer to Chapter 10 of the *Oxford handbook of clinical examination and practical skills*, Thomas and Monaghan (2007) Oxford University Press.

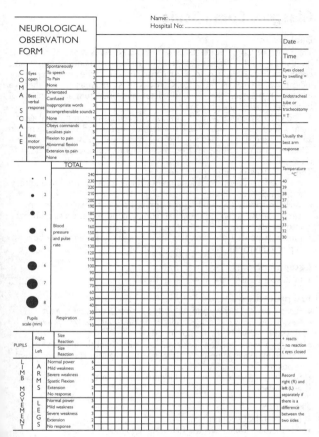

Fig. 16.1 Glasgow Coma Scale and neurological observation chart. Reprinted from *The Lancet*, vol. 304, Teasdate and Jennett, *Assessment of coma and impaired consciousnes—a practical scale*, p.81–4. Copyright (1974), with permission from Elsevier.

Glasgow Coma Scale

Background

The Glasgow Coma Scale (GCS) is a standard assessment of conscious level and is used to detect deterioration or improvement in the patient's condition (Fig. 16.1). The level of consciousness is the most important indicator of neurological change. Consciousness depends on the effective interaction between the cerebral cortex and brainstem and consists of two aspects; arousal and cognition.

The GCS is a component of a more comprehensive neurological assessment which also includes pupillary activity, motor and sensory function and vital signs. It provides an objective numerical measurement of conscious level on a continuum from worst = 3 (unconscious) to best = 15 (Fully alert).

The GCS assesses three specific responses:

- Eye opening (E)—indicates the brain's ability to be aroused by auditory and sensory stimulus.
- Verbal response (V)—indicates awareness the cognitive component of consciousness and the ability to comprehend and express thoughts into words.
- Motor response (M)—indicates the ability to understand and obey simple commands.

Equipment

- GCS score observation chart (Fig. 16.1).

Pre-procedure

- Review patient history and rationale for conducting assessment.
- Review previous recordings and discuss observations with previous assessor/patient notes as appropriate.
- Identify any pre-existing conditions that may affect the assessment. For example native/preferred language, hearing loss, speech and visual problems.
- Review medication history and identify any drugs that may affect the assessment.

Procedure

- Decontaminate your hands.
- Assess the patient using the following sequence:
  - Eye opening 📖 on p. 584.
  - Best verbal response 📖 on p. 585.
  - Best motor response 📖 on p. 586.
- The GCS is normally performed in conjunction with the measurement of vital signs; pupillary response and limb movement.
- Record results onto GCS chart and clearly document how you obtained the responses. Results should be documented by detailing the EVM scores, rather than stating a single GCS score. This provides a more comprehensive indication of the patient's assessment, e.g. E4 V5 M6 = GCS of 15.
- Decontaminate your hands.

‿ode of care.
- Documen‿nges to the doctor or nurse in charge.
- Report ‿

Practi‿nsistency and reliability always provide a bedside handover
- To‿s and demonstrate how the responses were elicited.
  ‿ion can occur rapidly in the patient with an acute
  ‿al disorder or injury. Close observation is necessary when
  ‿nt's condition warrants assessment of conscious level.
  of 8 and below requires assessment and management to
  a clear airway is maintained 📖 on p. 203/204.
  ‿signs can also indicate changing neurological status. For example,
  ‿ming incontinent or slow to initiate interaction.
‿lways chart the best response, this may be at the end of the
assessment process when the patient becomes more alert, e.g. after
having their vital signs recorded.

Pitfalls

- Failing to recognize that a change in conscious level can occur before
  there is any deterioration in other vital signs, e.g. pupillary response,
  blood pressure.
- Delegating GCS assessment to health care workers (HCWs) who are
  untrained or unfamiliar with the assessment processes.
- Failing to repeat the assessment with another HCW when you are
  unsure of the response.
- Assuming that a high GCS score means that the patient is at low risk.
  A drop of 2 points indicates significant deterioration in neurological
  status.

Eye opening

E4: eyes opened spontaneously without need for auditor,
stimulus.
E3: eyes opened in response to voice, normal to raised tone. 'sory
E2: eyes opened in response to painful stimulus.
E1: eyes do not open to any verbal, tactile or painful stimulus.

Procedure

- When assessing eye-opening response approach patient without
  speaking and observe for eye opening.
- If there is no eye opening speak to the patient using a normal tone at
  first, then more loudly.
- If the eyes do not open to voice, explain the procedure, obtain consent
  and gently touch/ gentle shake the patient.
- If the eyes do not open to voice or gentle shaking, a peripheral or
  central painful stimulus will be required.
- To apply a peripheral pain stimuli place a pen between the patient's 3rd
  and 4th fingers and apply pressure, gradually increasing in intensity over
  a few seconds.
- Central painful stimuli can be applied in a number of ways, including:
  - Pinch the trapezius muscle, where the neck meets the shoulder,
    between the thumb and two fingers. Squeeze and twist two inches
    of the muscle for no longer than 30 seconds.
  - Rub the sternum with the knuckles of a clenched fist, however this
    can cause bruising and tissue damage.
- Clearly document the level of response and how it was obtained,
  e.g. eyes open to gentle touch.
- Indicate on chart 'C' if the eye is closed by swelling.

Practice tips

- Using the patient's real or preferred name may evoke a response, for
  example calling 'Jim' rather than James.
- The familiar voice of a relative or friend may elicit a response from the
  patient.
- Always chart the best response; this may be at the end of the
  assessment process, when the patient may become more alert, for
  example, after the recording other vital signs.

Pitfalls

- Tissue damage/bruising caused by application of a painful stimulus
  where repeated assessment is required. Apply the painful stimulus for
  the minimum duration required to elicit a response.
- Avoid application of painful stimulus to the supra orbital notch. This can
  cause grimacing and eye closure rather than eye opening.
- When applying a peripheral painful stimulus, avoid applying pressure to
  the nail beds as this may result in damage to the peripheral circulation
  and nerves.

...al response

...—able to state who they are, where they are and the

...—able to speak in sentences but is disorientated and ...ely.

...words—intelligible words, often random or swearing, ...versation.

...sounds—unintelligible sounds or moaning, may ...timulus to elicit a response.

...oice, physical stimulation or painful stimulus.

Best verbal response
V5: Orientated, month, year.
V4:

...ell you their name, where they are and the month and year. ...o spontaneous vocalisation and no response to conversation/ ...ng, obtain consent, if possible, and gently touch or shake the

...ere is still no vocal response a peripheral or central painful stimulus ...ould be applied.

- To apply a peripheral pain stimuli place a pen between the patient's 3rd and 4th fingers and apply pressure, gradually increasing in intensity for no longer than 30 seconds.
- Central painful stimuli can be applied in a number of ways, including:
  - Pinch the trapezius muscle, where the neck meets the shoulder, between the thumb and two fingers. Squeeze and twist two inches of the muscle for no longer than 30 seconds.
  - Rub the sternum with the knuckles of a clenched fist, however this can cause bruising and tissue damage.
  - Applying thumb pressure to the supra-orbital notch. This is found by running a finger along the supra-orbital margin. This method is not recommended for patients with suspected facial fractures and can cause swelling and brusing when applied frequently.
- Clearly document the level of response and how it was obtained, e.g. moans and groans only to gentle touch.

Practice tips

- Inappropriate words, may denote a patient who is weary of interrupted rest and swears or refuses to respond to the assessors requests, this does not necessarily warrant a lower score than one who is confused.
- Indicate on chart 'T' if intubated or has a tracheostomy and 'D' if dysphasic.
- Always chart the best response; this may be at the end of the assessment process, when the patient may become more alert, for example, after recording other vital signs, e.g. pupillary response, blood pressure.

Pitfalls

- Inferring confusion from an inability to recall day of the week or date.
- Failing to recognize that there may be other reasons for an abnormal verbal response, for example dysphasia, foreign language speaker or deafness.
- When applying central painful stimulus avoid the sternal rub, if possible, as it can cause tissue injury and bruising.
- When applying a peripheral painful stimulus, avoid applying pressure to the nail beds as this may result in damage to the peripheral circulation and nerves.

Best motor response

M6: Obeys commands – e.g. "lift up your arms" or "p...
tongue".
M5: Localises to pain – purposeful movement to remove...
pain.
M4: Flexes to pain – flexes the arm at the elbow without wrist...
a painful stimulus or withdraws.
M3: Abnormal flexion to pain – flexes the arm with rotation of v...
M2: Extension – extends arm at elbow with inward rotation in r...
to a painful stimulus.
M1: No response to painful stimulus.

Procedure

- Explain procedure and, if possible, gain consent.
- Give the patient a simple command, e.g. "lift up your arm" or "poke
  out your tongue" and observe response. The patient should be
  able to respond appropriately to a minimum of two commands.
- If there is no response apply a central painful stimulus and observe
  movement of the upper limbs.
- Central PS can be applied in a number of ways including:
  - Pinch the trapezius muscle, where the neck meets the shoulder,
    between the thumb and two fingers. Squeeze and twist two inches
    of the muscle for no more than 30 seconds.
  - Rub the sternum with the knuckles of a clenched fist, however this
    can cause bruising and tissue damage
  - Apply thumb pressure to the supra-orbital notch. This is found by
    running a finger along the supraorbital margin. This method is not
    recommended for patients with suspected facial fractures and can
    cause swelling and bruising when applied frequently.
- Clearly document the level of response and how it was obtained.

Practice tips

- Observe the patient closely for spontaneous movements to avoid the
  unnecessary application of a painful stimulus.
- Painful stimuli should only be applied when eliciting limb movement
  in the unconscious patient.
- A central painful stimulus is one which elicits a response from the
  cerebral cortex.
- For the purpose of testing conscious level always record the best
  response from the best upper limb.
- Observe for upper limb weakness when applying a painful stimulus.
  For example, one arm may move more purposefully or flex, while
  the other may demonstrate a weaker response.
- Always chart the best upper limb response. This may be at the end
  of the assessment process, when the patient may become more alert,
  e.g. after recording other vital signs.

- If the patient is unable to open their eyes on command, the lid should be carefully raised to avoid tissue damage and swelling. Record with a **'c'** for closed on the GCS chart if there is severe ocular swelling and assessment of pupil response is not possible.
- Decontaminate hands.
- Report any abnormalities to doctor or the nurse in charge.

Practice tips

- Subtle changes in pupil shape, i.e. one pupil becoming slightly ovoid may indicate early pressure on the 3rd cranial nerve. Dilatation of a pupil is indicative of increased pressure on the same side as the effected pupil.
- The normal consensual light reflex is pupil constriction of the contra-lateral eye when a light stimulus is applied to the other eye.
- When assessing the pupil light response note the position of the eyeball, abnormal movements of the eye, and the position of the eyelid. The 3rd, 4th and 6th cranial nerves innervate the extra-ocular muscles involved in movement of the eyeball.
- The young tend to have larger pupils and their reaction to light is more rapid than that of the older person.
- Always provide a bedside handover and perform an assessment with the oncoming HCW to ensure consistency of assessment.

Pitfalls

- Failing to recognize that approximately 25% of the population have physiological anisocoria (non-pathological inequality in the size of their pupils).
- Not obtaining an adequate drug history. For example tropicamide, atropine and amphetamines cause pupil dilation, while drugs such as codeine and morphine can cause pupillary constriction.
- Patients suffering from photophobia may find this procedure particularly distressing.
- If the patient is blind due to a lesion of the optic nerve there will be no response to light, even if the 3rd cranial nerve is intact.

Assessment of limb movement

Background

Assessment of limb movement is normally included on the neurological observation chart (see Fig. 16.1) and is in addition to the assessment of best motor response obtained as part of the Glasgow Coma Scale. Limb movement and muscle power are tested by assessing the patient's muscle strength against the assessor's own resistance by pushing and pulling (see Table 16.1). Assessment of limb movement is used to detect developing hemiparesis or paralysis in the upper or lower limbs caused by:

- Compression of brain tissue by a space-occupying lesion.
- Raised intracranial pressure.
- Damage to the motor cortex.
- Damage to the motor pathways of the brain and spinal cord.

Damage to the motor cortex will usually cause a weakness on the opposite side of the body because the motor fibres cross over in the brain stem (decussation).

Table 16.1 Assessment of limb movement and power

Upper limbs are scored from 1 to 6	Lower limbs score from 1 to 5
6 = normal power	5 = normal power
5 = mild weakness	4 = mild weakness
4 = severe weakness	3 = severe weakness
3 = spastic flexion	2 = extension
2 = extension	1 = no response
1 = no response	

Equipment

- Nil specific.

Pre-procedure

- Review patient history and note any condition that may affect the result, for example arthritis.
- Review medication history and note any drugs that may affect limb movement and power.

Procedure

- Decontaminate your hands.
- Explain the procedure and, if possible, gain consent.
- The patient should be semi-recumbent and each limb should be assessed separately.
- Begin by looking at muscle size and symmetry; are there any abnormal or involuntary movements?

Assessment of limb movement in the conscious patient who is able to obey commands

- Hold the patient's wrist and ask them to pull their arm towards their shoulder whilst you pull in the opposite direction.
- Ask the patient to push your hand away, if there is any weakness they will not be able to overcome your resistance.
- Compare strength between left and right sides.
- To test the lower limbs, apply a downward pressure onto the patient's ankle and ask them to raise their leg off the bed. A normal response is present when the patient is able to overcome your force.
- Ask the patient to push his foot down against your hand (plantar flexion) and then attempt to push upwards whilst you push the toes in the opposite direction (dorsiflexion). Normal power is present when the patient is able to overcome the resistance applied by the assessor's hand.
- To test for mild weakness of the arms, ask the patient to close their eyes and hold their arms outstretched in front, with palms upwards for 20–30 seconds. If a weakness exists the arm will turn inward, as the palm starts to face downwards—this is known as pronator drift.

Assessment of limb movement in the patient who is unconscious or unable to obey commands

- Begin by observing for any spontaneous movements, for example a patient trying to remove an oxygen mask using a preferred hand may indicate weakness of the other hand. Confirm this by holding the preferred hand and observing to see if the other hand is used instead.
- Raise the patient's arms up straight by holding the hands/wrists and then release. The weak or paralysed arm will fall more quickly than the normal side. Note: be careful, the weak arm may strike the patient's face as it falls.
- Test the lower limbs by flexing the knees and position feet flat onto the bed. Let go of the knees and observe movement. A weak leg will fall into an extended position with the hip outwardly rotated, while the normal leg will remain flexed for longer before returning to its original position.
  - If the patient is unable to obey commands, assess limb movement by applying a peripheral pain stimulus. Using a pen, pressure should be applied to the side of the finger or toe adjacent to the nail bed while observing for movement. Spastic flexion or abnormal flexion of the arms is present when the patient responds to painful stimuli by flexing the arm at the elbow with rotation of the wrist resulting in a spastic posture. At this point the legs will be extended and internally rotated. This is sometimes described as decorticate movement and indicates damage within the cerebral hemispheres.
  - Extension occurs when the arm extends at the elbow with an inward rotation when the painful stimulus is applied. The legs are also extended with the feet plantar flexed. This is abnormal extension, sometimes described as decerebrate posturing, and is indicative of a lesion in the pons varoli or midbrain.

- Make patient comfortable.
- Decontaminate hands.
- Document findings and how responses were obtained.
- Report any abnormalities to the doctor or nurse in charge.

Practice tips
- The patient may not be able to respond to the assessor's commands, due to dysphasia, a language barrier or being uncooperative. In this instance the assessor should observe spontaneous movements first.
- The assessment should be proportionate to the size of the patient.
- Always provide a bedside handover and perform an assessment with the oncoming health care worker HCW to ensure consistency of assessment.
- Abnormal movements and altered muscle tone may also be noted at the time of assessment.
- Application of a peripheral painful stimulus should only be used when eliciting limb movements in the unconscious patient.

Pitfall
- Misinterpreting a limb response to a peripheral pain stimulus as being due to purposive motor cortex function when it may be due to a spinal reflex.

Vital signs in neurological assessment

Background

Measurement of the vital signs includes the recording of the temperature, pulse, respirations (TPR) and systemic blood pressure (BP). When used in conjunction with the assessment of conscious level, using the Glasgow Coma Scale, observation of the vital signs can disclose a rise in intracranial pressure (ICP) and deterioration in the patient's condition.

Raised intracranial pressure can be caused by tumours, bleeding or swelling of brain tissue. The regulatory centres for blood pressure, respiration and heart rate are situated within the brain stem. When ICP rises, cerebral blood flow is reduced causing ischaemia. This causes a reflex increase in systolic blood pressure and a corresponding slowing of the pulse (Cushing reflex). A widening of the pulse pressure may also occur as the body tries to maintain cerebral perfusion pressure and cerebral blood flow.

Equipment/procedure

- Temperature 📖 on p. 44
- Pulse 📖 on p. 52
- Respiration 📖 on p. 54
- Systemic blood pressure 📖 on p. 56

Practice tips

- When there is a decreased level of consciousness, record the TPR and BP first in order to rouse the patient and gain the best response to the GCS assessment.
- An elevated systolic blood pressure and widening pulse pressure with a bounding pulse and bradycardia are signs of raised intracranial pressure.
- Tachycardia can be due to hypoxia, raised ICP or other non-neurological causes, for example, traumatic haemorrhage.
- Cardiac arrhythmias can occur in patients with neurological conditions.
- Hypotension is rare in the presence of cerebral damage and usually occurs in the terminal stages.
- Airway protection is required if the GCS is 8 or below 📖 on p. 204.
- Assessment of respirations is a vital indicator of the patient's condition.
- Slowing of respiratory rate, which becomes more rapid and noisy, may accompany an acute rise in ICP.
- Increasing $PaCO_2$ can cause changes in the rate, rhythm, depth and pattern of respiration.
- Damage to the hypothalamus may affect the thermoregulation centre, and cause a rise in temperature.
- Pyrexia will increase the metabolic rate, which in turn results in an increased requirement for oxygen to an already compromised brain.
- Some drugs, for example, anticonvulsants, may induce a fever unrelated to infection.

Pitfall

- Failing to recognize that changes in the vital signs, such as bradycardia, are late indicators of raised ICP and neurological deterioration.

Abbreviated assessment of conscious level

Background

The **A**lert **V**oice **P**ain **U**nresponsive (AVPU) system is designed to detect the early warning signs of deterioration in primary assessment or emergency situations. It can be used by the inexperienced to rapidly assess conscious level, but should be not replace a full assessment using the Glasgow Coma Scale. The AVPU system uses a continuum of conscious level which measures responsiveness to no stimuli, auditory stimuli and painful stimuli.

Equipment

- Nil specific.

Procedure

- Explain the procedure and gain consent.
- Decontaminate hands.
- Alert: patient is awake, lucid and looking about.
- Voice: speak to the patient, e.g. ' can you hear me?', if there is no response gently shake the patient's shoulders— patient is drowsy, eyes are closed, but he responds to your voice.
- Pain: the patient is not alert, does not respond to your voice or touch, but responds to painful stimuli.
- There are two types of responses to painful stimuli, central and peripheral:
- A *central painful stimulus* is one which elicits a response from the cerebral cortex and is used to obtain a cerebral rather than spinal response.
- Central painful stimuli can be applied in a number of ways;
  - Pinch the trapezius muscle where the neck meets the shoulder, between the thumb and two fingers. Squeeze and twist two inches of the muscle for no longer than 30 secs.
  - Rub the sternum with the knuckles of a clenched fist, however this can cause bruising and tissue damage.
  - Applying pressure to the supra-orbital notch. This is found by running a finger along the supraorbital margin. This method is not recommended for patients with suspected facial fracture and can cause swelling and brusing.
- Peripheral painful stimuli should only be used when eliciting limb movements in the unconscious. To apply a peripheral pain stimuli place a pen between the patient's middle and ring fingers and apply pressure, gradually increasing in intensity over a few seconds.
- Unresponsive: the patient does not respond to any stimuli and is unconscious.
- Where the patient is unresponsive assess airway, breathing and cardiac function 📖 on p. 202, 364.
- Call for assistance as appropriate.
- Document findings.
- Decontaminate your hands.

Practice tips

- Assessment should be made by initially using the minimal amount of stimulus and increasing until a response is elicited.

Pitfalls

- Vigorous shaking of the shoulders in patients with possible cervical spine injury.
- Applying painful stimuli can result in damage tissue if too vigorous, for example, sternal rub, supra-orbital pressure, and direct nail bed pressure.

Epilepsy and seizure management

Background

Epilepsy is one of the most common serious neurological conditions, affecting at least 450 000 in the UK. Approximately 1000 die of epilepsy each year and 500 deaths per year occur in otherwise fit young people. Correct diagnosis and appropriate prescribing of anticonvulsants depend on effective observational skills. Lives can be saved if prompt action and reporting is undertaken.

A seizure is the manifestation of abnormal electrical activity in the brain and alteration in the level of consciousness. There are a wide variety of causes and type of seizure (see Table 16.2).

Table 16.2 Causes and type of seizure

Causes of seizures	Types of seizure
Genetic/chromosomal disorders	*Simple partial seizures*: no loss of awareness with motor, sensory or autonomic signs. Sometimes begin as a partial seizure which develops into a generalized seizure.
Birth injury	
Tumours	
Infections e.g. malaria, meningitis	
Head injuries	*Complex partial*: degree of impaired consciousness, symptoms are various, may have déjà vu, feel fearful or elated or experience hallucinations or nausea. Motor disturbances such as chewing or fumbling with clothing may occur.
Drugs/alcohol/toxins	
Metabolic disturbances	
Hypoglycaemia	
Hyperthermia/hypothermia	
Eclampsia	*Generalized seizures*: primary and secondary. convulsive or non-convulsive. Level of consciousness is always impaired includes: absence attacks, myoclonic, tonic, tonic/clonic and atonic seizures.
Degenerative/age	
Idiopathic (primary epilepsy)	
Triggers	
Emotional stress	
Lack of sleep	
Hormonal changes	
Flickering lights	
Alcohol withdrawal	

Equipment

- Oxygen and oral suctioning equipment if available.
- Seizure observation chart if available.

Pre-procedure

- If there is a known history or a high risk of seizures, the patient should be cared for in an area which is easily observed.
- If the patient is known to suffer with seizures obtain a full medical/social history and note type, pattern and frequency of seizures.
- Obtain a description of the usual manifestations of the seizures; the patient may experience a prodromal stage, lasting hours or days, when they may feel unwell or irritable.

- Establish if there are any seizure triggers, for example, sleep deprivation, alcohol, stroboscopic lighting.
- Obtain a medication history and any prescribed anticonvultants.
- Determine how the patient normally reacts/manages their seizures and establish the usual recovery time.
- Establish if the patient experiences any 'aura' prior to seizure onset. For example, the patient may experience stomach fullness, metallic taste, certain smells, flashing lights, or hear strange sounds.

Procedure

- Note the time that the seizure commences.
- Remain calm and reassure patient.
- Endeavour to maintain the patient's dignity.
- If patient is on the floor, remove furniture etc to reduce the risk of secondary injury.
- If patient is in bed prevent risk of further injury by applying padded cot sides and lowering the bed.
- Remove glasses and loosen restrictive clothing.
- Be careful of flaying limbs in the initial stage of seizure.
- If possible guide limbs to prevent injury, but do not forcibly restrict movement.
- Observe and note the characteristics of the seizure, including motor and sensory effects.
- Maintain a clear airway by turning patient into lateral position once the tonic (clenched jaw, and limb rigidity) stage has passed.
- Use position, oral suctioning or tissue to remove excessive secretions.
- Administer oxygen as appropriate 📖 on p. 304.
- Check capillary blood glucose level.
- Stay with the person until a conscious response is obtained.
- Note the time that the seizure ended.
- Check pupillary function, size and reaction to light 📖 on p. 588.

Post-seizure procedure

- Place in the recovery position 📖 on p. 388.
- Orientate and reassure patient.
- Meet any personal hygiene needs, for example , if incontinence has occurred.
- Provide mouth care and observe tongue for any bite damage 📖 on p. 420.
- Administer prescribed anti-inflammatory oral pellets to relieve any sore, swollen tongue.
- Make patient comfortable as they may want to sleep.
- On waking the patient may complain of headache and muscle pains. Administer analgesia as prescribed.
- Observe patient closely during the post-seizure (post-ictal) stage as they may fit again, be confused or disorientated or exhibit automatism or compulsive behaviour.
- Administer prescribed anticonvulsans.
- Establish and treat cause of seizure where possible.
- Be aware of, and assess for, the possibility of a head injury, bruising or fractures if the patient fell at the start of the seizure.

- Assess and monitor conscious level using the Glasgow Coma Scale 📖 on p. 582.
- Document details of seizure activity using a seizure observation chart if available.

Practice tips

- As the seizures starts a shrill cry may be heard as air is forced out through closed vocal cords. The jaw snaps shut as the tonic phase begins, the breath is held and the patient becomes cyanosed, teeth are clenched, legs extended and arms pronated. The pupils dilate and are unresponsive to light. The patient may be incontinent; this stage usually lasts for 15–30sec.
- The clonic stage may last for 30sec to 2min, with rhythmic violent shaking; the tongue may be bitten. There may be hyperventilation, frothing of saliva, sweating and tachycardia.
- At the end of the clonic stage the patient may be unconscious for approximately 5min; on waking they may be disorientated and amnesic.
- Partial seizures, focal motor or sensory seizures and subclinical seizures may not be easily recognized.
- The patient may have a mild pyrexia post-seizure, however the onset of seizures in an otherwise well-controlled epileptic may be due to an underlying infection.
- Some patients with or without true epilepsy may also suffer from pseudo seizures. These non-epileptic seizures can be very difficult to distinguish from true seizures.
- Electroencephalograph (EEG) recordings using telemetry equipment is used to monitor seizure activity for diagnostic purposes.

Pitfall

- Attempting to force something between the teeth during the tonic stage of seizure.

Status epilepticus

Background

Status epilepticus (SE) carries a significant mortality (22%) and is a medical emergency. It is characterized by tonic–clonic seizures that last for >30min or where there is no recovery before another seizure begins. A prolonged seizure is usually defined as lasting 5 or more minutes. Serial seizures are defined as 3 or more seizures in one hour. SE has a number of causes including cerebral tumour, head injury, drug overdose and drug withdrawal, hypoglycaemia, intracranial infection, electrolyte disturbance and non-compliance/modification of anti-epileptic drug therapy.

Equipment

- Oropharyngeal airway (OPA), e.g. Guedal airway.
- Bedside oxygen and oral suction.
- Prescription chart and anticonvulsant medication.
- Seizure observation chart if available.
- Cardiac monitor, pulse oximeter and glucometer.
- Sphygmomanometer, stethoscope and thermometer.
- Intravenous cannula and giving set.
- Padded cot sides.

Pre-procedure

- If there is a known history or a high risk of seizures, the client should be nursed in an area which is easily observed.

Procedure

- Assess airway, breathing and circulation (ABC).
- Manage as for general seizure 📖 on p. 598.
- Establish and maintain patent airway 📖 on p. 204.
- Administer oxygen via mask/nasal cannula 📖 on p. 304.
- Obtain immediate medical assistance.
- Establish intravenous access 📖 on p. 162.
- Record TPR, BP, SpO$_2$, and capillary blood glucose (CBG) 📖 on p. 46, 53, 54, 56, 296, 66.
- Establish ECG monitoring 📖 on p. 44.
- Obtain blood samples for U&E's, glucose, calcium, Magnesium, full blood count (FBC) and anti-epileptic drug levels 📖 p. 160.
- Administer anticonvulsant, e.g. lorazepam, diazepam, phenytoin, fosphenytoin.
- Establish and treat any underlying cause, e.g. hypoglycaemia.
- Perform regular neurological observations 📖 on p. 582.
- Alert anaesthetist and intensive care unit.
- Treat any complications.
- Initiate/re-establish long term maintenance of anti-epileptic drug theraphy.

Post-procedure

- Obtain blood samples for arterial blood gases, renal and liver function and toxicology as appropriate.
- Initiate intracranial pressure monitoring if appropriate.
- Perform chest X-ray.
- Consider CT brain scan and lumbar puncture (LP).
- Maintain comprehensive, contemporaneous records.
- Observe and monitor for complications (see Table 16.3).

Practice tips

- The first line anticonvulsant lorazepam is stored in the refrigerator. Bolus IV dose = 4mg.
- Established SE requires IV phenytoin infusion at a dose of 15–18mg/kg at a rate of 50mg per minute or fosphenytoin. Patients should be monitored for hypotension and cardiac arrhythmia.
- Fosphenytoin is prescribed as a phenytoin equivalent (PE) dose.
- 1.5mg fosphenytoin = 1mg phenytoin sodium.
- Hypoglycaemia should be treated with 50mls of 50% glucose.
- Where hypoglycaemia is suspected to be due to alcohol abuse or impaired nutrition; intravenous thiamine (250mg over 10min) and high-potency pabrinex® should also be given.
- Failure to respond to anticonvulsants may necessitate admission to an Intensive Care Unit (ICU) for sedation and intubation.
- Patients can present with non-epileptic status (functional seizures) which can be difficult to recognize. Features include fluctuating intensity of movements, resistance to examination, opisthotonus, atypical history, past psychiatric history. The EEG is normal during an attack.
- Non-convulsive status and partial status do not require the same treatment and should be treated as per general seizures 📖 on p. 598.

Table 16.3 Complications associated with SE and its management

Hypoxia	↑ ICP
Acidosis	Hypoglycaemia
Cardiac arrhythmia	Hyperthermia
Electrolyte disturbance	DIC
Hypertension and hypotension	Rhabdomyolosis
Pulmonary oedema	

Lumbar puncture

Background

While computed tomography scanning has reduced the need for lumbar puncture (LP) the examination of the cerebrospinal fluid (CSF) remains a valuable diagnostic tool. LP should be considered in cases of suspected infection, e.g. meningitis, subarachnoid haemorrhage (SAH), demyelinating and inflammatory disease e.g. multiple sclerosis (MS) and Guillain-Barré syndrome. It can also be used for the introduction of antibacterial therapy, anaesthetic and contrast medium for myelography. Additionally, LP is used to remove excess CSF in idiopathic intracranial hypertension. The procedure should only be performed following neurological assessment to identify any raised intracranial pressure (ICP) which is considered a relative or absolute contraindication to LP. In addition, LP should not be performed where there is uncorrected coagulopathy, thrombocytopenia, spinal cord trauma or local skin infection at the LP site. LP is also best avoided in confused or uncooperative patients and it is safer to obtain a CT scan before proceeding to LP in patients with focal neurological signs or papilloedema.

The procedure is performed by the medical staff and can usually be performed under local anaesthetic although a sedative, e.g. lorazepam or midazolam may be indicated in particularly anxious patients. LP is normally performed between the lumbar vertebrae, L3–L4 or L4–L5 and it is common practice to obtain manometric measurement of CSF pressure at the same time. Complications are rare, but can include dural, subdural or arachnoid bleeding secondary to needle trauma, headache and possible tentorial or uncal herniation.

Equipment

- Lumbar puncture kit or dressing pack.
- Skin cleansing agent, e.g. chlorhexidine, povidone Iodine (as per local policy).
- Sterile towel/drapes.
- Local anaesthetic, e.g. lidocaine 1%.
- Selection of 25, 23 and 21 gauge needles and 5 + 10mL syringe.
- Lumbar puncture needle (usually size 22G or 20G).
- Specimen tubes x 3 or 4.
- Wound dressing/plaster.
- Sharps bin.
- Sterile gloves.
- Apron/gown and mask.
- Marker pen as required.

Pre-procedure

- Explain the procedure and gain consent.
- Obtain and review the neurological history.
- Obtain medication history and in particular note any anticoagulants taken.
- Review full blood count and clotting screen results.
- Establish allergic status to skin cleansing agent, local anaesthetic etc.

Procedure

- The procedure is best performed by two people.
- Decontaminate hands.
- Check and confirm patient identity and consent.
- Position patient and identify preferred site/position for needle entry.
- The patient should be made comfortable with their head on a pillow in the lateral decubitus position with the patient's back as close to the edge of the bed as possible. The pelvis and shoulders should be at right angles to the bed with the legs drawn up toward the chin (see Fig. 16.2).
- Wash hands using surgical hand wash technique and put on apron, mask and sterile gloves.
- Apply sterile towels/ drapes and clean skin around chosen LP site. (An imaginary line drawn between the posterior superior iliac crests will bisect the vertebral column at the level of L3–L4 and facilitate identification of the chosen LP site).
- Check equipment and ensure that the stylet can easily be removed from the lumbar puncture needle.
- Infiltrate skin and subcutaneous tissues with local anaesthetic.
- Insert lumbar puncture needle perpendicular to the skin and in the direction of umbilicus.
- Advance needle slowly into the deeper tissues and ligaments.
- Once the needle is in deeper ligaments (approx 2cm) remove the stylus every few millimetres of needle advance to check for CSF flow. (The moment at which the needle passes through the dura mater and enters the subarachnoid space may be felt as a subtle 'give' or 'pop'.)
- Once CSF is obtained, perform CSF manometry as required (see below).
- Allow CSF to flow from needle into specimen tube (approx 1ml in each). Tubes should be labelled in numerical sequence from 1–4.
- Observe CSF (normal CSF is clear and colourless).
- Replace needle into stylet.
- Remove LP needle and stylet.
- Clean off any remaining skin preparation solution and apply dressing.
- Dispose of sharps and other clinical waste.
- Remove gloves and decontaminate hands.
- Label specimen bottles and send to laboratory for Gram staining, culture and sensitivity, glucose and protein levels, differential cell count and any special investigations, e.g. cytology, viral titr3 as required.
- Document episode of care.

CSF manometry

- Attach three-way tap and manometer to LP needle.
- Hold manometer vertically and open tap to allow CSF to enter manometer.
- Record pressure when CSF stops rising (normal 6–20 cm H_2O).
- Turn off three-way tap to LP needle and turn tap to allow the CSF to drain from the manometer into specimen tubes.
- Detach manometer.
- Replace stylet or obtain additional CSF sample.

Post-procedure

- Take blood sample for blood glucose level as required 📖 on p. 158. Normal CSF glucose level is approximately 60% blood glucose level.
- Make patient comfortable.
- The evidence and opinion on remaining flat post-procedure remains equivocal. As such, local policy should be followed.
- Monitor patient's condition.
- Observe wound site for signs of bleeding/seepage.
- Post-procedural headache usually develops after 24–72 hours. Treat with analgesia and adequate hydration.
- Pain at LP site due to local tissue trauma is not uncommon but usually resolves within 2 or 3 days. Give mild analgesia as required.

Practice tips

- As the patient cannot see what is happening it is important to reassure and communicate with the patient throughout the procedure.
- The site for needle entry can be marked prior to skin cleansing to aid subsequent needle insertion and positioning of sterile drapes/towels.
- Use the opportunity presented when infiltrating the skin and subcutaneous tissue with local anaesthetic to assess the depth and track to be taken by the LP needle.
- Where a cutting LP needle is used, e.g. Quinke needle, the bevel should be uppermost so that it divides, rather than cuts, the dural fibres.
- The use of atraumatic and 22 gauge needles or smaller is associated with less post-procedure headache.
- If bony resistance is felt withdraw the needle slightly and re-advance while pointing the needle slightly more cephalad.

Pitfalls

- Delaying antibiotic therapy in cases of suspected bacterial meningitis until LP is performed.
- Failing to properly remove skin cleansing agents, such as povidine lodine, that can cause skin irritation.

Table 16.3 Lumbar puncture findings

Finding	Normal	Finding and possible cause
Appearance	Clear and colourless	Cloudy/turbid—bacterial infection Uniform red blood staining—SAH<12 hours Yellow/straw colour(xanthochromia)—SAH >12 hours
Pressure	6–20cm H_2O	↑ SAH, infection
RCC	Zero	↑ SAH, trauma
WCC	<5mm³	↑ Infection
Protein	<450mg/L	↑ Infection, MS, SAH, Guillain–Barré syndrome
Glucose	2.5–4.0mmol/L	↓ bacterial infection

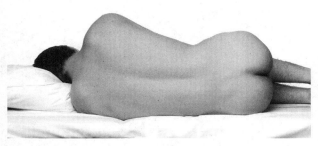

Fig. 16.2 Position of patient for lumbar puncture. Reproduced from Thomas and Monaghan (2007) *Oxford handbook of clinical examination and practical skills*. With premission from Oxford University Press.

Ear–nose–throat system

Brenda Clarke
Associate Lecturer,
Open University, UK

Frank Coffey
Consultant in Emergency Medicine, Emergency Department,
Nottingham University Hospitals NHS Trust, Associate Professor
and Consultant in Advanced Clinical Skills, School of Nursing,
Midwifery & Physiotherapy, University of Nottingham, UK

History-taking: the ear

Background
The ear has an essential role in both hearing and balance. It comprises three parts: the outer, middle, and inner ears. The patient might present with a symptom relating to the ear, such as earache or hearing loss, or the history might be part of a comprehensive health assessment.

Current health
Enquire about:
- Hearing loss—there are two types of loss: conductive and sensorineural. People can have a mixture of the two types. Patients with sensorineural loss usually have trouble understanding speech, particularly in noisy environments. There are many possible causes of hearing loss.
- Sensorineural causes include advancing age (presbyacusis), acoustic trauma (loud noise), infection, drugs, Meniere's disease, acoustic neuroma and neurological conditions such as stroke, multiple sclerosis or brain tumour. Conductive hearing loss can result from middle ear infection (glue ear in children), trauma, wax, foreign bodies, otosclerosis and perforated ear drum.
- Earache/pain in the ear (otalgia)—usually suggests a problem with the outer ear, such as otitis externa. If it is associated with symptoms of respiratory infection, the inner ear or middle ear may be affected as in otitis media.
- Fever, sore throat, cough, and nasal discharge/blockage—common in upper respiratory tract infections.
- Discharge from the ear (otorrhoea)—results from otitis externa or can be due to discharge through a perforated eardrum in otitis media or trauma.
- Tinnitus—a perceived sound that has no external stimulus, usually a ringing, whistling, or rushing noise.
- Popping sounds might originate in the temporomandibular joint.
- Vertigo—a perception that the environment is rotating or spinning. It points to a problem in the inner ear, peripheral lesions of the vestibular–cochlear (8th) cranial nerve, or lesions in the brain.
- Cerebrospinal fluid (CSF) otorrhoea—a clear, fluid discharge from the ear, which occurs in some fractures of the skull base.

Past history
- Enquire about past problems or operations involving the ears.
- Certain systemic conditions, such as measles, mumps, and meningitis, can cause deafness.

Family history
- Some ear–nose–throat (ENT) conditions have a hereditary or familial link. Ask, in particular, about deafness in the family.

Medications/allergies

- Certain medications can cause deafness, tinnitus, or problems with balance, eg erythromycin and vancomycin. Gentamicin and streptomycin can cause disabling ataxia and deafness by destruction of labyrinthine function.
- Enquire about drug allergies.
- Enquire about use of cotton buds which are significant causes of ear infection and trauma to the ear.

Social history

- Problems with hearing can impact significantly on the patient's life. Enquire about their social circumstances and support mechanisms. Hearing problems can be work-related (occupational deafness). Enquire about the nature of their work environment.

Habits

- Smoking and alcohol history.
- Enquire about illicit drug use and 'snorting'.

History-taking: the nose, sinuses, and throat

Current health

Symptoms and features to enquire about are:

- Nasal discharge (rhinorrhoea)—often associated with nasal congestion. In upper respiratory tract infections, it can be accompanied by sneezing, watery eyes, and a sore throat. Itchiness of the nose, throat, and eyes is more common with an allergic cause. Symptoms occurring when pollen levels are high or associated with specific contacts or environments suggest allergic rhinitis.
- Postnasal drip (a sensation of phlegm or mucus dripping down from the back of the nose or blocking the back of the nose or throat)—which can be caused by rhinitis, sinusitis or laryngopharangeal acid reflux.
- Nasal congestion/stuffiness or obstruction—is the congestion in both nostrils or limited to one side, suggesting a deviated septum, foreign body, or tumour?
- Loss of smell (anosmia).
- Facial pain or tenderness over the sinuses/localized headache—features of sinusitis.
- Epistaxis—bleeding from the nose.
- Sore throat—a common complaint, usually associated with a viral upper respiratory tract infection.
- Swallowing difficulties (dysphagia).
- Hoarseness—usually caused by diseases of the larynx but might result from pressure on the laryngeal nerve. It can also occur in hypothyroidism.
- Swollen glands or lumps in the neck—the cervical nodes are commonly enlarged in tonsillitis and pharnygitis. Malignancies should be considered. The thyroid is a common cause of swelling in the anterior neck.

Past history

- Enquire about previous problems or operations relating to the nose, throat, or sinuses, e.g. deviated septum from previous trauma. Bleeding disorders might contribute to epistaxis.
- Family history.
- Enquire about a family history of allergy.

Medications/drug allergies

- Certain drugs, such as oral contraceptives, can cause nasal congestion as a side-effect.
- Over-use of decongestants can make the symptoms of nasal blockage worse.

▶ Know whether a patient with epistaxis is on warfarin or any other anticoagulant therapy. Steroid inhalers, commonly used in the treatment of asthma, can cause hoarseness.

Social history

- The patient's living conditions, work, hobbies, and pets might all contribute to upper respiratory symptoms.

Habits

- Obtain a smoking and alcohol history.
- Enquire about illicit drug use and 'snorting'.

Physical assessment: the ear

Background
Examination of the ear involves assessing the external ear, including the pinna and external auditory meatus (ear canal), and tympanic membrane (eardrum) using an auroscope. More experienced personnel can use a Chiron lamp and head mirror.

Equipment
- Adequate light source.
- Auroscope.
- Variery of sizes of aural speculae.
- Headllight or Chiron lamp and mirror.
- Microscope.

Procedure
- Explain the procedure and gain consent.
- Position yourself comfortably at the same level as the patient.
- Inspect the back and front of the pinnae—look for abnormalities, such as bat ears (enlarged protruding ears), preauricular sinuses, accessory auricles (polypoid elevations of skin containg cartilage), microtia (small pinna) or anotia (absent pinna), haematomas, perichondritis, or 'cauliflower ears'.
- Look for dermatitis or eczema of the external ear and scars from previous surgery or trauma.
- Examine the mastoid area for tenderness, erythema and fluctuance. Mastoid tenderness in mastoiditis is a vital sign to elicit.
- Examine the external auditory meatus (ear canal). If only one ear is symptomatic, examine the unaffected ear first.
- Check that the auroscope is working and that the light source is bright.
- Select the appropriate size of aural speculum.
- Straighten the external auditory meatus by grasping the upper part of the pinna between the thumb and first finger and apply gentle traction in an upwards and backwards manner.
- Hold the auroscope, like a pen, in the right hand to examine the right ear and in the left hand to examine the left ear.
- Insert the auroscope gently into the patient's auditory canal, noting grimacing or complaints of pain. Observe the external auditory meatus for discharge, infection, foreign bodies, or abnormal anatomy.
- Any obstruction, such as wax or debris from otitis externa, should be removed by aural toilet or microsuction.
- The normal tympanic membrane (TM) is pearly grey and translucent and reflects light. The light reflex is in the shape of a cone and passes downwards and forwards. The handle of the malleus and the long process of the incus should be seen behind the TM. Observe the TM for the following:
  - Deviations in colour, retraction, or fullness.
  - ↑ vascularity.
  - Scars.
  - Perforation.
  - Discharge of blood, pus, or mucus.

   - Any evidence of aural polyps or cholesteatoma.
- Following examination, ensure that the patient does not feel dizzy before they mobilize.

Practice tips
- The patient might cough on insertion of the auroscope—this is a normal vagal reflex.
- Rest the little finger of your hand against the patient's face when using the auroscope. If the patient moves suddenly, your hand will also move to avoid trauma to the ear canal.
- A microscope should ideally be used when performing microsuction of the ear.
- During microsuction a patient might cough excessively or faint.

Pitfall
- Not pulling correctly on the pinna, making insertion of the auroscope difficult.

Use of a head mirror
The head mirror is a circular concave mirror with a central hole attached to a headband by an adjustable joint. A Chiron lamp is placed behind the patient's left shoulder and light is reflected from the mirror onto the patient's ear. The examiner views the patient through the central hole, which is placed close to their right eye. This method enables the examiner to have both hands free, so that one can be used to hold the aural speculum and the other used to hold an instrument, such as a probe or suction device.

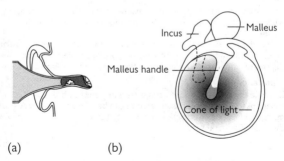

(a)   (b)

Fig. 17.1 (a) Position of the speculum in the ear; (b) diagram showing the eardrum as seen through an auroscope. Reproduced from Castledine and Close (2007) *Oxford handbook of general and adult nursing*. With permission from Oxford University Press.

Physical assessment: the nose

Background
Examination of the nose involves assessing the external, anterior, and posterior nose.

Equipment
- Adequate light source.
- Variety of sizes of Thudicum's nasal speculae.
- Headlight or Chiron lamp and mirror.
- Postnasal space mirrors.
- Suction.
- Nasendoscope.

Procedure
- Explain the procedure and gain consent.
- Position yourself comfortably at the same level as the patient.

The external nose
- Note the general condition of the skin—look for scars, deviation, or depressions.

The anterior nose
- Use a head mirror or headlight.
- Tilt the columella gently upwards to enable a good view.
- Insert a Thudicum's nasal speculum gently into the nose, with the blades held together until it is in position.
- In children, an auroscope can be used.
- Examine the septum, floor of the nose, and lateral wall.
- Note the appearance of the nasal mucosa, which should be pink and moist.
- Look for septal deformities, abnormal secretions, mucosal changes, ulcerations, foreign bodies, neoplasms, and septal haematoma in trauma.
- Check the patency of the nasal cavity by gently occluding each nostril, in turn, with a finger or thumb. Alternately, place a metal tongue depressor under the nose and note the pattern of misting.

The posterior nose
- Examine the posterior nose using a rigid or flexible fibreoptic nasendoscope; the rigid nasendoscope can be more traumatic. A small mirror (rhinoscopy mirror) can be inserted through the mouth to view the posterior nasal space.

Pitfalls

- Putting pressure on the bridge of the nose rather than the fleshy anterior part—there is a common misconception that this is the correct pressure point.
- Persisting with non-invasive measures in severe anterior bleeds or posterior bleeds if resuscitation and nasal packing (📖 on p. 620) are the priorities.

Nasal packing

Background

Nasal packing is used to control haemorrhage in epistaxis if simple measures have failed; it is also used after nasal surgery. Most epistaxes are anterior and can be controlled by anterior nasal packing. Traditional anterior nasal packing with ribbon gauze has largely been supplanted by preformed nasal tampons or epistaxis balloons. If posterior bleeding is suspected, posterior packing should be performed first using an epistaxis balloon.

Equipment

- Select the most appropriate one of the following nasal packs:
  - Merocel®—a dehydrated compressed sponge material that functions like a tampon and expands to fill the nasal cavity if soaked in blood or saline.
  - RapidRhino® —Gel-Knit™ material, containing an active haemostatic agent (carboxymethylcellulose) that creates a physiological clot within minutes.
  - Ribbon gauze impregnated with bismuth iodoform paraffin paste (BIPP).
  - Calcium sodium alginate (Kaltostat®)—an alginate-based material with haemostatic potential.
- Nasal speculum.
- Disposable apron/gloves.
- Headlight or Chiron lamp and mirror.
- Local anaesthetic spray.
- Tilley's nasal forceps.
- Vomit bowl.

Procedure

- Explain the procedure and gain consent.
- Ensure that there is intravenous (IV) access if the bleeding is severe.
- Monitor blood pressure and pulse for signs of hypovolaemic shock.
- Commence oxygen and intravenous fluids if the bleeding is severe or any signs of shock.
- Position the patient upright or leaning slightly forwards just below eye level.
- Protect the patient's clothing with a plastic apron.
- Give the patient a vomit bowl to spit out any blood that comes into the back of their mouth.
- Use a nasal speculum, headlight or Chiron lamp and head mirror to visualize the nasal cavity.
- The nasal speculum is used to spread the nares vertically, with the index finger resting on the nose for stabilization.
- Use suction to clear the nose of blood and identify any obvious bleeding points.
- Cautery should be performed if a bleeding point is identified.
- Apply a local topical anaesthetic spray to the nasal cavity.
- Insert the nasal pack of choice.

Merocel® nasal pack
- Hold the Merocel® at 45° and insert 1–2cm into the nasal cavity.
- Rotate the Merocel® into the horizontal plane and, with firm pressure, push it straight backwards into the nasal cavity until the entire tampon is inside the vestibule (warn the patient that this move will hurt).
- Secure the drawstring to the cheek.
- Assess the patient for further bleeding.
- Antibiotic cover is required if a Merocel® pack is left *in situ* for >24 hours.

Traditional anterior packing
- Grasp the BIPP ribbon gauze ~15cm from its end with the Tilley's nasal forceps.
- Place the ribbon as far back in the nasal cavity as it will go, ensuring that the free end is still protruding from the nose.
- Press the ribbon gauze in the nose down with the forceps closed.
- Grasp the ribbon 10cm from the nasal alae.
- Reposition the nasal speculum so that the lower blade holds the ribbon against the lower border of the nasal alae.
- Bring a second strip into the nose and press it down.
- Continue this process until there is no room left in the nose.
- Both ends of the ribbon gauze must protrude from the nose.
- If more than one piece of BIPP is used, they should be knotted together and the number of pieces recorded in the notes.
- Cover the nostril with a piece of gauze and secure with tape.
- Ensure that the patient is provided with a written advice sheet on actions to take in the event of further bleeding and measures to take to prevent further bleeding 📖 p. 622.
- Seek senior help if bleeding continues.
- Patients with nasal packs *in situ* must be admitted to hospital.
- Maintain good oral hygiene because nasal packing forces the patient to breathe through their mouth.
- Document the episode of care.

Practice tip
- Be prepared for the patient to faint during the procedure—ensure that a couch, oxygen, and personnel to assist are at hand.
- Monitor blood loss and consider use of colloids/plasma expanders.

Pitfall
- Being unaware of the risk of hypoxia, especially in sedated elderly patients with nasal packs—use pulse oximetry and humidified oxygen, if required.

Assisting with nasal packing

Background
Nasal packing(📖 on p. 620) is used to control haemorrhage in epistaxis. The main role of the assistant is to facilitate the procedure for the health care worker (HCW) performing the procedure and to observe and reassure the patient throughout.

Equipment
- Plastic apron for the patient and assistant, plus gloves for the assistant.
- Gown (with long sleeves), gloves and visor mask for HCW performing the procedure.
- Headlight or Chiron lamp and mirror.
- Suction, using nasal sucker.
- Local anaesthetic spray, with new nozzle.
- Thuddicum's nasal speculum.
- Tilley's nasal forceps.
- Vomit bowl and tissues.
- Nasal pack of choice—usually Merocel® or BIPP 📖 p. 620.

Procedure
- Position the patient sitting facing the HCW performing the procedure (HCW 1).
- Ensure that the patient understands the procedure and has given consent for it.
- Provide reassurance throughout the procedure.
- Give the patient a vomit bowl and tissues or swabs.
- Hold the patient's head still to prevent them from backing away.
- Ensure that there is intravenous (IV) access if the bleeding is severe.
- Perform regular blood pressure and pulse recordings and monitor blood loss. Observe the patient for signs of fainting or shock during the procedure.
- HCW 1 will pack the nose 📖 on p. 620.
- Assist HCW 1 by passing equipment and, if required, with suctioning the nose.
- At the end of the procedure, observe the patient for signs of further bleeding and monitor vital signs.
- Provide the patient with mouthwash, if required, and assist them with washing, if they have blood on them.
- Provide the patient with written and verbal instructions on how to prevent further bleeds and what to do if further bleeding occurs. They should avoid hot fluids and spicy foods and refrain from taking hot baths or showers while the pack is *in situ*. They should also avoid heavy lifting.
- Clean or replace the equipment used and leave the area clean and tidy.
- If the bleeding has been controlled, ensure that the patient is safe to travel home and has transport.
- If re-bleeding occurs before the patient leaves the department, seek senior clinical advice.

Removal of Merocel® and bismuth iodoform paraffin paste nasal packs

Background

Merocel® and BIPP nasal packs (📖 on p. 620) are commonly used for the treatment of anterior epistaxis. They are usually left *in situ* for 24–48 hours. Prophylactic antibiotics should be given if the nasal packs are present for more than 24 hours. When removing nasal packs, remember that the floor of the nose, formed by the roof of the mouth, is horizontal.

Equipment

- Disposable apron and gloves.
- Tilley's nasal forceps.
- 10mL syringe and saline (for Merocel® pack).
- Nasal speculum.
- Gauze squares.
- Vomit bowl.
- Ice.

Procedure

- Explain the procedure and gain consent.
- Ascertain what type of pack is *in situ*—if it is a BIPP pack, ascertain how many pieces of BIPP are present.
- Position the patient upright in bed or on an examination couch, with a vomit bowl at hand.
- Protect the patient's clothing with a plastic apron.
- Wear a plastic apron and gloves.
- Ask the patient to breathe through their mouth and spit out any blood in their mouth into the vomit bowl.
- Apply an ice pack to the bridge of the nose and ask the patient to hold it *in situ*.

Merocel® pack

- Instil 10mL of warm saline into the space between the pack and the wall of the nose from a syringe with no needle.
- Allow 10min before proceeding, to give time for the pack to soften.
- Grasp the pack firmly between the blades of a pair of Tilley's nasal forceps. Apply firm horizontal pressure and pull the pack out gently.

BIPP pack

- Gently pull the free end of the pack out horizontally using Tilley's nasal forceps. Allow the pack to fall into a receiver.

After pack removal

- After removal, check that there is no pack remaining by tipping the columellar up gently and shining a light into the nasal cavity. A nasal speculum can be used to aid visualization.
- In the event of bleeding, use the modified Trotter's manoeuvre 📖 p. 618.
- Record blood pressure and pulse.

- Advise the patient to remain in bed for 30min and summon assistance if further bleeding occurs. Ensure the patient knows the first aid management for epistaxis.
- Avoid putting a nasal bolster under the nose. It is better to allow air into the nose to avoid sepsis.
- Document the episode of care.

Chemical nasal cautery

Background

Cautery can be used to control an anterior nasal bleed if the bleeding point can be visualized. There are two types of cautery: chemical, using silver nitrate sticks; and electrocautery. The latter should only be attempted by trained and experienced clinicians.

Equipment

- Silver nitrate stick.
- Topical anaesthetic spray.
- Thudicum's nasal speculum.
- Headlight or Chiron lamp and mirror.
- Disposable apron and gloves.
- Eye protection.
- Vomit bowl.

Procedure

- Explain the procedure and gain consent.
- Seat the patient at the same level as yourself.
- Protect the patient's clothing with a plastic apron.
- Wear a gown (ideally with full-length sleeves), mask with visor, and gloves.
- Give the patient a vomit bowl to spit out any blood they feel at the back of their throat.
- Visualize the nasal cavity using a headlight or head mirror and Chiron lamp.
- Insert a Thudicum's nasal speculum gently into the patient's nostril.
- Using nasal suction, clear the nose of blood clots.
- Apply a topical anaesthetic spray, such as lidocaine, using a new nozzle for each patient.
- Visualize the bleeding point.
- Apply the silver nitrate stick to the area around the bleeding point on the mucosa.
- Then apply the silver nitrate stick to the bleeding point itself for ~10 seconds.
- Avoid contact between nitric acid and the skin, because it can cause a chemical burn.
- After the procedure, warn the patient that they might suffer some bleeding in the days following nasal cautery, while the mucosa heals.
- Advise the patient not to pick at the clots.
- Document the episode of care.

Practice Tip

- Following the procedure scabs can be softened with Vaseline® or Naseptin® cream. Advise the patient of this.

Pitfalls

- Septal perforation is a risk if cautery is applied to both sides of the septum at the same level and time.
- Squeezing the nares/nostrils together following cautery can cause nasal adhesions.

Assisting with nasal cautery

Background
Chemical cautery or electrocautery is used to control anterior nasal bleeds if the bleeding point can be visualized.

Equipment
- Plastic apron for the patient and assistant, plus gloves for the assistant.
- Gown (with long sleeves), visor mask, and gloves for the health care worker (HCW) performing the procedure.
- Headlight or Chiron lamp and mirror.
- Suction, using nasal sucker.
- Local anaesthetic spray, with new nozzle.
- Thudicum's nasal speculum.
- Insulated speculum for electrocautery.
- Silver nitrate sticks.
- Electrocautery unit, with forceps if required.
- Nasal packing forceps.
- Vomit bowl and tissues.
- Choice of nasal packs in case cautery fails.
- Blood pressure monitor and pulse oximeter.

Procedure
- Position the patient sitting facing the HCW performing the procedure (HCW 1).
- Ensure the patient understands the procedure and has given their consent for it.
- Provide reassurance throughout the procedure.
- Give the patient a vomit bowl and tissues or swabs.
- Hold the patient's head still, if required.
- Observe the patient for signs of fainting and shock during the procedure.
- Assist HCW 1 by passing equipment and, if required, with suctioning the nose.
- At the end of the procedure, observe the patient for signs of further bleeding and monitor vital signs.
- Provide the patient with mouthwash, if required, and assist them with washing if they have blood on them.
- Provide the patient with written and verbal instructions on how to prevent further bleeds and what to do if a further bleed occurs.
- Clean or replace the equipment used and leave the area clean and tidy.
- If the bleeding has been controlled, ensure that the patient is safe to travel home and has transport.
- If re-bleeding occurs before the patient leaves the department, seek senior clinical advice.

Removal of a foreign body from the nose

Background

Nasal foreign bodies occur predominantly in preschool children. A variety of objects, including food particles, parts of toys, paper, and disc batteries, can be implicated. Symptoms might include unilateral foul-smelling nasal discharge, unilateral nasal obstruction, unilateral vestibulitis, or epistaxis. Only attempt to remove the foreign body if it is near the nasal vestibule and easily visualized. The method of removal depends on the nature of the foreign body. Non-invasive methods should be attempted first if the patient is cooperative. The commonest method is simply is to ask the patient to blow their nose with the unaffected nostril occluded.

Equipment

- Auroscope.
- Headlight or Chiron lamp and mirror.
- Thudicum's nasal speculae.
- Tilley's nasal forceps.
- Jobson's horn probe.
- Nasal suction.

Procedure

- Explain the procedure and gain consent.
- If the patient is a child, ask a parent or colleague to hold their head.
- Visualize the foreign body in the nostril with a light, using a nasal speculum if necessary.
- Tilley's nasal forceps can be used to remove irregularly shaped or soft compressible objects.
- Solid objects can be removed using a bent probe, Bart's wax hook, or a flange-tipped suction catheter connected to suction.
- After successful removal, always carefully re-inspect the nasal cavity to check for a second foreign body and any evidence of trauma or infection.
- Care must be taken to avoid aspiration of the foreign body by pushing it further back into the posterior nasopharynx.
- If aspiration seems a significant risk, removal should take place in the operating theatre with the airway protected.
- Document the episode of care.

Practice tips

- In young children, a useful non-invasive technique is to occlude the unaffected nostril while the parent blows a puff of air into the child's mouth.
- Disc batteries present a special challenge—seek senior advice. They can cause tissue destruction on contact with moisture in the nasal cavity. Right-angle hooks are the method of choice for these.

Pitfalls

- Missing foreign bodies because of inadequate examination.
- Pushing a foreign body posteriorly, leading to aspiration.
- Failing to re-inspect the nasal canal following removal of a foreign body.
- Failing to refer or seek senior help early for unsuccessful removal attempts or in special circumstances, such as disc batteries.

Removal of a foreign body from the ear

Background

Patients commonly present with foreign bodies in their ears. Symptoms include pain, discharge, and deafness. The method of removal depends on the nature of the foreign body. Deeply embedded foreign bodies might need to be removed under general anaesthetic.

Equipment

- Auroscope.
- Aural speculae of appropriate sizes.
- Headlight or Chiron lamp and mirror.
- Wax hook.
- Crocodile forceps.
- Microsuction.

Procedure

- Explain the procedure and gain consent.
- Examine the ear with an auroscope to visualize the foreign body.
- Select an appropriate size of speculum.
- A headlight or Chiron lamp and head mirror enables the examiner to have both hands free.
- Cotton wool or soft objects can be removed using crocodile forceps.
- For bead-shaped objects, pass a Bart's wax hook beyond the foreign body and gently pull out.
- Insects can be drowned by filling the ear canal with olive oil; they can then be removed by suctioning or syringing.
- Stop the procedure if it is causing trauma.
- Document the episode of care.

Practice tips

- If a headlight or Chiron lamp and mirror are unavailable, have an assistant to pull back the pinna to open the ear canal.
- Entonox might be prescribed to children to assist with removal. This should not be used if the ear drum is perforated.
- Patients can be distressed by the noise of an insect in the ear canal. If there is a delay before seeing the patient, olive oil should be inserted on arrival to drown the insect before definitive assessment and management.

Pitfalls

- Attempting to remove insects with crocodile forceps, which might result in dismemberment of the insect.
- Syringing vegetable matter, such as peas, beans, or nuts, causing them to swell.
- Using crocodile forceps on round objects, pushing them further into the ear canal.
- Not removing disc batteries from ears promptly. If left *in situ* they can cause tissue damage.
- Using medical glue to try and remove objects. This is not to be recommended.

- Failing to refer on or seek senior help early for unsuccessful removal of an object or in special circumstances, such as disc batteries. Persistence in removal attempts causes ↓ patient cooperation and ↑ risk of trauma.
- Failing to recheck the ear canal after removal of a foreign body, which can lead to missed or retained foreign bodies.

Ophthalmology

Keith Knox
Charge Nurse, Eye Casualty Department, Head and Neck
Directorate, Nottingham University Hospitals NHS Trust, UK

History-taking

Background

Systematic history-taking helps to identify symptoms on which a diagnosis, or list of potential diagnoses, can be made. Eye problems could be the manifestation of a systemic disease. Obtaining information regarding past or existing eye and systemic conditions can be crucial in making a correct diagnosis. A careful history can identify aspects of the examination that require special attention or additional investigations. The history should be holistic.

Presenting complaint

- Assess for severe pain due to:
  - Corneal abrasions.
  - Foreign bodies.
  - Sclerosis.
  - Acute glaucoma.
- Assess for less severe pain due to:
  - Conjunctivitis (inflammation of the conjunctive which is the delicate transparent membrane which lines the eyelids and the eyeball).
  - Keratoconjunctivitis (dryness of the cornea).
  - Optic neuritis (inflammation of the optic nerve).
  - Postoperative procedures.
  - Trigeminal neuralgia.
  - Referred pain.
  - Migraine and tension headaches.
  - Post laser treatment
  - Shingles.
- Assess for irritation and sensitivity and observe for:
  - Foreign body sensation.
  - Crusty debris.
  - Redness.
  - Entropion (inversion of the eyelid resulting in the lashes being in contact with the eyeball).
- Take details of any trauma, which can indicate the type of injury sustained and investigations needed, e.g. X-ray in hammer and chisel injury to exclude intraocular foreign body.
- Assess for presenting visual symptoms—see Box 18.1.
- Assess if symptoms are sudden (e.g. central retina artery occlusion or retinal detachment) or slow (e.g. cataract).
- Ask how visual symptoms impact on working, driving, reading, and watching TV.

Ocular history

Ask about:
- Contact lens wear.
- Previous ophthalmology care.
- Previous eye surgery.
- Childhood squint (amblyopia).

Medical history

Ask about:
- Diabetes mellitus—associated with diabetic retinopathy.
- Ankylosing spondylitis—associated with acute anterior ueveitis.
- Rheumatoid arthritis—associated with keratoconjunctivitis.
- Sarcoidosis—associated with ueveitis.
- Renal disease and hypertension—associated with retinal vein occlusion and papilloedema.
- Hyperthyroidism—associated with protrusion of the eyes (proptosis/ exophthalmos).
- Multiple sclerosis—associated with optic neuritis.

Drug history

Ask about:
- Steroids—long-term use can be associated with cataracts, eye infections and glaucoma.
- Chloroquine—associated with blurred vision.
- Anticoagulants—associated with blurred vision.
- Sulfonamides—associated with yellow eyes.
- Antidepressants—associated with blurred vision.
- Side-effects from previous eye drop medication.
- Previous drug allergies.

Family history

Check for:
- Glaucoma.
- Retinal disease.
- Strabismus (squint).
- Cataract.
- Tumour.
- Autoimmune disease.

Practice tip
- Previous eye surgery might indicate a future problem or place the patient at a greater risk of infection.

Box 18.1 Visual symptoms: details to establish

Type of disturbance
Previous experience of similar symptoms
Monocular or binocular
Speed of onset
If patient is complaining of visual loss, the presence and type of visual field loss
Associated symptoms—e.g. floaters, blurred vision, abnormal flashes of light, rainbow colours/halos around bright lights, irritation, discharge, changes in vision, dark spots in the visual field or distortion of straight lines
Photophobia (difficulty in adapting from dark to light conditions)
Effect on daily living
Specific worries

The ophthalmic examination

Background

History-taking should be followed by a systematic assessment of the visual system and an eye examination using basic equipment (Box 18.2, Fig. 18.1). This identifies signs that, in addition to the patient's symptoms, will help determine the diagnosis.

A fundamental clinical examination includes:

- Assessment of facial symmetry.
- The outer eye.
- The inner eye.
- Colour sensitivity.
- Visual acuity.
- Visual fields to confrontation.

Procedure

Facial asymmetry

With the patient relaxed and looking straight ahead compare the:

- Features of the face around each eye—are they the same?
- Position of the eyelids of each eye—are they the same?
- Position of each eye on the patient's face —are they the same?

Examination of the outer eye

With the patient relaxed and looking straight ahead observe for:

- Lid swelling, inflammation, bruising, or eyelash damage.
- Redness and discharge.
- Corneal clarity, trauma, or ulceration.

Examination of the inner eye

With the patient relaxed and looking straight ahead observe:

- The anterior chamber for clarity, hypopyon (accumulation of pus), and hyphaema (small bleed).
- Pupil responses—shape, symmetry, response to light, and accommodation.
- Red reflex (Bruckner test) is undertaken by asking the patient to sit in a dimly lit room, and hold the ophthalmoscope about two-thirds of an arm's length away. Ask the patient to look at the light of the ophthalmoscope and turn the dial until you see the reflex.
- Optic disc, macula, and peripheral retina (detailed examination would require an ophthalmologist).

Colour sensitivity

- The basic method of assessing colour sensitivity is to ask the patient to look at a red target, e.g. a pen top, with one eye closed and then repeat the process with the other eye closed. Ask if the redness is the same in both eyes or does the redness look paler in one eye compared with the other?

Eye movement

- Ask the patient to look in the 9 directions of gaze (Box 18.2) and observe both eyes
- Observe for restricted movement in either eye.

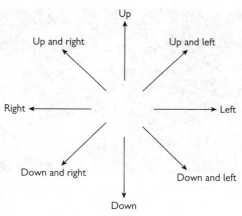

Fig. 18.1 Primary directions of gaze.

Practice tip

- Examination of the cornea should always include the use of topical fluorescein sodium (2%; drops or impregnated strip) used in conjunction with blue light.

Box 18.2 Basic equipment

1. Ophthalmoscope
2. Occluder with a pinhole cover
3. Pen torch, with blue filter for pen torch if ophthalmoscope does not contain blue filter
4. Basic occluder
5. Cotton buds
6. Sterile saline drops (used to moisten cotton bud when removing debris from the eye)
7. Sterile fluorescein drops to stain the cornea
8. Fluorescein-impregnated strips used to stain the cornea

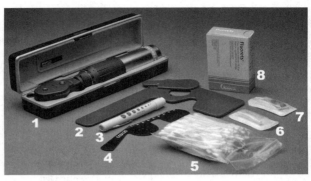

Fig. 18.2 Basic equipment.

Assessing visual acuity

Background

Visual acuity can be measured using a standard Snellen's chart (Fig. 18.3). The Snellen's chart has nine rows of letters, each with a number beneath it. The number beneath each row indicates the distance, in metres, at which a patient with no refractive error should be able to read that row. If, for example, a person undergoing the test can read only the top line, this would be recorded as 6/60. This indicates that the patient can only read at 6m what someone with no refractive error would be able to read at 60m. Hence, the top number (6) refers to the distance from the chart, whereas the bottom number refers to the row of letters read.

Equipment
- Snellen's chart.
- Eye occluder.

Procedure
- Explain the procedure and gain consent.
- Stand or sit the patient 6m from the chart.
- Cover the patient's left eye using the occluder and ask the patient to read from the chart, beginning with the top letter.
- Note the number above the lowest row of letters that the patient can read and record the vision for that eye as 6 over that number—e.g. 6/9.
- If the patient gets more than 2 letters wrong, assume they can only read the line above.
- Repeat the exercise, covering the right eye.
- Document the episode of care.

Practice tips
- If the patient wears distance glasses, these should be worn.
- If the room is small, a reverse chart can be used with a mirror and the patient situated 3m from the mirror.
- The chart should be illuminated.
- If the patient can only read so far down the chart, an occluder with pinholes can be placed in front of the eye being tested, to see whether this improves vision.
- If the patient cannot read the chart at 6m, bring them closer to the chart—either 3m then 1m. Vision should then be recorded as 3/x or 1/x.
- If no letters can be read at 1m, hold your fingers ~30cm from the eye and ask the patient to count them. If the patient is successful, this would be recorded as 'count fingers' (CF-1m).
- If fingers cannot be counted but hand movements can be detected, this would be recorded as 'hand movements' (HM).
- If the patient cannot see hand movements, a light should be shone into the eye (using a pen torch). Depending on the outcome, this would be recorded as 'perception of light' (PL) or 'no perception of light' (NPL).
- If the patient is experiencing difficulties in reading, check their literacy.

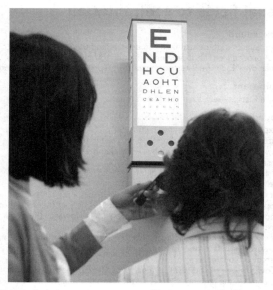

Fig. 18.3 Snellen's chart.

Visual fields to confrontation

Background

Large defects of the visual field can be detected using a simple confrontational procedure. The examiner compares the patient's visual fields with his/her own. Each eye is tested separately, so one eye must be covered.

Equipment

- A red target—e.g. a hat pin or pen top.

Procedure

- Explain the procedure and gain consent.
- Sit at the same level and directly opposite the patient, 1m apart.
- Ask the patient to cover one eye with a hand.
- Instruct the patient to look directly at you.
- Ask the patient, 'Can you see all of my face?'—this detects gross defects.
- In the absence of gross defects, use a target (e.g. a red hat pin or pen top) or use your fingers (Figs 18.4 and 18.5)—instruct the patient to look directly at your corresponding eye and not towards the target you are holding.
- Bring the target or your fingers inwards, from your peripheral vision towards your face, and ask the patient to say when they can see the target or your fingers.
- Covering one of your eyes, compare your field of vision with the patient's—the patient's right eye with your left eye and then the patient's left eye with your right eye.
- Record visual fields as the patient sees them (Fig. 18.6).
- Document the episode of care.

Practice tip

- Move the target slowly, equidistant between you and the patient.

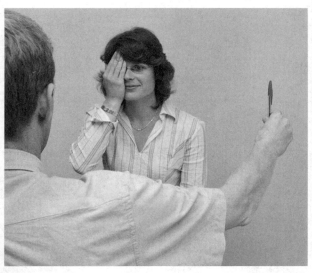

Fig. 18.4 Examination using a red target.

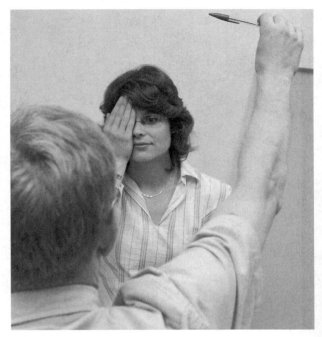

Fig. 18.5 Examination using peripheral finger movements.

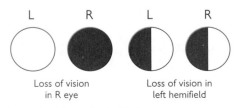

L   R   L   R

Loss of vision
in R eye

Loss of vision in
left hemifield

Fig. 18.6 An example of drawing the visual fields.

Detecting strabismus (squints)

Background
One method of detecting the presence of a squint is to observe the corneal light reflex, i.e. light reflected by the cornea from a light source directed at the eye. 'Cover tests' are used to detect the presence of a squint or manifest squint.

Equipment
- Pen torch.
- Occluder.

Procedure

Corneal Hirschberg reflection test—corneal reflex
- Explain the procedure and gain consent.
- Sit at the same level and directly opposite the patient.
- Instruct the patient to look straight ahead into the distance.
- Using a pen torch at an arm's length, shine light in front of their eyes aiming towards the bridge of their nose.
- Observe where the reflection of the pen torch lies with respect to the cornea (corneal reflex position).
- Document the episode of care.

Practice tips
- The corneal reflex position should be central bilaterally.
- A squint might be present if the corneal reflex position lies at the inner margin of the pupil (exotropia) or if it lies at the outer margin (esotropia).

Procedure

Cover–uncover test—to detect a squint
- Explain the procedure and gain consent.
- Observe whether one eye is favoured for fixation by looking for facial asymmetry—craniofacial abnormalities or head tilt.
- Using a target, ask the patient to fixate on it.
- For a few seconds, occlude the eye that seems to be fixating.
- While you cover the eye, watch the uncovered eye to see whether it moves to take up fixation.
- Remove the occluder and see whether the original eye again takes over fixation. If so, it is the preferred eye for fixating and the other eye has a squint.
- Do this for near (30cm) and distance (6m) vision.
- Movement of the eye inwards confirms exotropia and outwards confirms esotropia.
- Document the episode of care.

Procedure

Alternate cover test—to detect a latent squint

- Explain the procedure and gain consent.
- Ask the patient to fixate on a target held in front of them.
- Cover one eye and then quickly move the cover to the other eye.
- Repeat this quickly several times.
- Observe the movement of the occluded eye while it is uncovered.
- If it moves inwards to fix on the target, the patient has a latent exophria.
- If it moves outwards to fix on the target, the patient has a latent esophoria.
- Do this for near (30cm) and distance (6m) vision.
- Document the episode of care.

Using the direct ophthalmoscope

Background

The light source is directed into the patient's eye through a mirror and focused by a series of lenses. The illuminated retina is viewed through a sight hole in the mirror. A rotating disc of lenses can be rotated to account for the observer's and patient's refractive errors (Fig. 18.7). The image produced has a field of view of ~6°.

Equipment

- Ophthalmoscope.

Procedure

- Explain the procedure and gain consent.
- Select lens at '0' to start.
- Ensure there are no patterned or coloured filters in the aperture.
- Decontaminate your hands.
- Switch the room lights off or dim them.
- Ask the patient to fix on a distance target—to the left when you examine the right eye and vice versa.
- Examine the patient's right eye with your own right eye whilst trying to keep your left eye open.
- Place your hand on the patient's forehead so that your fingers are splayed but your thumb is on the right upper lid.
- Stand at arm's length from the patient, to the side of the eye you are examining and looking through the sight hole of the ophthalmoscope, while directing the light towards the pupil to view the red reflex.
- Follow this reflex until your forehead rests on your thumb.
- While you move towards the patient, rotate through the lenses, as necessary, to maintain focus.
- When the retinal details are clear, examine the optic disc (use the disc as a navigation aid).
- Examine the blood vessels from the disc.
- Ask the patient to look up, down, right, and left, to examine the retina.
- Finally, ask the patient to look directly into the light beam, to examine the macula and fovea.
- Document the episode of care.

Practice tips

- If the patient wears glasses remove them before the procedure or if they wear contact lenses, leave them on.
- Examine the right eye first (this helps when documenting findings).
- Ensure you are very close to the patient, almost cheek to cheek.

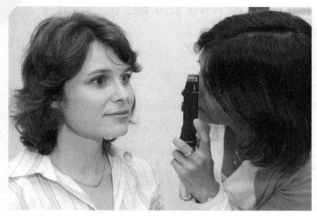

Fig. 18.7 Using the ophthalmoscope.

Removal of hard and gas permeable contact lenses

Equipment
- Container.
- Sterile water.

Procedure
- Explain the procedure and gain consent.
- Decontaminate your hands.
- Using one hand, open the patient's eyelids wide and beyond the margin of the contact lens.
- Using the index finger of the other hand, apply gentle pressure temporarily at the outer canthus, to pull the lids taught.
- Ask the patient to blink and be ready to catch the lens as the patient's blinking action forces the lens off the cornea.

Removal of soft contact lenses

Equipment
- Container.
- Sterile water.

Procedure
- Explain the procedure and gain consent
- Decontaminate hands
- Using one hand, open the patient's eyelids wide and ask the patient to look towards their nose.
- Using the index finger of your other hand, gently make contact with the edge of the lens at the edge of the cornea, carefully sliding the lens temporally a few millimetres.
- Gently pinch the part of the lens you have moved upwards between thumb and forefinger and lift it from the eye.

Insertion of contact lenses

Procedure
- Explain the procedure and gain consent.
- Decontaminate your hands.
- Place the lens, with the cup facing upwards, on your index finger.
- Using the index finger of your other hand, lift up the patient's upper lid and ask the patient to look straight ahead.
- Pull down the patient's lower lid using the middle finger next to your index finger with the lens on it.
- Now, with the lids open and the patient looking straight ahead, bring the lens slowly towards the cornea until contact is made (Fig. 18.8).
- Ask the patient to close the eye and the lens will centre itself.

Practice tip
- Always remove lenses when using fluorescein dye.

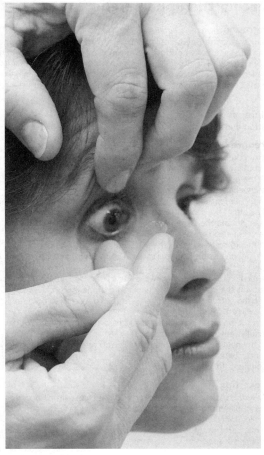

Fig. 18.8 Insertion of contact lens.

Everting the upper eyelid

Background

Everting the upper eyelid should form part of any examination of a patient with a red eye. It is also performed to remove foregin bodies from under the upper eyelid. The procedure can be performed using a slit lamp, with the patient sitting in front of you. If you are not using a slit lamp, the procedure is best performed by standing behind the patient with the patient seated.

Equipment

• Cotton-bud applicator.

Procedure

• Explain the procedure and gain consent.
• Decontaminate your hands.
• Ask the patient to sit on a chair.
• Stand behind the patient, facing their back.
• Ask the patient to tip their head backwards slightly and look down.
• Take hold of the patient's eyelashes of the upper lid between the forefinger and the thumb of your left hand (if you are right-handed, and vice versa if you are left-handed).
• Pull the lid down towards the cheek so that it is taut.
• Holding the cotton-bud applicator in your other hand, use one end to apply pressure to the lid above the tarsal plate.
• Lift the lid upwards and backwards, as if over the end of the cotton bud, removing the cotton bud when eversion of the lid is achieved.
• Place the cotton bud on the lashes at the lid margin, to hold the lid in the everted position (Fig. 18.9).
• Examine the tarsal conjunctiva for signs of injury and if appropriate carefully remove any foreign body.
• Ask the patient to look upwards while you release the lid. The lid will then flip back into position.
• Document the episode of care.

Practice tips

• Advise the patient that the procedure could feel a little uncomfortable.
• Ask the patient to keep looking down until you have completed your examination.
• Do not perform this procedure if a penetrating injury or corneal thinning is suspected.

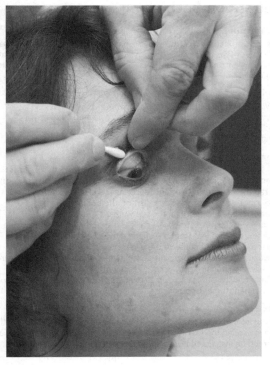

Fig. 18.9 Everting the upper eyelid.

Hot spoon bathing

Background

This is a procedure you can advise patients to perform if they have a chalazion or stye in an eyelid. The procedure can help inflammatory material to discharge from the affected area, bringing relief and early resolution of the problem.

Equipment

- Wooden or hard plastic cooking spoon.
- Eye pads and bandage (or clean handkerchief and bandage).
- Adhesive tape.
- Large basin.

Procedure

- Explain the procedure and gain consent.
- Pad the cup end of the spoon with the eye pads or handkerchief and wrap the bandage around this, securing it with the adhesive tape.
- Pour hot water into the basin (just off the boil).
- Soak the padded spoon in the hot water.
- Leaning slightly over the bowl, raise the spoon from the water and hold it a few centimetres from the affected eye, with the eyelids closed (so that the heat can be felt on the eyelids) to avoid scalding.
- Instruct the patient not to press the heated padded spoon on their lids.
- While the padding cools, soak it again in the hot water.
- Carry out the procedure for 20 minutes twice or three times daily.
- Document the episode of care.

Practice tip

- If the lesion begins to discharge, the patient can be advised to gently press around the lesion to encourage discharge. However, the patient should be instructed not to squeeze the lesion.

Removal of an artificial eye

Background

The prosthetic eye is fitted following either enucleation or evisceration, during which the patient's eyelids remain unaffected. An artificial eye must be removed for certain reasons, as follows:

- To enable healing.
- To treat infection.
- To remove debris or foreign bodies.
- Before surgery, to prevent loss.
- To assess false pupil.
- According to the patient's preference.

Equipment

- Container to place the prosthesis in.

Removal of the prosthesis

- Explain the procedure and gain consent.
- Decontaminate your hands.
- Ask the patient to look straight ahead.
- Gently pull down the lower lid so that you can see the edge of the prosthetic eye.
- Ask the patient to look upwards.
- Place a fingertip just beneath the bottom edge of the prosthesis, which you will now be able to see.
- Lever the eye forwards and it will fall from the socket.
- Document the episode of care.

Practice tip

- Be prepared to catch the prosthesis.

Insertion of an artificial eye

Procedure
- Explain the procedure and gain consent.
- Decontaminate your hands.
- Lift up the upper lid using one hand.
- Hold the prosthesis the correct way round (with the most pointed side towards the nose).
- Gently push the eye into the top of the socket beneath the upper lid (Fig. 18.10).
- Transfer the finger holding the upper lid to the prosthesis, to stop it from falling from the socket (if necessary).
- Using your other hand, pull down the lower lid and the bottom edge of the prosthesis will slip inside the bottom lid.
- Check that the prosthesis is positioned correctly and that the patient has no discomfort.
- Document the episode of care.

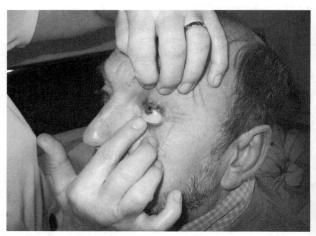

Fig. 18.10 Insertion of a prosthetic eye.

Haematology

Martyn Bradbury
Clinical Skills Network Lead, School of Nursing and
Community Studies, Faculty of Health and Social Work,
University of Plymouth, UK

Blood transfusion guidance based on McClelland D.B.L. (Ed) (2007) Handbook of
Transfusion Medicine, 4th edition, HMSO, London.

Sample collection

Background

Pre-transfusion compatibility testing is the first step in the transfusion process and the point at which patient and pre-transfusion checks begin. Before sample collection, a full explanation of the blood-transfusion process, including benefits and potential risks, should be given to the patient. A record of this should also be made in the patient's case notes.

Equipment

- Blood-transfusion request form.
- Vacuum tube, e.g. Vacutainer® and needle/holder.
- Tourniquet.
- Sharps bin.
- 2% chlorhexidine gluconate in 70% isopropyl alcohol skin-cleaning solution.
- Patient record/case notes.
- Non-sterile gloves.

Procedure

- Decontaminate your hands.
- Explain the procedure and gain consent.
- Enter a record of the discussion in the patient's case notes.
- Complete the request form, including:
  - Patient's full name.
  - Date of birth.
  - Gender.
  - Patient identification/hospital number.
  - Location of the patient.
  - Number and type of blood products required.
  - Any special requirements—e.g. gamma irradiation.
  - Any past obstetric history.
  - Any previous transfusion history.
  - Diagnosis and reason for the transfusion.
  - Date and time the blood component is required.
  - Signature of the health care worker (HCW) requesting the test.
- If possible, ask the patient to verify their identity by stating:
  - Full name.
  - Date of birth.
- Confirm the patient's identity by checking the patient's name band against the hospital record/request form, and confirm:
  - Full name.
  - Date of birth.
  - Patient identification/hospital number.
- Obtain a venous blood sample 📖 on p. 160.
- Discard the sharps using clinical waste disposal.
- Make the patient comfortable.

Label the sample bottle, including:
  • Patient's full name.
  • Date of birth.
  • Patient identification/hospital number.
  • Gender.
  • Date and time of sample collection.
  • Signature of the HCW obtaining the sample.
• Place the sample in a specimen bag with the request form.
• Transport the sample to the blood laboratory.
• Decontaminate your hands.
• Document episode of care.

Practice tips

• The sample should be labelled at the patient's bedside once the sample has been collected.
• Pre-printed labels should not be used to label specimens.
• If the identity of a patient cannot be established, e.g. a patient with multiple trauma in the emergency department, the patient's gender and emergency identification number should be used.
• Blood sampling is an aseptic procedure and, as such, sterile gloves might be used as part of the sampling procedure in some clinical areas.
• If an alcohol-impregnated swab is used as the method of skin cleansing, the swab should be applied to the skin for a minimum of 30sec and allowed to dry fully before the blood sample is taken.

Pitfalls

• Obtaining venous blood samples from more than one patient at a time.
• Labelling blood sample bottles other than at the patient's bedside.

Further reading

www.transfusionguidelines.org.uk

www.learnbloodtransfusion.org.uk

Collection of blood from storage

Background

This procedure should only be carried out by suitably trained staff and according to local policy. Blood should not be removed from storage until the patient is ready for the transfusion and only one unit should normally be removed at a time. Consent for the transfusion should be verified before removal of the blood component from the blood-transfusion refrigerator.

Equipment

- Prescription chart.
- Collection slip or other documentation (according to local policy).
- Transportation box/carrier (according to local policy).

Procedure

- Explain the procedure to the patient (if the patient is conscious) and gain consent for the transfusion.
- Check and confirm the prescription.
- The staff member collecting the blood component should then locate the required blood product in the storage refrigerator and verify the following details from the collection slip against the blood component:
  - Patient's full name.
  - Date of birth.
  - Gender.
  - Patient identification/hospital number.
- Remove the unit from storage and complete the register, including:
  - Patient's identification number.
  - Donation number of the blood component removed.
  - Name of the staff member removing the blood component.
  - Date and time of removal.
- Transport the unit to the ward/clinical area for transfusion.
- The HCW receiving the blood on the ward should sign a collection slip to acknowledge receipt of the blood component.

Practice tips

- Ensure a patent venous cannula is in situ before removing the blood component from storage.
- The intravenous cannula should be secured with a clear dressing, to enable direct observation.
- Blood collection slips should be retained for a minimum of 1 month post-transfusion.
- Staff removing blood from storage should receive training and be assessed as competent in blood-transfusion processes every 3 years.

Pitfalls

- Removing blood product from storage before it is required.
- Storing blood in ward refrigerator prior to use.
- Delegating collection of blood products to HCWs who have not received appropriate training.

Further reading

www.transfusionguidelines.org.uk

www.learnbloodtransfusion.org.uk

Pre-transfusion checks

Background

Because this is the last stage in the component-checking procedure, it is the most crucial step in preventing the transfusion of ABO-incompatible blood. Local policy will dictate whether checking by a single person or two people is required. Final checks should always be made at the patient's bedside. Strict asepsis should be observed during the setting-up procedure.

Equipment

- Prescription chart.
- Blood component for transfusion.
- Infusion pump, as appropriate.
- Blood warmer, as required.
- Compatible blood administration set, with integral 170/200 micron micro-aggregate filter.
- Non-sterile gloves.

Procedure

- Confirm the patient understands the procedure and reaffirm consent.
- Check and confirm the prescription.
- Decontaminate your hands.
- Obtain and record the patient's temperature, pulse, blood pressure, and respiratory rate on p. 42.
- Make a visual inspection of the blood component for signs of the following:
  - Discolouration and haemolysis.
  - Leakage.
  - Clumping of cells.
  - Presence of gas bubbles.
- If possible, ask the patient to verify their identity by asking them to state their:
  - Full name.
  - Date of birth.
- Check and confirm the details on the patient's identity band against the prescription and blood component, and verify:
  - Patient's full name.
  - Date of birth.
  - Patient identification/hospital number.
  - Blood component and any special requirements, according to the prescription.
  - Details on the blood component are the same as those on the identity band.
- Check the compatibility label/tag against the label on the blood component and ensure there is an exact match for the following:
  - Blood group.
  - Unique donation number.
- Ensure the patient is comfortable and expose the cannulation site.
- Decontaminate your hands.
- Put on gloves.
- Attach the administration set to the blood component and prime the infusion line on p. 172.

- Attach the infusion line to the intravenous cannula 📖 on p. 176.
- Regulate the infusion rate.
- Ask the patient to report any new symptoms.
- Record the date and start time of the transfusion in the patient's case notes.
- Record the administration on the prescription chart.
- Ensure the call bell is within reach.
- Dispose of equipment using clinical waste disposal.
- Wash your hands.
- Record the administration and document the episode of care.
- Monitor the response to the transfusion.

Blood warmers

The routine use of blood warmers is usually unnecessary. However, blood warming is indicated in patients who have cold agglutinins, are hypothermic, undergoing surgery, or receiving >100mL of blood/minute.

Note

When using a blood warmer follow the the the equipment manufacturer's instructions regarding use.

Practice tips

- The patient's case notes and blood-compatibility form should not be used as part of the immediate pre-transfusion checking process.
- Infusion lines can be primed with 0.9% sodium chloride solution before the administration of blood, although this is not a necessity.
- Infusion of red blood cells should be completed within 4 hours of their removal from storage.
- Infusion of platelets should be completed within 30 minutes of their removal from storage.
- Observations associated with blood transfusion should ideally be recorded separately from routine observations.
- Transfusion should only be undertaken when the patient can be observed and where resuscitation facilities are available.
- Patients receiving blood-component therapy on a regular basis might be issued with a photo-identification card, which can be used as part of the pre-transfusion checking process in place of the name band.
- Staff involved in the transfusion of blood components should receive training and be assessed as competent in blood-transfusion processes every 3 years.

Pitfalls

- Transfusing blood through an IV line that contains glucose solution.
- Adding drugs to a blood component or the administration line.
- Transfusing blood during the night or out of normal hours.
- Warming blood by using improvised methods e.g. radiator or microwave.

Transfusion monitoring

Background
Monitoring and observation of the patient during the transfusion process is essential to ensure the safe transfusion of blood components. An adverse reaction to the transfusion of blood components is a potentially serious sequelae and might occur at any time during the transfusion process. However, acute transfusion reactions usually occur within the first 15min of the transfusion.

Equipment
- Observation chart.
- Thermometer.
- Sphygmomanometer and stethoscope (as required).
- Watch with a second hand.

Procedure
- Obtain and record the patient's temperature, pulse, blood pressure, and respiratory rate after 15min of transfusion 📖 on p. 42.
- Observe the cannula site for early signs of extravasation and inflammation.
- Ensure the patient is comfortable and monitor for new symptoms and signs e.g.:
  - Headache.
  - Palpitations.
  - Shortness of breath.
  - Dizziness.
  - Pruritus.
  - Nausea and vomiting.
  - Pain.
  - Hypotension.
  - Rash.
  - Oliguria.
- Monitor the infusion rate.

Practice tips
- The frequency of observation, after the first set of observations at 15min, is determined by local policy. However, if there is any change in the patient's condition, the temperature, pulse, blood pressure, and respiratory rate must be recorded immediately.
- Transfusion administration sets should be changed at the end of the transfusion or every 12 hours if the patient is receiving multiple transfusions.
- Each new unit of blood component should be treated as if it is the first and all pre-transfusion processes should be followed.
- Observations associated with the blood transfusion should be recorded separately from routine observations.

Pitfall
• Failing to monitor the patient closely enough during the first 15min of blood transfusion.

Further reading
www.transfusionguidelines.org.uk

www.learnbloodtransfusion.org.uk

Managing acute transfusion reactions

Background

Complications associated with the transfusion of blood components might or might not have an immune origin and can occur immediately or after a time delay (Table 19.1). An acute haemolytic reaction is, perhaps, the most severe and immediate of the acute reactions.

Table 19.1 Adverse transfusion events

	Immune	Non-immune
Immediate	Acute haemolytic reaction (AHR) Anaphylaxis Febrile reactions Allergic reactions Transfusion-related acute lung injury (TRALI)	Bacteraemia/septic reaction Circulatory overload
Delayed	Delayed haemolytic reaction Post-transfusion purpura	Transmission of infection Haemosiderosis

Procedure

If an acute transfusion reaction is suspected, the following actions should be performed as a matter of urgency:

- Stop the transfusion.
- Seek urgent medical/senior advice.
- Obtain and record the patient's temperature, pulse, blood pressure, respiratory rate on p. 42 and oxygen saturation (SpO_2) on p. 302.
- Monitor the patient's urine for the presence of haemoglobinuria.
- Ensure a health care worker (HCW) remains with the patient.
- Use the decision-making tree to decide on the appropriate treatment/ action (Fig. 19.1).
- Maintain accurate and contemporaneous records.
- Retain all blood components and documentation.
- Report the reaction using local reporting procedures.
- Report nationally to Serious Adverse Blood Reactions and Events (SABRE).

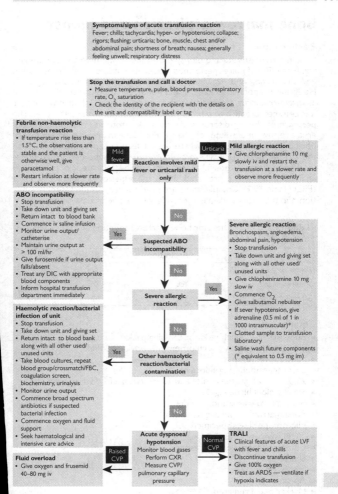

Symptoms/signs of acute transfusion reaction
Fever; chills; tachycardia; hyper- or hypotension; collapse; rigors; flushing; urticaria; bone, muscle, chest and/or abdominal pain; shortness of breath; nausea; generally feeling unwell; respiratory distress

Stop the transfusion and call a doctor
- Measure temperature, pulse, blood pressure, respiratory rate, O_2 saturation
- Check the identity of the recipient with the details on the unit and compatibility label or tag

Reaction involves mild fever or urticarial rash only

Mild fever →

Febrile non-haemolytic transfusion reaction
- If temperature rise less than 1.5°C, the observations are stable and the patient is otherwise well, give paracetamol
- Restart infusion at slower rate and observe more frequently

Urticaria →

Mild allergic reaction
- Give chlorphenamine 10 mg slowly iv and restart the transfusion at a slower rate and observe more frequently

No ↓

Suspected ABO incompatibility

Yes →

ABO incompatibility
- Stop transfusion
- Take down unit and giving set
- Return intact to blood bank
- Commence iv saline infusion
- Monitor urine output/catheterise
- Maintain urine output at > 100 ml/hr
- Give furosemide if urine output falls/absent
- Treat any DIC with appropriate blood components
- Inform hospital transfusion department immediately

No ↓

Severe allergic reaction

Yes →

Severe allergic reaction
Bronchospasm, angioedema, abdominal pain, hypotension
- Stop transfusion
- Take down unit and giving set along with all other used/unused units
- Give chlorpheniramine 10 mg slow iv
- Commence O_2
- Give salbutamol nebuliser
- If sever hypotension, give adrenaline (0.5 ml of 1 in 1000 intramuscular)*
- Clotted sample to transfusion laboratory
- Saline wash future components
(* equivalent to 0.5 mg im)

No ↓

Other haemolytic reaction/bacterial contamination

Yes →

Haemolytic reaction/bacterial infection of unit
- Stop transfusion
- Take down unit and giving set
- Return intact to blood bank along with all other used/unused units
- Take blood cultures, repeat blood group/crossmatch/FBC, coagulation screen, biochemistry, urinalysis
- Monitor urine output
- Commence broad spectrum antibiotics if suspected bacterial infection
- Commence oxygen and fluid support
- Seek haematological and intensive care advice

No ↓

Acute dyspnoea/hypotension
Monitor blood gases
Perform CXR
Measure CVP/pulmonary capillary pressure

Raised CVP →

Fluid overload
- Give oxygen and frusemid 40–80 mg iv

Normal CVP →

TRALI
- Clinical features of acute LVF with fever and chills
- Discontinue transfusion
- Give 100% oxygen
- Treat as ARDS — ventilate if hypoxia indicates

Fig. 19.1 Acute transfusion reactions: a management algorithm. Reproduced from the *Handbook of transfusion Medicine*, with permission.

Bone marrow aspiration and biopsy

Background

Bone marrow aspirate and biopsy (also called bone marrow aspirate and trephine—BMAT) are performed to enable microscopic investigation and the staging and evaluation of haematopoietic conditions e.g. non-Hodgkin's lymphoma, leukaemia, and non haematopoietic conditions such as myelotoxic drug and radiation damage and pyrexia of unknown origin. It is common practice to perform both procedures at the same time. The presence of clotting disorders and thrombocytopenia is variously considered a relative or absolute contraindication. Bone marrow aspiration should not be undertaken at sites where bone infection is present, or radiation therapy has been given. The procedure can usually be performed under local anaesthetic although a sedative may be indicated in particularly anxious patients. The preferred site is the superior posterior iliac crest (PIC) (Table 19.2). Complications are rare, but can include bleeding, infection, and tissue/organ damage secondary to needle trauma.

Table 19.2 Suitable sites for bone marrow aspiration and biopsy sites in adult

Site	Aspiration	Biopsy
Posterior iliac crest (PIC)	Yes	Yes
Anterior iliac crest	Yes	Yes
Sternum	Yes	No

Equipment

- Bone marrow puncture kit or dressing pack.
- Skin cleansing agent e.g. chlorhexidine, povidine Iodine.
- Sterile towel/drapes.
- Local anaesthetic, e.g. lidocaine 1%.
- 25, 23 and 21 gauge needles and 10 mL syringe for local anaesthetic.
- Small scalpel blade e.g. 11.
- Bone marrow aspiration needle.
- Bone marrow trephining needle.
- Microscope slides/specimen pot.
- 20 mL syringe for aspiration.
- Gauze and tape/wound dressing.
- Sharps bin.
- Sterile gloves.
- Apron/gown.
- Marker pen if required.

Pre procedure

- Explain the procedure and gain consent.
- Obtain medical history.
- Obtain medication history and in particular any anticoagulants taken.
- Review full blood count and clotting screen results.

- Establish if there is any allergy to skin cleansing agent or local anaesthetic.
- Allow patient an opportunity to empty their bladder.

Procedure

- Decontaminate hands.
- Check and confirm patient identity.
- Confirm consent.
- Position patient and identify site/position for needle entry. For PIC the patient should be made comfortable in the lateral position with the site of aspiration/biopsy uppermost. The lower leg is usually kept straight with the upper leg flexed at the knee (as for recovery position).
- Wash hands using surgical hand wash technique.
- Put on apron and sterile gloves.
- Clean skin around aspiration site.
- Apply sterile towels/drapes.
- Check equipment and ensure that the stylet can easily be removed from the needle.
- Infiltrate skin, subcutaneous tissues and periosteum with local anaesthetic.
- Use scalpel to make a small incision in the skin.
- Insert aspiration needle through incision and advance until bone resistance is felt.
- Apply pressure and a 90° clockwise/anticlockwise rotation to advance the needle through the cortical bone. (As the harder cortical bone is traversed the needle will usually be felt as a subtle 'give' as it enters the softer bone marrow cavity. The patient should experience this as a sensation of pressure rather than pain.)
- Advance needle 1cm into bone marrow cavity.
- Carefully remove stylet and attach syringe.
- Aspirate 1–2 mL of bone marrow. (The patient should be forewarned that they may experience a sharp pain as the bone marrow is aspirated.)
- Remove needle.
- Apply pressure to site until bleeding stops.
- Prepare and label slides/specimens.
- Perform bone marrow biopsy as required.
- Clean off any remaining skin preparation solution and apply dressing.
- Dispose of sharps and equipment using clinical waste disposal.
- Wash hands.
- Document episode of care.
- Send specimen to laboratory for analysis.

Bone marrow biopsy

As for bone marrow aspiration. Then:

- Insert biopsy needle through incision and advance to periosteum.
- Apply pressure and a 90° clockwise/anti-clockwise rotation to advance the needle through the cortical bone.
- Advance needle 1.5–2cms into bone marrow cavity to obtain sample.
- Rotate needle through 360° to dislodge sample.
- Slowly remove needle using a clockwise/anti-clockwise rotating action.

- Apply pressure to site until bleeding stops.
- Use sterile probe/stylet to remove specimen into specimen pot.
- Clean off any remaining skin preparation solution and apply dressing.
- Dispose of sharps and equipment using clinical waste disposal.
- Wash hands.
- Document episode of care.
- Send specimen to laboratory for analysis.

Post procedure
- Make patient comfortable.
- Patient should remain supine for 30–60min post procedure.
- Observe wound site for signs of bleeding/bruising.
- Give analgesia as required.
- Wound should be kept dry until dressing is removed after 12–24 hours.
- Ask patient to report any bleeding/tenderness post discharge.

Practice tips
- Use the opportunity presented when infiltrating the skin and subcutaneous tissue with local anaesthetic to assess the distance from the skin to periosteum.
- The site for needle entry may be marked prior to skin cleansing to aid subsequent needle insertion and location and positioning of sterile drapes/towels.
- In very anxious patients an oral or IV anxiolytic/sedative, e.g. lorazepam or midazolam, may be helpful.

Pitfalls
- Performing bone marrow biopsy on confused or uncooperative patients.
- Giving inadequate local anaesthetic. The patient should experience a sensation of pressure rather than pain as the needle is advanced through the bone.
- Failing to reassure and explain the procedure to the patient as it is performed. Remember, the patient cannot see what is happening.
- Failing to remove cleansing agents properly at the end of the procedure. Cleaning agents, such as povidine iodine, can cause skin irritation.

Index